Multidisciplinary Approach to Rehabilitation

Multidisciplinary Approach to Rehabilitation

Edited by

Shrawan Kumar, PH.D., D.SC., F.ERG.S.

Professor of Physical Therapy, University of Alberta, Edmonton

With 18 contributing authors

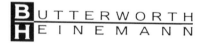

Boston Oxford Auckland Johannesburg Melbourne New Delhi

Copyright © 2000 by Butterworth–Heinemann

℟ A member of the Reed Elsevier group

Library of Congress Cataloging-in-Publication Data
Multidisciplinary approach to rehabilitation / [edited by] Shrawan Kumar.
   p. ; cm.
  Includes bibliographical references and index.
  ISBN 0-7506-7067-3
  1. Medical rehabilitation. 2. Health care teams. I. Kumar, Shrawan.
  [DNLM: 1. Rehabilitation—organization & administration. 2. Patient Care Team. WB 320 M961 2000]
  RM930 .M854 2000
  617'.03--dc21

                          99-056946

British Library Cataloguing-in-Publication Data
A catalogue record for this book is available from the British Library.

The publisher offers special discounts on bulk orders of this book. For information, please contact:

Manager of Special Sales
Butterworth–Heinemann
225 Wildwood Avenue
Woburn, MA 01801-2041
Tel: 781-904-2500
Fax: 781-904-2620

For information on all Butterworth–Heinemann publications available, contact our World Wide Web home page at: http://www.bh.com

10 9 8 7 6 5 4 3 2 1

Printed in the United States of America

To my parents, Tribeni and Dhairyavati Shankar, for their abiding love and shaping of my life

To my wife, Rita, the love of my life, for her love and support

To my children, Rajesh and Sheela, who have given me boundless joy and pride

Contents

Contributing Authors   ix
Preface   xi

1. Rehabilitation Settings   1
   Gilson J. Capilouto

2. Teamwork in Rehabilitation   27
   Donna Latella

3. Team Ethics in Rehabilitation   43
   Dick Sobsey

4. Clinical Reasoning and Decision Making   63
   Joy Higgs and Mark Jones

5. Case Management   87
   Donna L. Smith

6. Attitudes Toward Disability   109
   Roseanna Tufano

7. Cultural Diversity and Health Behavior   123
   Renè Padilla

8. Team Approaches to Geriatric Rehabilitation   155
   Janet E. McElhaney and Marion C. E. Briggs

9. Sexuality in Rehabilitation: Options and Alternatives   177
   Benita Fifield and Shaniff H. Esmail

10. Functional Assessment   209
    Deanne Scoville Anderson

11. Rehabilitation Ergonomics   243
    Shrawan Kumar

12. Vocational Rehabilitation and Work Hardening   261
    Muriel Westmorland

13. Supervision of Service Delivery in the Rehabilitation Disciplines   285
    Paul Hagler

14. Administrative and Legal Issues   319
    Ron Scott

15. Rehabilitation Professionals as Consultants to
    Business and Industry   329
    Jean Bryan Coe

16. Health Promotion   351
    Vivien Hollis

    Index   369

Contributing Authors

Deanne Scoville Anderson, B.S.
Adjunct Faculty, Department of Occupational Therapy, Quinnipiac College, Hamden, Connecticut; Director of Rehabilitation, Harborside Healthcare—The Reservoir, West Hartford, Connecticut

Marion C. E. Briggs, B.S., P.T.
Principal, Seeds of Corporate Consciousness, Edmonton, Alberta; Research Associate, John Dossetor Health Ethics Centre, University of Alberta, Edmonton; Special consultant, Eastern Virginia Medical School

Gilson J. Capilouto, M.S., C.C.C.-S.L.P.
Assistant Professor of Physical Medicine and Rehabilitation, Medical University of South Carolina, Charleston

Jean Bryan Coe, Ph.D., M.P.T., O.C.S.
Retired Colonel, Army Medical Specialist Corps, and Retired Director, U.S. Army—Baylor University Graduate Program in Physical Therapy, U.S. Army Medical Department Center and School, Fort Sam Houston, Texas

Shaniff H. Esmail, M.S., B.S.O.T., B.A.
Assistant Professor of Occupational Therapy, University of Alberta, Edmonton

Benita Fifield, M.S., B.S.O.T., A.C.S.E.
Professor Emeritus of Occupational Therapy, University of Alberta, Edmonton

Paul Hagler, Ph.D.
Professor and Director, Centre for Studies of Clinical Education, University of Alberta, Edmonton

Joy Higgs, B.S., Grad. Dip. Phty., M.H.P.Ed., Ph.D.
Professor, School of Physiotherapy, University of Sydney, Lidcombe, Australia

Vivien Hollis, Ph.D., M.S., T. Dip. C.O.T.
Professor and Chair of Occupational Therapy, University of Alberta, Edmonton

Mark Jones, B.S., Cert. Phty., Grad. Dip. Adv. Manip. Ther., M.App.Sc.
Senior Lecturer and Coordinator of Postgraduate Programs in Manipulative Physiotherapy, University of South Australia, Adelaide, Australia

Shrawan Kumar, Ph.D., D.Sc., F.Erg.S.
Professor of Physical Therapy, University of Alberta, Edmonton

Donna Latella, M.A., O.T.R./L.
Assistant Academic Clinical Coordinator and Assistant Professor of Occupational Therapy, Quinnipiac College, Hamden, Connecticut; Occupational Therapist, Hospital of St. Raphael, New Haven, Connecticut

Janet E. McElhaney, M.D.
Associate Professor, Glennan Center for Geriatrics and Gerontology, Eastern Virginia Medical School, Norfolk

Renè Padilla, M.S., O.T.R./L.
Associate Professor and Vice-Chair of Occupational Therapy, Creighton University, Omaha, Nebraska

Ron Scott, J.D., L.L.M., M.S.B.A., P.T., O.C.S.
Chair, Physical Therapy Department, Lebanon Valley College, Annville, Pennsylvania

Donna L. Smith, R.N., M.Ed., C.H.E.
Associate Professor, Faculty of Nursing and Department of Public Health Sciences, University of Alberta, Edmonton

Dick Sobsey, R.N., Ed.D.
Director, J. P. Das Developmental Disabilities Centre, University of Alberta, Edmonton

Roseanna Tufano, L.M.F.T., O.T.R./L.
Academic Coordinator and Assistant Professor of Occupational Therapy, Quinnipiac College, Hamden, Connecticut

Muriel Westmorland, O.T.R., Dip. C.B.S., M.H.S.
Associate Professor and Associate Dean of Health Sciences and Director, Faculty of Health Sciences, McMaster University, Hamilton, Ontario

Preface

The umbrella of rehabilitation is large and encompasses many disciplines. Because many of these are established disciplines in their own right, their coming together under rehabilitation is, at times, multidisciplinary; at others, interdisciplinary; and at yet others, transdisciplinary. The overriding principle that binds them together is the client's comfort, welfare, and readaptation to his or her environment with the new reality of impaired structure and function. In this context, the disciplines themselves may undergo an adaptation to suit the purpose of rehabilitation. Thus, the blend of disciplines under the rehabilitation umbrella is unique and purpose driven. Whereas different branches of rehabilitation have emphasized different aspects for rehabilitation (i.e., physical, occupational, or speech), the client is always multidimensional and may need more than one service. For some time, because of specialization in different aspects, there had been attenuation in communication between various professionals. It has become increasingly clear that to achieve the goal of rehabilitation, it is desirable that professionals work in teams, bringing their expertise to bear on the needs of the client. Such an approach may be multidisciplinary, interdisciplinary, or transdisciplinary. Hence, there is a need for an entry-level book on the multidisciplinary approach to rehabilitation. This book enables entry-level professionals to recognize the needs of their clients and to sensitize them for the future. With these goals in mind, the current book was conceived and developed.

This book has endeavored to be a comprehensive source of current multidisciplinary ideas. However, there may be some gaps. Nonetheless, the book takes a student from the initial steps of introducing rehabilitation settings to acting as rehabilitation professionals as consultants to business and industry, with everything in between. In the first chapter, Capilouto defines rehabilitation, introduces the reader to the rehabilitation team, and describes various rehabilitation settings, including inpatient, transitional care, home health care, assisted living facilities, and outpatient rehabilitation. In the second chapter, Latella describes the teamwork in rehabilitation. She defines a rehabilitation team and its purpose, dynamics, and advantage to all parties concerned. The third chapter is dedicated to team ethics in rehabilitation. In this chapter, Sobsey takes the reader through numerous real-life ethical dilemmas dealing with issues such as ethical responsibility of rehabilitation teams and euthanasia.

Having described rehabilitation settings, the teamwork involved, and the ethical dilemmas in dealing with clients, the book proceeds to address more specific issues. In Chapter 4, Higgs and Jones describe clinical reasoning and the decision-making process that occur in clinical practice. They examine the nature of clinical reasoning and decision making, common errors in the process, and the nature of multidisciplinary clinical decision making. They discuss conceptual and practical differences between independent and collaborative decision making. They also discuss the implication of bringing together different models of clinical reasoning in the management of individual client cases. Smith discusses case management in Chapter 5. Case management is a process used to improve integration of services. In this chapter, Smith describes the origin of case management and the terminology used and provides a definition of case management. In addition, through examples, the author shows the operation of case management and the role of the case manager.

In Chapters 6 and 7, some of the subjective issues of attitudes, cultural diversity, and health behavior are explored. First, Tufano addresses these issues primarily from two points of view: (1) health professional perspective and (2) client perspective. She traces the basic sources from society that influence and shape perceptions and convictions toward persons with disability. She also summarizes popular theories and models in health care, assisting the reader to recognize the significant formulations that he or she makes about wellness, normalcy, and illness. She discusses common reactions and anxieties associated with disability. In the next chapter, Padilla describes cultural diversity and health behavior. Here, she develops an understanding of culture and the culture-learning process. She also describes the dimensions of culture and their impact on health behavior. Padilla discusses the strategies rehabilitation professionals may use to understand the cultural perspective of clients and to provide treatment with cultural sensitivity and relevance for their greater good.

The demographic shift of recent years and its projected accentuation is a cause of concern to all health care professionals. The phenomenon of aging is also accompanied with frailty and functional impairment. McElhaney and Briggs address the issue of geriatric rehabilitation in Chapter 8, particularly for people 85 years of age and older. They argue that the cornerstones in geriatrics include multidimensional, multidisciplinary, and holistic assessment of individuals; the multidisciplinary team approach to management of acute change; and the support to maintain independence. In Chapter 9, Fifield and Esmail deal with the issue of sexuality among persons with disability. The authors indicate that physical and mental differences associated with different disabilities, as well as personal attitudes and values, may prohibit, change, or present difficulties for some sexual behaviors. They argue that it is important that individuals have alternative behaviors from which to choose if they wish to do so. The authors make a strong case that to present sexual alternatives to their clients, helping professionals may first have to assess their own sexual attitudes and values and acquire the necessary information. They argue that it is only when the professionals are able to communicate in a nonjudgmental manner that the client learns to trust and seek assistance. Given the prevalence of problems among persons with disability, it is an important area to enhance the quality of life.

The cluster of Chapters 10, 11, and 12 focuses on assessment of function, enhancement of function, and vocational rehabilitation. In the functional assessment chapter, Anderson begins with the increasing need for such assessment because of rapid change in the health care system as well as demographic change in the society. The author defines function, gives a clinical perspective, and describes the components of functional assessment. Thereafter she describes assessment of function with contextualized observation using a common language. The author follows this with descriptions of standardized functional assessment and finishes the chapter with implementation of functional assessment and documentation advice. Chapter 11 is dedicated to development of the rationale and philosophy of ergonomics in rehabilitation. I explore the natural link between ergonomics and rehabilitation. I consider the origin of fields and their philosophies and goals. On the basis of the foregoing, I draw out the parallelism between these two disciplines as well as their divergence. I argue that ergonomics complements rehabilitation. This is illustrated in principle as well as through studies I carried out. In essence, I argue that incorporation of ergonomics in rehabilitation arenas enhance the extent of rehabilitation and thereby the quality of life of the client. Westmorland, in Chapter 12, describes vocational rehabilitation by a review of literature, outlines the multiple factors affecting return to work, and depicts the dynamic equilibrium between person, occupation, and environment. She describes the vocational rehabilitation plan under subheadings of work site assessment, work hardening, career- or job-related testing, simulated work experience, vocational retraining, modified work trial, work site modifications, and job-seeking advice or placement. The chapter presents case studies to exemplify the approach and strategies.

In Chapters 13 and 14, supervision of service delivery in rehabilitation disciplines and administrative and legal issues are discussed. Hagler describes how little attention has been paid to a very important function of clinical supervision in Chapter 13. This chapter brings together information from diverse sources, such as health sciences, education, and business management, to provide a template to structure the supervisory process. Scott begins the administrative and legal issues section with a description of legal environment in Chapter 14. Subsequently, he describes the theory issue of malpractice and various liabilities. Finally, patient-informed consent to health care intervention is presented.

In Chapter 15, Coe discusses the role of rehabilitation professionals as consultants to business and industry. The author argues that with the rapid change in health care and its delivery system, rehabilitation professionals are required increasingly to play the role of consultant. Therefore, she states, it is important for rehabilitation professionals to understand the consulting process and develop specific nonclinical competencies. Specifically, program planning, training, and program evaluation are important tools for rehabilitation professionals as consultants. As such, it is important for them to pursue continuing educational opportunities in the fields of business, safety, adult education, and human resource development. Coe argues that such efforts result in improved consultation with business and industry to help organizations control work injury rates and reduce their costs as well as injuries in their companies. In Chapter 16, Hollis makes a case that the best rehabilitation is prevention of disease and disability by healthy lifestyle and choices. This strategy, in addition to adding years to life, adds life to years. She characterizes health promotion by a number of guiding values, including social justice, empowerment, and equity. Hollis makes a case that a holistic notion of physical, mental, social, and spiritual well-being are probably the broad determinants of health. She emphasizes that there is ongoing debate on semantics, and perhaps it is time to practice the principles earnestly.

This book has been written to draw the attention of entry-level professionals to broader aspects in rehabilitation that affect their clients and hence themselves. Increasingly there needs to be greater interaction among different rehabilitation professionals. It is hoped that this book will contribute toward achieving that goal by providing a substantive platform for interaction. Any advancement in this direction will be a huge reward for those who have put their efforts into making this book a reality.

SHRAWAN KUMAR

CHAPTER 1

Rehabilitation Settings

Gilson J. Capilouto

Defining Rehabilitation

Medical *rehabilitation* exists to enhance the functional capabilities of persons who experience activity limitations as a result of impairment in body structure or body function. (This is the proposed nomenclature by the World Health Organization to replace the previous terms and definitions of *impairment, disability,* and *handicap.* For more information, go to http://www.who.org; ICIDH-2 Beta-1 Field Trial.) Impairments may be the result of trauma (head injury, spinal cord injury), illness (multiple sclerosis), or a chronic health condition (diabetes). Congenital impairments are considered within this definition because they are "acquired" at birth. The goal of rehabilitation is for persons to achieve the greatest level of independence, to participate fully within their communities, and to limit their dependence on health systems as well as social systems.

Rehabilitation services became most visible around the time of World War II, when the need for restorative care was heightened by returning veterans and victims of the polio epidemic. Since then, the field of rehabilitation has broadened to serve a large number of people across a variety of settings. At this time, there is a documented rise in the demand for rehabilitation services as a result of several factors (Kaye et al., 1997; Figure 1.1).

The universal trend toward health consciousness has led to a rapidly growing population of older persons. Increased age brings a concomitant increase in the potential for disease or injury, thereby increasing the need for rehabilitation. In addition, improved perinatal care has increased the survival of disabled children and likewise the need for rehabilitation. There is evidence that the number of traumatic injuries resulting from violence, con-

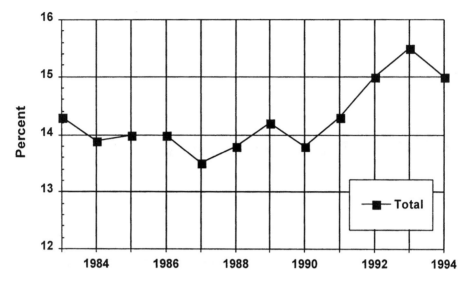

FIGURE 1.1. Proportion of U.S. population with activity limitation, 1982–1994. (Adapted from Kaye, H.S., LaPlante, M., Carlson, D., & Wenger, B. [1997]. Trends in disability rates in the United States, 1970–1994, #17. Disability Statistics Abstract [On-line data]. Available: http://dsc.ucsf.edu/abs/ab17.html)

flict, and motor-vehicle accidents is also climbing steadily, and victims of trauma are very often in need of rehabilitation services. All of these factors contribute to medical rehabilitation evolving into a billion dollar industry that is expected to exceed $45 billion by 2000 (DeJong and Sutton, 1995).

Rehabilitation Team

Successful rehabilitation requires the participation of multiple disciplines. In addition to the patient and caregiver(s), rehabilitation teams typically include *physiatrists* (fi ze a' trists; physicians specializing in physical medicine and rehabilitation), physical and occupational therapists, speech-language pathologists, nurses, psychologists, social workers, and assistive technology specialists. Recreation therapists, rehabilitation engineers, vocational counselors, orthotists, and prosthetists are also essential components of a multidisciplinary team (Figure 1.2).

It is important to have a working understanding of the terminology used to differentiate the way in which rehabilitation teams interact. The term *multidisciplinary* refers to teams of health professionals operating within a traditional medical model in which the physician acts as the care team leader. Team members working within this model share their respective goals for the patient but are not necessarily affected by what each team

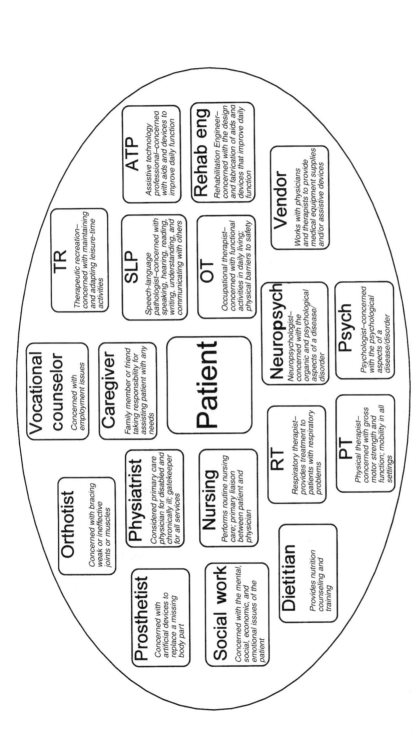

FIGURE 1.2.   The rehabilitation team: A diagram of the potential rehabilitation team members with a brief description of their general area of expertise. Note that each team has been represented equally because at any given time various members could have a primary role. The encapsulating circle is used to capture the idea that communication is occurring among all members of the team.

member may be doing. For instance, in the course of a care conference, the occupational therapist may explain that the patient is using an adapted utensil during mealtime, while the physical therapist may report using a specific technique to assist the patient in transferring from the bed to the chair. This dialogue between team members is important and valuable, even though it does not alter their respective approach to treatment. Multidisciplinary teams are often the model of choice on acute medical/surgery floors, although this is not always the case.

As in the case of multidisciplinary teams, *interdisciplinary* team members also share their respective goals for the patient. However, carry-over of goals is expected to be supported by all team members throughout the day. Using the above scenario, once team members learned that the patient was using an adapted utensil, anyone working with the patient at mealtime would be expected to support that recommendation and see that it was carried out by the patient. Likewise, once instructed in the physical therapist's procedures for transfers, the nurses, occupational therapists, caregiver(s), and anyone else in contact with the patient would follow the same procedures. Interdisciplinary teams differ from multidisciplinary teams in that all members are considered equal. Interdisciplinary teams are a required component of accredited hospital-based rehabilitation programs.

Transdisciplinary teams focus on task-specific treatment, each from the standpoint of their respective disciplines. All of the patient's activities are designed to approximate what occurs in the course of a typical day, such as getting up, self-grooming and hygiene, dressing, and eating breakfast. Consequently, each discipline strives to contribute to enhancing the patient's functional ability within a given activity. If you happened to walk into a facility using a transdisciplinary approach to rehabilitation, it might take some time before you could determine who was the physical therapist, the occupational therapist, or the speech-language pathologist. As patient length of stay has shortened, the interest in transdisciplinary rehabilitation has grown. Many rehabilitation administrators view this approach as the most efficient way to assist the patient in achieving maximum function in a limited amount of time. In a great many of the facilities supporting transdisciplinary approaches to rehabilitation, physical and occupational therapists and speech-language pathologists treat patients in one large area as opposed to individual departments or separate rooms.

The disciplines represented within a team may vary throughout the rehabilitation process according to the needs of the patient at any given time and the disabling condition or impairment. For instance, a dietician may be an integral part of the team and work closely with the occupational therapist and speech-language pathologist in remediating feeding and swallowing difficulties resulting from a stroke. However, as the patient's abilities in that area improve, the dietician's presence on the team may diminish. In contrast, there might be instances when a patient's dietary practices or nutritional needs would not be a concern, in which case there would be no need for a dietician on the team. The important thing to remember is that to support all of the patient's needs, it is essential that service providers work together to support one another's goals and treatment techniques. It is for this reason that interdisciplinary teamwork is considered the cornerstone of effective rehabilitation.

Rehabilitation Settings

Rehabilitation services are provided in a variety of settings. The purpose of this chapter is to describe many of those settings and to offer a glimpse into the way(s) rehabilitation might look within each of them. It is important to understand that clear-cut definitions for each potential setting are difficult to come by for a number of reasons. First, the scope of services within each setting can vary from community to community and even from facility to facility. For example, larger metropolitan communities may offer more specialty services within a particular rehabilitation setting than are available in a smaller, more rural community setting. Second, the level(s) of service provided within a particular setting may also vary between facilities and communities. *Level of service* refers to the intensity with which the patient is expected to participate. Levels of service could range from 1 to 3 days per week of treatment to as many as 7 days per week of treatment, and from 1 hour to 8 hours a day. It is important to keep in mind that levels of service are often driven by reimbursement regulations that are subject to rapid change and that make rigid descriptions of the various rehabilitation settings difficult at best. In response to this dilemma, the Health Care Financing Administration (HCFA) is proposing an "integrated payment system for post-acute services" which would, in essence, make reimbursement for rehabilitation services "setting-neutral" (Eli Rehad Report, April 1997). In this way, payment would be standardized for specific treatments regardless of the setting in which the services were delivered. Although the merits of such a system are debatable, it is certain that changes in the current reimbursement structure would affect the entire rehabilitation industry.

Health care facilities offering rehabilitation services are subject to a myriad of standards by which they are expected to operate. The standards may vary according to the specific setting in which services are delivered. *Licensure* of a facility is set by individual states and consequently is directed by state governments. Issues of licensure include the physical nature of the facility (e.g., accessibility), fire safety, and cleanliness. In some settings, such as inpatient facilities, licensure might also require meeting minimum standards for equipment and personnel (Shi and Singh, 1998).

Certification allows a rehabilitation facility to receive payment from the Medicare and Medicaid programs. This is a federal mandate and is based on conditions of participation developed by the U.S. Department of

Health and Human Services. Conditions include specific directives on aspects of care, such as maintenance of clinical records and physician involvement in planning and delivery of care.

Health care organizations receive *accreditation* through the Joint Commission on Accreditation of Healthcare Organizations (JCAHO), which sets standards of operation for health facilities ranging from inpatient hospital facilities to substance abuse programs to home health agencies. In addition to accreditation, facilities specifically providing rehabilitation services are subject to an additional accreditation process administered by the Commission on Accreditation of Rehabilitation Facilities (CARF). CARF standards are designed to promote the delivery of quality rehabilitation service and include a wide range of programmatic regulations, such as the qualifications of rehabilitation personnel, clinical record management, patient rights, and patient education and training.

Inpatient Rehabilitation

Inpatient rehabilitation refers to rehabilitation services that are provided in a hospital atmosphere (von Sternberg et al., 1997). Inpatient rehabilitation may take the form of an acute rehabilitation unit within a community hospital, a freestanding rehabilitation hospital, or a rehabilitation unit within a medical academic center. In many instances, the setting of a hospital-based medical rehabilitation program may dictate the ancillary services available to patients. For example, in an academic medical center, patients often have access to a larger variety of consultants and specialty services than are normally offered in a traditional community hospital. However, there are certainly examples of community hospitals that offer as comprehensive an array of specialties as an academic medical center. To further illustrate comparison between the options, consider that often a freestanding hospital-based rehabilitation program may be unequipped to provide some of the diagnostic and evaluative procedures needed for rehabilitation patients, and as a result may transport patients to other facilities to have certain procedures completed. Again, this is not always the case, because there are examples of freestanding rehabilitation facilities offering an extensive choice of services. The point to keep in mind is that inpatient rehabilitation facilities do not always look the same, even though there is a general set of standards by which they all have to operate.

Patients admitted to acute rehabilitation units require on-site physician and nursing services and need to be able to tolerate at least 3 hours of ancillary health-related services, such as physical therapy, occupational therapy, speech-language pathology, therapeutic recreation, and psychological counseling/intervention. Accredited hospital-based rehabilitation units have a medical director trained as a physiatrist or a medical doctor with specific experience in rehabilitation. The medical director serves the

Case Study 1

Mrs. B is a 67-year-old woman with left middle cerebral artery cerebrovascular accident (CVA) manifested in right hemiparesis and aphasia. She presents with no comorbidities contraindicated for rehabilitation. Premorbid status includes working as a housewife and being independent in basic and instrumental activities of daily living (ADLs). Her current level of function includes the report that she is continent and independently walks to the bathroom. She is independent in upper extremity (UE) self-care and dependent in lower extremity (LE) self-care. She communicates via gestures and speech, although her speech is only moderately intelligible and characterized by dysarthria. Her receptive language abilities appear to be functionally intact. She has a supportive husband in good health, who plans to be the primary caregiver on the patient's release. Mrs. B will return to a single-family dwelling with a two-step entrance and a handrail. The financial aspects of care were discussed with the husband, and coverage is not an issue. This patient would benefit from admittance to the rehabilitation unit to receive needed therapies.

Terminology key: ADLs = basic ADLs include eating, dressing, grooming; instrumental ADLs include shopping, preparing a light meal, light housework; aphasia = disruption in receptive or expressive language abilities; comorbidities = associated diseases; hemiparesis = one-sided paralysis; LE self-care = self-care involving the lower extremities (e.g., donning socks and shoes); dysarthria = slow, laborious speech; UE self-care = self-care involving the upper body (e.g., brushing hair, brushing teeth, applying makeup).

unit for a minimum of 20 hours per week. In addition to the medical director, the attending physicians are available 24 hours a day, 7 days a week. There is an approximate 1 to 10 nurse to patient ratio on hospital-based rehabilitation units (Jones and Foster, 1997). The average length of stay for patients treated on inpatient rehabilitation unit(s) varies according to the admitting diagnosis. Generally speaking, patient stays range from 1 week to approximately 4 weeks (J. E. Warmoth, oral communication, September 10, 1998). Intake begins with an evaluation of the patient while he or she is still in acute care. A preadmission assessment includes information regarding the patient's diagnosis, prognosis, morbidity, comorbidity, premorbid level of function, social status, mental status, and ability to tolerate the intensity of comprehensive inpatient rehabilitation (Joint Commission on Accreditation of Rehabilitation Facilities, 1998).

In Case Study 1, once the decision is made to transfer Mrs. B to inpatient rehabilitation, the admission and orientation process begins. Ideally,

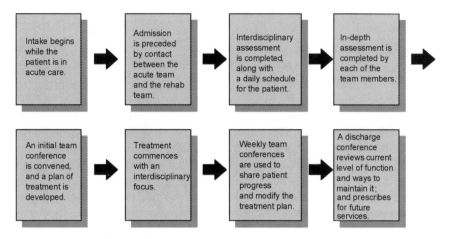

FIGURE 1.3. Sample flow chart for comprehensive integrated inpatient rehabilita-

before the patient even enters the unit, the acute care team would have communicated the patient's strengths and abilities to the rehabilitation care team (Figure 1.3). Once Mrs. B is brought to the unit, the care team begins its individual assessments. The initial assessments are administered using an interdisciplinary assessment tool. The purpose of such an approach is to ensure that the patient is not forever repeating the same information to the various members of the team. Generally speaking, the initial assessments are a fairly cursory view of the patient's current level of function. Using the daily schedule developed for the patient, individual team members move to complete more detailed evaluations to develop long- and short-term patient goals.

After completion of more in-depth assessments, an initial team conference is convened so that team members can share their goals for Mrs. B and a treatment plan can be developed. Always keep in mind that Mrs. B and Mrs. B's caregivers are actively contributing to the development of her goals. The treatment plan also includes an estimated time frame for accomplishing the goals, so discharge planning begins immediately. Team discussion around discharge might include answering the following: What equipment does Mrs. B require to maintain the highest level of independent functioning? What, if any, barriers exist to Mrs. B's independence at home or in the community? What are the plans for Mrs. B's follow-up medical care? Will she require continued therapy at the time of discharge? If so, what is the most appropriate referral, outpatient or home health therapy?

After the admission meeting is completed and a plan of treatment is developed, the various team members initiate treatment. Interdisciplinary team conferences are held so that the members of the team can update one another on progress, discuss any problems or concerns, and upgrade their respective goals—for example developing new short-term goals or possibly changing long-term goals. In addition, team conferences may be used to discuss any assistive aids or devices being recommended for Mrs. B, as well as the status of family education regarding Mrs. B's care after discharge. The frequency of team conferences varies across programs and across patients. However, according to the 1998 Medical Rehabilitation Standards Manual (Joint Commission on Accreditation of Rehabilitation Facilities, Section 3.CIIRP.-109), this frequency should be directly related to the patient's needs.

The interdisciplinary nature of Mrs. B's treatment should be obvious. If one considers how much these team members have in common with respect to their skills and abilities, it is easy to imagine the many ways they might collaborate on Mrs. B's behalf: the physical therapist and the occupational therapist might travel to the home to complete an assessment of Mrs. B's environment and identify strategies and equipment that could minimize physical barriers to her independence; the speech-language pathologist and psychologist may conduct numerous joint treatment sessions with Mrs. B, because she may be frustrated and depressed about her difficulties communicating; the speech-language pathologist and assistive technology specialist may collaborate with the rehabilitation engineer on inexpensive ways to facilitate Mrs. B's speech intelligibility over the telephone. These are just a few of the ways in which interdisciplinary rehabilitation teams work together in comprehensive integrated inpatient rehabilitation programs.

The discharge conference for Mrs. B would include all team members and would focus on a general overview of her current functional capabilities, including ways she and her caregivers could foster her current level(s) of independence. The discharge conference would also be a time for addressing any unanswered questions regarding Mrs. B, for example, questions about her prognosis and chances for having a second stroke or questions about any medications she might be taking. At the time of discharge, arrangements are made for the delivery and setup of any equipment that has been ordered, along with instructions for medical follow-up. Follow-up visits to the physician are the benchmark for seeing that Mrs. B maintains the skills she has acquired in inpatient rehabilitation.

Rehabilitation Services in Transitional Care

The term *transitional care* is a broad one. It encompasses a range of rehabilitation services that would best be described as intermediate. The terms *skilled nursing facility, subacute care,* and *transitional care unit* are often used interchangeably when in fact they may be very different (Jones and Foster, 1997). Each of these settings has one thing in common, regardless of the varying degrees of service that might distinguish them from one another: the care received is considered to be postacute. For the purposes of this chapter, we use the term *subacute care* to represent this portion of the rehabilitation industry because it is the term in widespread use at this time.

Rehabilitation-based subacute programs combine rehabilitation and convalescent services (Sultz and Young, 1997). Examples of rehabilitation-oriented subacute programs are varied and could include stroke rehabilitation, orthopedic rehabilitation, brain injury rehabilitation, pulmonary rehabilitation, neuromuscular rehabilitation, or general rehabilitation (Kelly, 1996). Subacute rehabilitation units may exist as a skilled nursing floor in a hospital, as a freestanding facility, or as part of a skilled nursing facility. In some instances, a subacute care unit may be part of a long-term-care facility such as a nursing home. Patients admitted to subacute care units have stabilized medically after their acute episode, but they are not yet able to go home or be admitted to a comprehensive rehabilitation program (PM&R in Practice, 1995). Daily physician visits and 24-hour nursing care are not required by these patients, and they may even be tolerating some physical, occupational, or speech-language therapy. However, compared with inpatient rehabilitation units, the treatment pace is slower, and in contrast to acute rehabilitation, the minimal tolerance level is 1–3 hours. JCAHO specifies that patients admitted into subacute rehabilitation should not require "high technology monitoring or complex diagnostic procedures" (Tellis-Nayak and MacDonnell, 1995).

Patients admitted to subacute rehabilitation might include those in need of gait training after a hip replacement, patients being weaned from ventilators, patients with tracheostomies, and patients who are comatose. Licensed subacute facilities have a medical director trained as a physiatrist, a medical doctor with experience in rehabilitation, or a general medical doctor with board certification in family medicine or internal medicine. The medical director serves the unit 1–3 days per week but is available 24 hours a day, 7 days a week. According to Jones and Foster (1997), the typical patient to nurse ratio in the subacute rehabilitation setting varies from 8 to 1 to 10 to 1, depending on the location of the facility (hospital versus freestanding facility). The permitted length of stay in a subacute care facility is 90 days. However, some reports indicate that lengths of stay are on average less than 45 days (Haffey et al., 1995). As in the case of inpatient rehabilitation, intake begins while the patient is in acute care. The preadmission assessment should include information regarding the patient's diagnosis, prognosis, morbidity, comorbidity, premorbid level of function, social status, mental status, and ability to tolerate the treatment (Joint Commission on Accreditation of Rehabilitation Facilities, 1998).

In Case Study 2, once it has been decided that the patient's needs can be met by the receiving subacute facility, the admission process continues. In well-coordinated facilities, communication between care teams occurs before the patient's transition to the new setting. Because of the minimal tolerance level of patients admitted to subacute rehabilitation, the first day's activities may differ to some degree from what was previously

Case Study 2

Mr. J is an 87-year-old man with congestive heart failure (CHF), who recently fell and broke his hip while at home. He underwent a total hip arthroplasty and is being seen to consider rehabilitation. Premorbid status includes the report that before his fall, he was living alone and was independent in basic ADLs and dependent in instrumental ADLs. He received Meals on Wheels and required assistance when he left his home. His endurance is reportedly poor because of his tendency toward CHF, and he reports failing eyesight. His current level of function includes the finding that he is nonambulatory and is dependent in transitional movements as well as LE self-care. Despite his advancing age, he is remarkably lucid and coherent. His receptive and expressive language skills appear to be intact, as do his cognitive function and hearing. He has been widowed for 20 years and has two sons and one daughter. His oldest son and his daughter live out of state. His remaining son is supportive but is having financial difficulties. Mr. J resides in a trailer with two steps, no hand rail, and no ramp. His postacute disposition is of concern. He would benefit from admission to the subacute rehabilitation unit. Because of his fragile cardiac reserve, he could not tolerate the aggressive 3-hours-per-day treatment regime expected in the rehabilitation unit. However, he would benefit from physical and occupational therapies.

Terminology key: Arthroplasty = plastic repair of a joint; nonambulatory = not walking; transitional movements = movements such as sit-to-stand, stand-to-sit.

described for inpatient rehabilitation. Nonetheless, Mr. J's first day provides for an orientation to his new surroundings and the completion of an interdisciplinary assessment. In his case, the initial assessment would then be followed by in-depth physical and occupational therapy assessments.

An initial team conference is convened to establish the patient's long- and short-term goals, with estimated time frames and initial plans for discharge. All of this information is used to develop the patient's plan of care. Once the plan of care is established, any recommended treatment begins. The ongoing nature of Mr. J's treatment looks very similar to that described for inpatient rehabilitation. However, the pace is less intense (Figure 1.4). As in inpatient rehabilitation, regular team conferences are held to discuss Mr. J's progress and the status of his plan of care. Once Mr. J successfully achieves his treatment goals, he is ready for discharge. Team discharge plans for him might include returning home with a walker, referral to home health for nursing services, personal aide assistance, and continued physical and occupational therapy. In addition, dis-

Patient: Mr. J				Week of: 00/00/00		
	MONDAY	TUESDAY	WEDNESDAY	THURSDAY	FRIDAY	TEAM
9:00	OT					Physician:
9:30	LE self-care					
10:00		OT	PT		OT	Case Manager:
10:30		IADL	Mobility aid	PT/OT	IADL	
11:00		group	training	Co-test	group	Nurse:
11:30						
12:00						PT:
12:30						
1:00	Healthy			Healthy	PT/OT	OT:
1:30	living	OT		living	home	
2:00	group	Basic ADLs		group	assessment	SLP:
2:30						
3:00			Team			Other:
3:30			conference			
4:00						

FIGURE 1.4. Sample schedule for Mr. J—subacute rehabilitation. (ADLs = activities of daily living; IADL = instrumental activities of daily living; LE = lower extremity; OT = occupational therapy; PT = physical therapy; SLP = speech/language pathologist.)

charge plans might also include establishing a "lifeline" service in case of an emergency.

Home Health Rehabilitation Services

Home health rehabilitation services refer to restorative services provided in a patient's home. The patient who is considered to be homebound is experiencing "a normal inability to leave home" (Sections 1814[a] and 1835 [a][2][a] of the Social Security Act). The reasons a person might not be able to leave home include the effort required by the patient to leave, a psychiatric condition that presents as fear of leaving the home, or the safety risk of leaving the home unattended. It is important to keep in mind that being "homebound" does not mean that a patient never leaves his or her residence. It is considered acceptable for patients to receive home health care and still go out for a visit to the doctor, to attend church or synagogue, or to get a needed haircut. However, trips from home should be infrequent and relatively short if a patient is to maintain homebound status. We traditionally think of home health services as being delivered to the elderly. However, a large portion of the home health

Case Study 3

Mrs. C is a 78-year-old woman with diabetic peripheral vascular disease and an LE open wound. She receives insulin twice daily. She lives with her 84-year-old husband who is supportive and in good health, but who is unable to provide the necessary care. Mrs. C has a daughter who lives at home and works full-time. Mrs. C is in need of wound care 3 times per day and education regarding her medicine regime and twice-a-day insulin injections. She requires assistance with basic ADLs. In addition, she may require physical therapy services because of the decreased endurance resulting from her long stay in acute care. Mrs. C is home-bound because neither she nor her husband drives. In addition, Mrs. C's reduced endurance and LE wound present a safety risk. Mrs. C would benefit from home health services to meet the above needs, and she has been referred to the ABC Home Health Agency. She is scheduled to go home in 2 days, and the agency has been notified of this date.

industry today includes services to patients of all ages, including infants and small children.

To qualify for home health services, patients must meet the following criteria:

1. Require intermittent skilled nursing; and/or
2. Require physical therapy; and/or
3. Require speech-language pathology services; and
4. Be essentially homebound; and
5. Be under the care of a physician who agrees to sign orders on their behalf.

Home health regulations state that occupational therapy services can be introduced only after one of the other skilled services has been initiated. However, this does not preclude occupational therapy from staying in the home, once the other services have been discharged. Additional assistance provided by comprehensive home health agencies includes social work and personal aide services.

Referral for home health services comes from physicians, other agencies, and the community at large. As with other rehabilitation settings, referral may also begin while the patient is still in acute care. The hospital discharge planner is a vital member of the acute care multidisciplinary team and is instrumental in determining postacute placement. If a discharge planner decides that a patient would benefit from home health services, he or she discusses that recommendation with the other members of the team, including the physician. Once everyone is in agreement, the discharge planner contacts a home health agency. Initially, the discharge planner describes the patient over the phone, and home health agency personnel determine whether their particular agency can support all of the patient's needs. It is important to keep in mind that home health agencies vary considerably in the nature of the skilled service they can provide. The following scenario helps to paint a picture of the type of patient who might benefit from home health services.

In Case Study 3, once Mrs. C goes home, the initial agency visit is arranged. In many cases, the initial visit is scheduled within 72 hours of the patient's return home, although this can vary among agencies. However, in Mrs. C's case, the initial visit would need to take place on the day she returns home because she is in need of daily insulin injections and daily wound care. During the initial visit, the attending registered nurse (RN) performs a "head-to-toe" physical examination, prioritizes the patient's educational needs pertaining to her condition(s), and, along with the physician, determines the need for additional services. In addition, the RN assesses the availability of caregivers in terms of the burden of caregiving (e.g., the number of hours of care required per day) and the ability of the caregiver(s) to provide the necessary care. The RN also examines the patient's home and community environments to insure that both are safe and adequate for the delivery of home care.

During the RN's initial visit, it would be necessary for Mrs. C's caregiver to demonstrate both the proper administration of insulin injections and the proper procedures for performing wound care. In addition, the RN would need to assess the caregiver's knowledge of Mrs. C's medicine regime. The frequency of nursing visits would then be dependent on the caregiver's availability and current level of knowledge and skill in providing the necessary care. For illustration purposes, let's say that Mrs. C's daughter has expressed her willingness to care for her mother and has successfully demonstrated the ability to provide her mother's insulin injections and wound care. However, she works full time, so she is only available to provide wound care in the morning and evening. It would be necessary for the RN to maintain a frequency of daily visits to meet the patient's needs. Because there is a limit to the amount of daily skilled nursing that can be provided in the home health setting, the RN would need to refer Mrs. C's case to the home health agency's social worker so that he or she could help in identifying any community resources available to provide wound care.

Earlier, the patient's reduced strength and endurance was described, as well as her dependency in LE self-care. To address these needs, the RN would request physician referral for additional services including physical therapy and personal care assistance. In general, evaluations for additional services are completed within 72 hours of a referral and require at minimum the attending physician's verbal orders. In the case of physical therapy, once the need for services is determined, the physical therapist would prioritize Mrs. C's goals, determine the frequency of physical therapy visits, and determine the ability of the caregiver(s) to assist with a home exercise plan. Given the age of Mrs. C's husband and the number of responsibilities already imposed on the daughter, the therapist might decide that an alternative plan is needed. Based on patient needs and scheduling preference, the home health aide would also complete an initial visit. For example, in Mrs. C's case, the nurse might recommend three aide visits per week to assist with basic and instrumental ADLs (grooming, hygiene, fixing a light meal, picking up Mrs. C's prescriptions). Through interdisciplinary communication, the physical therapist would discover that an option for providing Mrs. C's home exercise program would be to instruct the aide in how to administer the plan. In this way, the home health aide could complete the exercise plan during her weekly visits. Herein lie the advantages of interdisciplinary rehabilitation. Everyone on the team is vested in the rapid recovery of the patient, and all team members work collaboratively toward that end. Without this type of communication and interaction, Mrs. C's recovery might take substantially longer and yield fewer positive outcomes.

As one might predict, interdisciplinary communication can be more difficult in the home health care setting than in many of the other settings described in this chapter. The nature of home health service delivery is such that various team members are on the road for substantial amounts of time, and rarely are two service providers in the home simultaneously. Consequently, collaboration and communication about patients frequently require creative uses of available resources. Interdisciplinary conferencing is often accomplished via voice mail, written notes throughout the patient's chart, phone calls between service providers, and, in some instances, face-to-face care conferences. As demonstrated above, the value of this communication is crucial to the well-being of the patient.

There is no "average" length of time home health services are provided, because patient needs vary greatly. In the past, home health care continued until all of the patient's goals were achieved as long as coverage criteria were met. However, HCFA has proposed changes in reimbursement regulations that would dictate the number of home health visits a patient could receive, irrespective of their rehabilitation needs. HCFA has proposed that it will use those saved dollars toward coverage of adult daycare services. Consequently, a substantial growth in adult daycare facilities is expected over the next year (J. E. Warmoth, oral communication, October 11, 1998).

However, at this time, a regulatory provision of discharge from home health is that a skilled service must be the last service out of the home. This means that a paraprofessional or personal aide would not be allowed to physically make the last visit. Instead, a service such as skilled nursing or allied health would determine the need for discharge and communicate that recommendation to the physician. Discharge planning might include a visit from the agency social worker with information about community resources available to the patient and directives for follow-up medical care.

Rehabilitation Services in Assisted-Living Facilities

Assisted living is a level of care that falls between independent living and nursing home care. Services include personal care assistance, medication management, health promotion and exercise programs, and limited health care services. Estimates of the number of assisted-living facilities (ALFs) operating in the United States range from 30,000 to 40,000 (Eli Rehab Report, June 1997). The number of people being served by ALFs is reported to be about 1 million (Shi and Singh, 1998). The Assisted Living Federation of America (http://www.alfa.org) describes the typical resident of an ALF as being 83 years old or older, female, and either widowed or single.

The assisted-living industry has been reported to be the fastest growing portion of the elderly housing market (Pynoos, 1996). ALFs offer opportunities for older people to "age in place," a term used to describe the elderly's desire to remain in home- and community-based settings. In addition, assisted living is an attractive and cost-efficient alternative to nursing home care and home health care. In some areas of the country, patients are being discharged to an ALF when they are not independent enough to return home but are too independent for a nursing home (Rehab Continuum Report, April 1998). Benefits include three prepared meals per day; transportation whenever it is needed; assistance with bathing, dressing, toileting, and walking as needed; and 24-hour security and staff. Social and recreational activities are also common features of ALFs. ALFs may be referred to as personal care homes, sheltered housing, residential care, continuing care retirement communities, catered living, board and care, or domiciliary care (http://www.aoa.gov/Housing/al.html). There is some question as to the validity of defining assisted living so broadly, because the actual services provided can vary significantly across different settings (Harrington, 1994).

ALFs are quickly becoming an attractive option for the delivery of rehabilitation services. Generally speaking, ALFs do not hire rehabilitation personnel to provide treatment for their residents. Instead, rehabilitation services tend to be arranged on an individual basis. Often, rehabilitation services in ALFs are provided by home health agencies, because an ALF is the equivalent of a residence from a reimbursement prospective (Rehab Continuum Report, 1998). To provide a more complete continuum of health care services than is typically seen in assisted living, some developers have opted to link their residences with comprehensive outpatient rehabilitation facilities (CORFs). By doing so, residents have access to more physician-directed care, such as diagnostic and therapeutic services (Eli Rehab Report, June 1997).

Case Study 4

O. F. is a 94-year-old woman diagnosed with emphysema. She requires around-the-clock personal aide services with intermittent-skilled nursing. She is independent in UE self-care but dependent in LE self-care. She is also dependent in instrumental ADLs. She has been widowed for more than 20 years and continues to live in the home she shared with her husband. She has a large family network, but many of her friends have died. She has recently become depressed as she spends a great deal of time alone. It is difficult and tiring for her to leave home. She is remarkably lucid and coherent and enjoys telling her grandchildren and great-grandchildren stories of her childhood. Although the cost of her current care has not been an issue, her family has become increasingly concerned over her depression. After a family discussion, it was decided that O. F. would move into an ALF only minutes away from her home and in close proximity to her family. That way, she could continue to live independently and receive the assistance she needed. A nursing center is part of the complex, should she ever need it. She would also benefit from occupational therapy consultation for LE self-care aids and devices.

It should be pointed out that regulation and licensing of ALFs varies considerably from state to state (http://www.alfa.org/). In fact, a recent survey by the American Seniors Housing Association found that 14 states had no rules or regulations governing continuing care (Moss, 1998). ALFs can opt for accreditation by the Continuing Care Accreditation Commission, but this process is voluntary. Groups concerned with the potential risks in nonregulated continuing care are working toward federal legislation to oversee these types of facilities. The following case study illustrates the benefit of the assisted-living option for older persons.

In Case Study 4, treatment for O. F. does not look particularly different from what was described for home health. At this time, there are no specific models for team-based intervention in the assisted-living environment. However, as this setting becomes more visible in the rehabilitation industry, multidisciplinary, interdisciplinary, and transdisciplinary models need to be developed.

Outpatient Rehabilitation Services

Outpatient rehabilitation services are services that do not necessarily follow an inpatient hospitalization (Sultz and Young, 1997). Ambulatory rehabilitation is provided in a number of settings, including outpatient hospital programs, freestanding rehabilitation clinics, private practice, and CORFs.

Hospital-based outpatient rehabilitation programs typically offer physical therapy, occupational therapy, and speech-language pathology services. To remain competitive, many hospitals have elected to set up satellite outpatient rehabilitation facilities in their communities. However, billing practices and reporting mechanisms are such that they are still considered hospital-based services (Gill, 1995). According to a 1995 Outpatient Utilization Profile report from HCIA, Inc. and Arthur Andersen, LLP, hospital-based outpatient rehabilitation departments provide only 3.18% of all ambulatory rehabilitation services (Gill, 1995). The patients seen in hospital-based programs tend to present with more catastrophic diagnoses, such as spinal cord injury, traumatic brain injury, or neurologic conditions. Only 25% of the hospital-based rehabilitation programs treat pediatrics, and the children served almost always fall into a category of catastrophic diagnosis (Gill, 1995).

Freestanding facilities make up the large majority of outpatient rehabilitation providers. In the past, these facilities were operated by small corporations owned by private practice clinicians. Recently, however, there has been a shift toward ownership and management by large companies such as HealthSouth and NovaCare. Many of these facilities offer physical therapy, occupational therapy, and speech-language pathology services, but a majority only provide physical therapy services. According to statistical data from HCFA, Medicare providers of outpatient physical therapy increased from 386 in 1980 to 2,302 in 1996.

Private practice, single-therapy clinics, and physician-based rehabilitation facilities do not make up as large a portion of the rehabilitation services industry as they did in the past. The 1990s have been described as a "feeding frenzy," as managed-care forced small rehabilitation practices either to affiliate with or to sell to larger providers, and the larger providers moved to acquire the smaller practices, expand their geographic area, and attract managed-care contracts (Eli Rehab Report, April 1997). The physician anti-self-referral law, expanded in 1993, prohibited doctors from referring Medicare or Medicaid patients for any health care service to a facility or organization in which the physicians might have a financial interest. Physical therapy was among the health services specifically mentioned in the legislation, known as Stark II, after Representative Fortney "Pete" Stark, D-CA (PM&R in Practice, 1998). Consequently, a great number of physician-owned practices have also been forced to sell.

CORFs are a relatively new player in the field of rehabilitation services. A CORF is distinguishable from the other ambulatory rehabilitation settings in a number of ways. A CORF offers a more comprehensive array of services than is typically seen in outpatient rehabilitation. In addition to physical, occupational, and speech-language therapy services, social work, psychological services, and rehabilitation nursing are also reimbursable within a CORF designation. Another difference between a CORF and a traditional outpatient program is the CORF utilization of interdisciplinary

Case Study 5

M is an 8-year-old boy who presents with cerebral palsy manifested in spastic quadriplegia. He is accompanied by his mother and father, who both served as informants in the initial interview. M is nonambulatory, dependent in all of his basic ADLs, and nonverbal. He is currently fitted in a manual wheelchair with customized features. He is fed via a gastrostomy tube, although, per his mother's report, he is beginning to tolerate some pureed foods. M's parents report that he primarily uses vocalizations and gestures to communicate as well as other nonsymbolic forms of communication: pushing away unwanted objects, turning his head when he is bored or uninterested, smiling and laughing to denote pleasure, and pouting to denote disappointment. M attends his neighborhood school where he is mainstreamed in a second grade class. He receives physical, occupational, and speech-language services in the school. He has been referred to this outpatient center for recommendations regarding assistive technology in the areas of electronic mobility, increased independence in basic ADLs, and augmentative communication.

Terminology key: Assistive technology = aids and devices designed to enable persons to be more functional in their daily lives; augmentative communication = aids or devices that facilitate a person's expressive communication when speech or writing is difficult; gastrostomy = feeding tube surgically inserted into the stomach; mainstreamed = placed with nondisabled peers; nonverbal = unable to use speech as a primary means of communication; spastic quadriplegia = all four limbs are affected.

team goals, as opposed to the more typical discipline-specific treatment plans and sessions (Rehab Continuum Report, 1997). According to some analysts, establishing a CORF is an important move for communities with a large Medicare population who are being released from the inpatient setting somewhat earlier and a bit sicker (Rehab Continuum Report, 1997).

The types of patients one might serve in an outpatient therapy setting vary significantly. Some practices exist to serve only those persons with sports injuries or hand injuries, while others provide treatment for any rehabilitation need. The following illustration is but one example of an outpatient case.

In Case Study 5, in M's case, rehabilitation must be interdisciplinary. Because of the need to integrate a number of assistive aids and devices, M's therapists must be working with him together, or the results could prove costly and ineffective. It is certainly easier to treat cases such as M's in rehabilitation settings where all three disciplines are represented. However, M's treatment could be delivered by three individual therapists from three separate facilities. The problem comes in sorting out reimbursement issues and time lost for travel between agencies. This scenario is certainly one that is being seen less frequently.

Summary

Rehabilitation services and programs exist in a variety of settings. The ways in which services are delivered depend to some degree on where patients are seen. This is a significantly volatile time for health care in general and rehabilitation in particular. Recently, Congress moved to capitate Medicare reimbursement for outpatient services at $1,500 dollars for each of the three disciplines: physical therapy, occupational therapy, and speech-language pathology. In addition, there is a trend toward reimbursing all nonoutpatient rehabilitation services (inpatient, subacute, home health) equally, regardless of the setting. It has been proposed that those cost savings should in turn be used to cover some of the expenses involved in providing adult daycare.

It is likely that these changes will have a serious impact on the ways in which rehabilitation services are delivered. The proliferation of subacute facilities observed in the 1990s will probably be replaced with significant growth in the number of adult daycare centers. Rehabilitation providers will move toward restructuring and will redefine their programs in ways that allow for a seamless continuum of care and a single point of entry. For allied health workers, the result of these changes mean less time available to rehabilitate. Treatment will be forced to move away from a multidisciplinary orientation toward an interdisciplinary or transdisciplinary frame of reference. Therapists will have to work collaboratively to effect the same level of patient change within a significantly shorter period of time. It is also likely that we will see an increased interest in the evaluation of and recommendation for assistive aids and devices, because we will be obliged to identify what our patients can do, rather than what they are unable to do. Many argue that the proposed changes facing rehabilitation will most likely result in the need for additional care/services, greater risk of repeated injury or new injury, reduced levels of functional ability and quality of life, and ultimately, increased costs (Eli Rehab Report, 1997). It is certain the impact will be unprecedented.

Application Activities

1.   Contact a local inpatient rehabilitation facility and ask permission to sit in on a team care conference. Then, do the same for a subacute program. Compare and contrast the meetings and the roles of the individual team members. How did the role of the patient vary between settings?

How did the role of the caregiver differ? Did the nature of the information shared between rehabilitation service providers vary between settings? If so, how?

2. Organize a group of allied health students from your training program. Conduct a brainstorming session designed to identify those areas of care you each have in common. Then discuss ways you might use that information in developing cotreatment sessions. Discuss ways you might use that information in a transdisciplinary rehabilitation program.

3. Arrange an observation session with a therapist in an outpatient rehabilitation facility that serves both children and adults. Take note of how the facility is physically arranged. Are there opportunities for interdisciplinary communication? If not, how is that accomplished? How do the sessions between children and adults differ? How do the therapists track patient progress and billable hours? What differences do you see between rehabilitation services delivered in this setting versus your experience with inpatient and subacute rehabilitation?

Key Terms

Activity: Limitation in daily activities

Goal: General statement of intent or purpose

Impairment: Problems in body structure or body function

Inpatient rehabilitation: (1) Rehabilitation unit within a community hospital; (2) Rehabilitation within an academic medical center; (3) Freestanding rehabilitation hospital

Interdisciplinary: Professionals share what they are doing with respect to the patient and the various members support one another's treatment goals within the context of their own treatment session

Long-term goal: Expected level of performance when therapy services are terminated

Multidisciplinary: Professionals from various disciplines share what they are each doing with respect to the patient

Outpatient rehabilitation: (1) Housed within a community; (2) Freestanding facility; (3) Private practice; (4) Comprehensive outpatient rehabilitation facility

Participation: Restrictions on participation in society

Short-term goal: Steps to successful completion of long-term goals

Skilled nursing: A nursing service that must be provided by a registered nurse (RN) or a licensed practical nurse (LPN) under the supervision of an RN to be safe and effective

Subacute rehabilitation: (1) Delivered in a specialized unit of a community hospital; (2) Delivered in a unit within a long-term care facility; (3) Delivered within a skilled nursing facility; (4) Delivered in a free-standing facility

Transdisciplinary: A task-specific approach to treatment in which professionals work in teams to contribute to the patient's functional ability within the context of a specific activity

Study Questions

1. Compare and contrast the inpatient rehabilitation setting and the subacute rehabilitation setting in terms of medical criteria for admission, level(s) of care, and length of stay. Describe the different ways rehabilitation service delivery might look in each setting.

2. Define and give examples of *multidisciplinary, interdisciplinary,* and *transdisciplinary* approaches to rehabilitation. Discuss each approach in terms of its implications for inpatient, subacute, and home health rehabilitation.

3. Predict how site-neutral reimbursement for rehabilitation services may affect the growth and direction of the rehabilitation industry.

4. Discuss some of the challenges to interdisciplinary collaboration in the home health rehabilitation setting. What are some of the dangers in a lack of interdisciplinary communication? Identify some of the ways you might overcome the barriers to communication unique to home health service delivery.

5. Differentiate *licensure, accreditation,* and *certification* in terms of purpose, governing body, and implications for rehabilitation service delivery.

6. Describe an ALF. What are the advantages and disadvantages of this addition to the rehabilitation market?

7. How does outpatient rehabilitation differ from the other rehabilitation settings described in this chapter?

8. Discuss the relationship between issues of reimbursement and the delivery of rehabilitation services in the various settings. Predict ways in which you think rehabilitation service delivery may change over the next decade.

Acknowledgments

I acknowledge the help of Dr. James E. Warmth, Medical University of South Carolina, and Mrs. Mary Lou Waitschies, RN, St. Francis Xavier Home Health, for their assistance in developing this chapter.

References

CORF designation a way to offer more medically related services through assisted living. (1997, June). Eli Rehab Report IV, (6), 3851–3852.

DeJong, G., & Sutton, J. P. (1995). Rehab 2000: The evolution of medical rehabilitation in American health care. In P. K. Landrum, N. D. Schmidt, & A. McClean, Jr. (Eds.), Outcome-oriented rehabilitation: Principles, strategies, and tools for effective program management (pp. 3–42). Gaithersburg, MD: Aspen Publishers.

Despite "feeding frenzy" of last few years, market for selling rehab clinics remains strong. (1997, April). Eli Rehab Report IV, (4), 3808–3810.

Gill, H. S. (1995). The changing nature of ambulatory rehabilitation programs and services in a managed care environment. Archives of Physical Medicine and Rehabilitation, 76(Suppl. 12), SC10–SC11.

Haffey, W. J., Cayce, L. E., & Hallman, L. E. (1995). Outcome-oriented subacute rehabilitation. In P. K. Landrum, N. D. Schmidt, & A. McClean, Jr. (Eds.), Outcome-oriented rehabilitation: Principles, strategies, and tools for effective program management (pp. 125–146). Gaithersburg, MD: Aspen Publishers.

Harrington, A. K. (1994). Assisted living in alternative residential environments. In S. B. Goldsmith (Ed.), Essentials of long-term care administration (pp. 296–316). Gaithersburg, MD: Aspen Publishers.

HCFA supporting post-acute bundling over rehab pps. (1997, April). Eli Rehab Report IV, (4), 3801–3802.

Is a CORF in your facility's future? The marketplace may demand it. (July, 1997). Rehab Continuum Report, 6, 89–93.

Joint Commission on Accreditation of Rehabilitation Facilities. (1998). Medical rehabilitation standards manual. Tucson, AZ: Author.

Jones, A. M., & Foster, N. (1997). Transitional care: Bridging the gap. MEDSURG Nursing, 6(1), 32–38.

Kaye, H. S., LaPlante, M., Carlson, D., & Wenger, B. (1997). Trends in disability rates in the United States, 1970–1994, #17. Disability Statistics Abstract [On-line data]. Available: http://dsc.ucsf.edu/abs/ab17.html

Kelly, M. W. (1996). Hospital perspective on subacute care. In M. W. Kelly (Ed.), Subacute care services: The evolving opportunities and challenges (pp. 108–128). Chicago: Irvin Professional Publishing.

LaPlante, M. P. (1996). Health conditions and impairments causing disability, #16. Disability Statistics Abstract [On-line data]. Available: http://dsc.ucsf.edu/abs/ab16.html

Looking for land mines on the CORF battlefield: Here are items to consider before joining the fray. (1997, July). Rehab Continuum Report, 6, 91–92.

Medical University of South Carolina. (1998). Medicare Part B 1998 updates workshop (p. 17). Charleston, SC: University Medical Associates.

Moss, M. (1998, October 8). For retirees, moving into continuing care offers no guarantees. The Wall Street Journal, pp. A1, A8.

Physiatrists react to Stark II proposed regulations. (1998, April). PM&R in Practice, 6(3), 2–3.

Providing home care to assisted-living patients. (1998, April). Rehab Continuum Report, 7, 50–51.

Pynoos, J. (1996). Housing and the continuum of care. In S. J. Williams (Series Ed.) & C. J. Evashwich (Vol. Ed.), The continuum of long-term care (pp. 109–124). New York: Delmar Publishers.

Shi, L., & Singh, D. A. (1998). Delivering health care in America: A systems approach. Gaithersburg, MD: Aspen Publishers, Inc.

Sultz, H. A., & Young, K. M. (1997). Health care USA: Understanding its organization and delivery. Gaithersburg, MD: Aspen Publishers.

Tellis-Nayak, M., & MacDonnell, C. M. (1995). Joint commission and CARF accreditation for subacute care. In K. M. Griffin (Ed.), Handbook of subacute health care (pp. 205–220). Gaithersburg, MD: Aspen Publishers.

The evolution of subacute care: An overview. (1995, Summer). PM&R in Practice, 3, 1–4.

von Sternberg, T., Hepburn, K., Cibuzar, P., Convery, L., Dokken, B., Haefemeyer, J., Rettke, S., Ripley, J., Vosenau, V., Rothe, P., Schurle, D., & Won-Savage, R. (1997). Post-hospital sub-acute care: An example of a managed care model. Journal of the American Geriatrics Society, 45(1), 87–91.

Suggested Readings

Anderson, K. (1993, January). Is it still home sweet home care? Business and Health, 42–46.

Barr, K. W., & Briendel, C. L. (1995). Ambulatory care. In L. F. Wolper (Ed.), Health care administration: Principles, practices, structure and delivery (2nd ed.) (pp. 547–573). Gaithersburg, MD: Aspen Publishers.

Burns, J. (1993, December 13). Subacute care feeds need to diversify. Modern Healthcare, 34–38.

Burns, J. (1994, April 25). Sorting out subacute care. Modern Healthcare, 28–32.

Burns, J. (1995, May 22). Outpatient chains keep on growing. Modern Healthcare, 82–86.

Dey, A. N. (1997). Characteristics of elderly home health care users: Data from the 1994 National Home and Hospice Case Survey (Advance Data from Vital and Health Statistics No. 279). Hyattsville, MD: National Center for Health Statistics.

England, B. (1989). The rehabilitation environment. In England, B., Glass, R. M., & Patterson, C. H. (Eds.), Quality rehabilitation: Results oriented patient care (pp. 11–18). Chicago: American Hospital Publishing.

Fein, E. B. (1996, February 19). Region's hospitals have seen the future, and it's an outpatient clinic. The New York Times, p. B1.

Gans, J. S. (1983). Hate in the rehabilitation setting. Archives of Physical Medicine and Rehabilitation, 64, 176–179.

Grebin, B., & Kaplan, S. (1995, December). Toward a pediatric subacute care model: Clinical and administrative features. Archives of Physical Medicine and Rehabilitation, 76(Suppl. 12), SC16–SC20.

Haffey, W. J., & Welsh, J. H. (1995, December). Subacute care: Evolution in search of value. Archives of Physical Medicine and Rehabilitation, 76(Suppl. 12), SC2–SC4.

Kane, M. (1989). The home care crisis of the nineties. The Gerontologist, 22, 24–31.

Kane, R. A., & Wilson, K. B. (1993). Assisted living in the United States: A new paradigm for residential care for frail older persons. Washington, DC: American Association of Retired Persons.

Lellis, M. (1994). Who provides more cost effective care—rehab hospitals or SNFs? National Report Subacute Care, 2, 5–6.

Liu, K., Manton, K., & Liu, B. (1985). Home care expenses for the disabled elderly. Health Care Financing Review, 7, 51–57.

Lowell-Smith, E. G. (1994). Alternative forms of ambulatory care: Implications for patients and physicians. Social Science and Medicine, 38(2), 275–283.

Meili, P. (1993, April/May). The rehabilitation market. Rehabilitation Management, 96–102.

Micheletti, J. A., & Shlala, T. J. (1995). Understanding and operationalizing subacute services. Nursing Management, 26(6), 49–56.

Neu, C. R., & Harrison, S. C. (1988). Posthospital care before and after the Medicare prospective payment system. Santa Monica, CA: Rand Corporation.

Ory, M. G., & Duncker, A. P. (Eds.). (1991). In-home care for older people. Newbury Park, CA: Sage Publications.

Pallarito, K. (1992, February 24). Charting the rapid rise of subacute care. Modern Healthcare, 52–56.

Pynoos, J., & Liebig, P. (Eds.), Housing frail elders: International policies, perspectives and prospects. Baltimore: The Johns Hopkins University Press.

Ross, B. (1992). The impact of reimbursement issues on rehabilitation nursing practice and patient care. Rehabilitation Nursing, 17(5), 236–238.

Shaughnessy, P. W., & Kramer, A. M. (1990). The increased needs of patients in nursing homes and patients receiving home health care. New England Journal of Medicine, 322, 21–27.

Smith, J. R., & Shiner, P. Transforming nursing practice: Acute care to community. Home Health Care Management and Practice, 8(6).

St. Martin, E. E. (1996). Community health centers and quality of care: A goal to provide effective health care to the community. Journal of Community Health Nursing, 13(2), 83–92.

Tilson, D. (Ed.). (1990). Aging in place: Supporting the frail elderly in residential environments. Glenview, Ill: Scott, Foresman and Company.

Troop, J. E. (1994). The development of subacute services: Struggling to complete the continuum. Strategic Health Care Market, 4.

Wolk, S., & Blair, T. (1994). Trends in medical rehabilitation. Reston, VA: American Rehabilitation Association.

Zolk, I. K. (1990). Disability and the home-care revolution. Archives of Physical Medicine and Rehabilitation, 71, 93.

CHAPTER 2

Teamwork in Rehabilitation

Donna Latella

According to Kouzes & Posner (1987), a team is "a group of equally important people collaborating, developing cooperative goals, and building trusting relationships to achieve shared goals." It is a group of people who hold a specified task that requires collaboration of its members. Team collaboration is a process that evolves over time. A productive team demonstrates the ability to be task specific and goal oriented. Specific to health care, the professionals work in a client-centered environment.

This chapter provides entry-level and practical information on teamwork in rehabilitation to answer the following questions:

- What is a team?
- What is the purpose of a health care team?
- Where do teams practice?
- Why are teams effective in a rehabilitation setting?
- What are the benefits of working in a team?
- What types of team approaches are there?
- Who are team members?
- How does a health care professional become part of a team?
- How does a health care professional create a new team?

History of Health Care Teams

In the past, health care was typically delivered by a sole provider. The emphasis was on sickness and cure rather than wellness, prevention, and patient/family involvement. According to Keith (1991), I. Brown, an historian, described three periods in the evolution of team care. In the first period, before World War II, there was only minimal use of the team, although recognition of its need was beginning.

In the second period after the war, the rapid expansion of knowledge in medicine and the creation of new specialty areas in health care made it evident that efforts were needed to coordinate services. Initial endeavors of a team approach occurred at the Montefiore Hospital in New York during the 1940s, when home care services were delivered by an interdisciplinary team. This team consisted of a social worker, nurse, and physician. From the 1940s to 1960, the delivery of care was termed *comprehensive care*, and other members were added to the primary health care team, such as psychologists; dieticians; medical technologists; and physical, occupational, and speech therapists. This approach intended to serve the social and physical needs of the patient.

The third period began in the 1970s, when interdisciplinary team development became federally funded to support training of staff in team settings.

With the development of teams came the shift toward treating clients holistically and a broad approach to client care. This broad approach attempts to address the client's physical, psychological, social, educational, cultural, spiritual, and vocational needs within the framework of the family and community. Today, collaboration with many professionals and coordination of care in a team approach is essential, particularly because clients often have multiple diagnoses, deficits, and issues.

Purpose of Teams

When thinking of a team approach, the first analogy that comes to mind is the flock of geese flying together in the V formation. Each member of the flock has its own important position in the formation. His or her destination cannot be reached unless each member holds formation, so no one may falter. The flock is as strong as its weakest link. Therefore, each goose is as important and vital to the task as the next.

In most health care settings, the team approach and each member is vital to client progress and success. The general purpose of a health care team is client-focused care, with each individual having specialized goals. According to Kemp et al. (1990), "Teams often evolve from the necessity of integrating a broad array of information into a plan of action or a course of treatment." Therefore, it is the team's responsibility to provide a high quality of care in an efficient manner. This is accomplished through collaborative tasks such as communication, evaluation, decision-making, problem solving, brainstorming, and networking.

The expertise of each team member allows for the team to look at the *whole* person versus the diagnosis or dysfunction in isolation. According to Purtillo and Haddad (1996), "The idea of the health care team is that all team

TABLE 2.1
Rehabilitation Teams: Benefits to Patients

Patient-centered environment
Coordination of care
Patient treated holistically
Increased trusting relationship between health care practitioners, patient, and family
Increased lines of communication between all parties involved
Increased patient/family education
Increased knowledge of the rehabilitation process
Ability to incorporate wellness and prevention into plan of care
Patient may be able to function independently longer
Increased knowledge of illness, progress, and discharge options
Involvement of patient and family in goal setting, treatment planning, and discharge
    options
Decreased inpatient stays
Efficient follow-up care on discharge

---

members are more equal. All are working together cooperatively and efficiently toward the professional *and* institutional goal of client management." This holistic approach may lead to prevention of further illness, which may include educating clients in wellness. These efforts work to achieve the client's goals: efficient client care and decreased health care costs.

Benefits of Working in a Team

According to Ling (1996), "Effective teams have been shown to significantly outperform individuals working alone with increased productivity, work quality, accountability, and job satisfaction." Working as a team in a rehabilitation setting provides many benefits to the clients involved (Table 2.1). Health care providers often find increased job satisfaction. In general, health care benefits as well (Tables 2.2 and 2.3).

Many new and experienced health care professionals choose to work in a client-centered environment because they are people oriented. Entering health care as a new practitioner is challenging. Therefore, it is often recommended to begin one's career as part of a health care team to learn and grow alongside other professionals of the same and different disciplines. According to Purtillo and Haddad (1996), "The team itself should become a means of support, growth and increased effectiveness for the health professional who wants to maximize his or her strengths as a person, while performing the necessary professional tasks."

One example is when a health care professional must make important recommendations to the client or family, particularly regarding life-threatening situations. For example, the speech therapist may need to recommend alternative methods of nutrition when a dysphagia evaluation

TABLE 2.2
Rehabilitation Teams: Benefits to the Health Care Provider

Increased communication between health care providers
Building of knowledge and respect for other disciplines
Building of trusting, working relationships
Learning environment for entry-level practitioners and in general
Goal-oriented environment
Professional growth
Opportunities to expand leadership skills
Involvement in group process
Collaboration and brainstorming of ideas, recommendations, and solutions
Feedback and affirmation leading to increased confidence
Motivating environment
Personal self-analysis, growth, and development
Opportunities to practice techniques
Opportunities to learn new skills
Opportunities to practice effective speaking techniques
Opportunities to increase ability to listen, give support, confront, and give feedback

TABLE 2.3
Health Care Teams: General Benefits to Health Care

Comprehensive care
Efficient mode of health care delivery
Cost-effectiveness
Increased productivity
Increased work quality
Increased job satisfaction, which may lead to employee retention and assist with
    recruitment
Decreased inpatient stays
Help in meeting the needs of expanding managed care
Help in competition for business

determines that "by mouth" feeding may be unsafe for the client. It is reassuring to have team members offering their thoughts, suggestions, affirmations, and expertise, especially when such a recommendation may be devastating to the client and family.

Those who choose to work as independent health care practitioners may find this environment isolating. Patient safety issues are also of greater concern. For example, an independent home-care practitioner or consultant (not employed by an agency) may enter a home situation when the client is experiencing a serious medical condition, and more than one person is needed to assist. As part of a team, it is more likely that a high-risk client will be seen by more than one practitioner at a time to ensure safety and client success.

There are health care professionals who do find satisfaction and success in working independently, however. Some of the benefits may be efficiency of work, making a more flexible schedule, and being one's own boss. In most cases, an independent practitioner has some communication with others to clinically manage client care.

Challenges, obstacles, and conflicts are part of becoming a team member, but the benefits for the patient certainly outweigh the risks.

Becoming a Team Member

It may be challenging to enter an already established team. A new team member must work for and earn the respect, trust, acceptance, and understanding of the team. This relationship is one that must be nurtured over time.

A new team member must also learn the group goals and process. He or she must adhere to the policies, procedures, and rules. It is important that the roles, responsibilities, personalities, and leadership qualities of each team member be learned, respected, and accepted. Specific skills for effective teamwork include:

- Cooperation
- Adherence to group rules
- Sensitivity to others
- Ability to work in a group effort
- Ability to take on roles as needed
- Ability to communicate
- Ability to give support
- A positive attitude
- Knowledge of group process
- Empathy
- Ability to confront
- Organization
- Flexibility
- Self-confidence
- Self-awareness
- Commitment
- Ability to problem solve
- Knowledge of boundaries
- Knowledge of team member roles

When starting out as a new team member, it is perfectly acceptable to sit back, listen, and observe for the first few meetings before giving input. It is also an excellent opportunity to familiarize oneself with the existing clients as well as the team.

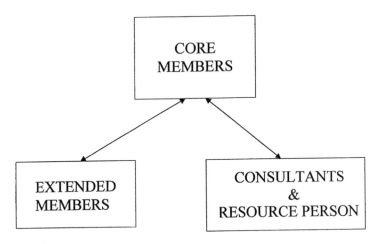

FIGURE 2.1. Example of a typical team.

Team Members

The number of team members may vary depending on the needs of the rehabilitation setting and the clients (Figure 2.1). The average size of a team is five members. Usually, the team leader is the physician or physiatrist, who may have the title of medical director, although leadership may be passed from one member to another during team meetings. In the medical model, the physician leads the team by guiding the medical treatment with rehabilitation. In the absence of the physician, a case coordinator may provide linkage between the physician and team members.

Typically, a head nurse or primary nurse represents either the facility or a specific unit. Either the nurse or a social worker may act as the discharge planner or case manager. Responsibilities may include conducting the initial client/family interview, obtaining client history and pertinent medical insurance and financial information, assessing the client's present mental status/safety issues, and determining early on the possible discharge options.

This information is key to report to the team members so that the team as a whole is steered toward appropriate evaluation tools, goals, treatment plans, and discharge recommendations specific to their discipline. After each discipline has completed its tasks, findings are reported back to the team. Then, initial goals and treatment plans may be meshed collaboratively, or individually, depending on the team approach (see "Team Approaches" section).

These and other typical team members are listed in Table 2.4. The mix of staff usually varies depending on the rehabilitation setting, needs of the client, diagnosis, goals, and complexity of discharge plans. For exam-

TABLE 2.4
Typical Team Members

Physician/physiatrist
Physician specialist
Physician's assistant
Nurse
Nurse specialist/practitioner
Certified nursing assistant
Social worker
Occupational therapist
Physical therapist
Speech therapist
Recreational therapist
Dance therapist
Art therapist
Respiratory therapist
Dietician
Psychiatrist/psychologist
Chaplain
Prosthetist
Home health aide
Optometrist
Dentist
Pharmacist
Exercise physiologist
Athletic trainer
Teacher
Insurance company representative
Counselor
Orthotist

---

ple, clients in a long-term-care facility may not require an occupational or physical therapist on their team, although it is highly likely that a client in subacute rehabilitation who is being discharged home will.

Team Settings

The team approach may be seen in many types of rehabilitation settings. In general, teams are used in inpatient, outpatient, home care, schools, and community programs. Table 2.5 lists specific settings that typically use a team approach.

Within these rehabilitation settings, virtually any diagnosis or client need may be addressed through the use of a team approach. Facilities may vary in types of diagnosis they see; age of clients; goals; and specific program mission/goals, expertise, demographics, or market niche.

TABLE 2.5
Typical Team Settings

Acute care
Subacute care
Long-term care
Outpatient clinic
Hospice
Home health care
School
Adult daycare
Partial day program
Community-based setting
Assisted living
Transitional care

Team Approaches

The three team approaches are *multidisciplinary, interdisciplinary,* and *transdisciplinary.* Sometimes these terms are used interchangeably, but they have specific meanings (Kemp et al., 1990). These types of team approaches differ in their philosophy, structure, leadership, goal-setting, and goal-attainment strategies.

Multidisciplinary Approach

In a multidisciplinary approach, the representatives of each discipline submit their own findings and recommendations, set their own disciplinary-specific goals, and work within the disciplinary boundaries to achieve these goals independently. Communication regarding the client's progress or attainment of goals is direct or indirect to the rest of the team. The team's outcome is the sum of each discipline's efforts. For example, the social worker may be exploring Meals on Wheels for the client on discharge, whereas the dietician is concerned for the client's need for a puree diet. Communication between team members is necessary for success and overall well-being of the client.

Interdisciplinary Approach

To achieve success with the interdisciplinary approach, collaboration augments communication. The team identifies goals and strives to avoid duplication of services and conflict of goals. Teams are involved in problem solving beyond the scope of their own discipline. Once the team goals are set, each discipline works toward goal attainment within their own discipline. There is collaboration when goals overlap discipline boundaries. For example, the recreation therapist may engage a client in a gardening activity for the pursuit of leisure interests, whereas the occupational therapist's outcome of a gardening task may be for upper extremity strength and coordination. The two therapists may collaborate for one of them to choose a different task or for both to be specific in documenting their final outcome or goal for the same activity.

Transdisciplinary Approach

The transdisciplinary approach maximizes the strength of team members and minimizes duplication of services. One team member is chosen to be the primary therapist or leader, depending on the specific needs of the client. For example, a nurse may be the primary therapist/leader for a client whose treatment or reason for admittance is to stabilize psychiatric medications. Other team members contribute information and recommendations through the primary therapist/leader.

This approach is now being attempted with hopes of increasing cost-effectiveness of client care delivery. The view is that one team member can accomplish the task at hand, regardless of his or her discipline, decreasing time spent in joint collaboration.

With this approach, cross-training of team members is required, and flexibility is needed because the boundaries are blurred. A popular example is seen with the expanding role of the certified nursing assistant (CNA). In many settings, the CNA's job description may be expanded to perform established therapeutic exercise regimes with clients, clean patient rooms, and pass meal trays.

Guidelines for Creating a New Team

Health care teams typically evolve either informally, by chance, or formally, with a specific purpose or goal at hand. The optimal time to create a new team is when a new rehabilitation program or unit is opening. The key factor in establishing this team is the needs of the clients.

There is no ideal mix of professionals, although the smaller, the better, according to Kemp et al. (1990). The following are guidelines for the levels of inclusion of team members.

First Level

Core members are those team members who work together on the same unit everyday, such as physicians, nurses, social workers, and physical and occupational therapists. This first level is responsible for developing team process and deciding how to include other disciplines in assessment and treatment of each client. The core members are also responsible for creating all operational guidelines and establishing the physical setting of team meetings (Figure 2.2).

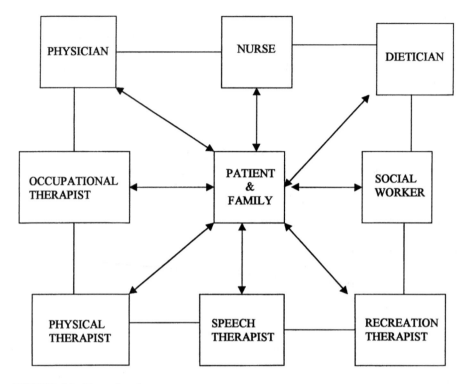

FIGURE 2.2. Team levels.

Second Level

Extended members are team members who may work in multiple clinical sites or units, usually because their particular discipline does not have full-time needs in one location. These members may include dieticians, pharmacists, psychiatrists/psychologists, speech therapists, and dentists.

Third Level

Involvement of *consultants* and *resource persons* is decided by the core members as appropriate and necessary. Consultants may be asked to only discuss with or send their evaluations and recommendations to the core team. Examples of consultants may be specialized physicians such as neurologists and oncologists, specialized nurses representing hemodialysis or geriatrics, and exercise physiologists. Resource persons are not usually part of client-centered meetings. They typically specialize and assist in team development, communications, or conflict management. An example may be a representative from the human resources department specializing in role delineation.

Clients

A major question may be whether to include the client in the team meeting. Typically, clients are not involved because of issues such as team conflicts, lack of understanding medical terminology used, and the risk of frightening the client. It is recommended that one team member represents the values, goals, and viewpoints of the client. Rounds and family meetings are usually the settings in which client and family involvement is encouraged with the primary care team. In these settings, joint goal setting may occur, as well as client/family education.

Stages

Teams progress through stages of evolution. Members must help one another function at every stage. At each stage of evolution, the team must accomplish tasks, problem solve, and answer new questions that may arise, while always keeping in mind the needs and desires of the client involved. Stages of evolution include:

1. *Getting started.* Getting started is a formal stage of development and interaction. Members are getting to know one another, the task at hand, and the overall group process that is emerging. In this stage, it is vital for trust to build.
2. *Truly beginning.* Formality decreases in this stage. Priorities are established, interpersonal interactions begin, and the culture of the group emerges. Conflict is common now, and each team member is challenged and evaluated. The team's goals have been established.
3. *Designing the plan.* The group works on strategies to achieve its goals through specific steps, timelines, and deadlines. Roles and responsibilities are assigned and apparent.
4. *Doing.* Strategies are carried out. The team is driven. There is trust, respect, and commitment seen at this stage.

Team Meetings

Team meetings may take many forms. Meetings are typically held in a room large enough for all members, such as a conference room, lounge, or staff area. Privacy and confidentiality are vital. On the other hand, teams may consider client rounds to be their meeting time. The advantage to this type of meeting is that it allows the client to be involved, ask questions, and see and be seen by the team members at one time.

Team meetings may be referred to by different names, such as patient care planning meetings, team conferences, discharge planning meetings, pupil-personnel-team meetings, and client rounds.

According to Heruti and Ohry (1995), the rehabilitation team's success depends greatly on effective meetings, which should be productive, stimulating, and goal-oriented. Communication is key to success. The meeting must be organized properly for group process to occur. Typically, each discipline takes a turn reporting on the current status of the client. Discussion may occur during this reporting or after everyone has reported.

Team meetings are held at regular times, and frequency may vary from daily to weekly to monthly, depending on the intensity and pace of the rehabilitation setting.

Considerations for the Future

Health care is an ever-changing and growing delivery system. As with any system, it has its strengths and weaknesses. Although hospital stays have declined and clients are recovering more quickly, cost-effectiveness will always be a concern. Therefore, it is unknown whether the team approach to rehabilitation will continue to be an effective means of managing client care. Additional issues to consider are managed care, possible restructuring of health care delivery, and alternative treatment modes.

Health care providers must work to provide the most cost-effective service, not only to advocate for the profession, but also to meet the needs of clients. It is hoped that the future will continue to prove the need for teamwork in health care to best meet the needs of everyone concerned.

Study Questions

Please read the following three case studies and discuss the questions/issues listed below for each case:

1. Apply and discuss how each of the three team approaches would work on this case.

2. Which team member should be the case manager? Why?

3. Which team members may act as core members in this case? Extended members? Consultants or resource persons?

4. What is the role delineation for each member above?

5. What factors are relevant to each team member?

6. What are possible discharge options?

7. Which team members may be needed for follow-up on discharge?

Case Studies

Case Study 1

Mrs. B is a 79-year-old woman who was admitted to Memorial Hospital on April 27, 1998, with a diagnosis of right hip fracture secondary to a fall at home. A right total hip replacement was performed on April 28, 1998, and the patient is on total hip precautions.

Medical history: Insulin-dependent diabetes mellitus, high blood pressure, myocardial infarction in 1988, and cataract surgery in 1995.

Social history: Widow who lives alone in senior housing, is independent with functional activities (activities of daily living, instrumental activities of daily living), and takes public transportation. Patient has one son who lives 1 hour away and helps out occasionally. The son states that his mother is often forgetful. For example, within the past year she has forgotten to turn the oven off several times.

Cognitive status: While in the hospital, the patient was oriented to self and year only, and had several bouts of confusion, in particular regarding her condition and locale. Mrs. B was discharged from the hospital to the local subacute nursing home on May 10, 1998.

Mrs. B reports her fall occurred while getting into the bathtub. She was found on the floor by a neighbor who had been ringing the doorbell for several hours after the patient did not show up for the weekly bingo game. It is reported that the patient's bathroom has an emergency pull cord, although the patient did not remember to use it.

Case Study 2

Danielle, a 5-year-old girl born after an uncomplicated, full-term pregnancy, labor, and delivery, is experiencing developmental delay and abnormal gait.

Medical history: There was no history of neonatal abnormalities. Danielle did well at home with no reports of serious illness, injuries, hospitalizations, or problems.

Developmental history: Appropriate milestones included sitting at 7 months, ambulating at 1 year, and speaking her first words at 11 months of age. Danielle's mother noted, however, that her sentences were never structured, and it was extremely difficult to understand her. Relatives and friends noticed that the child appeared "uncoordinated," as she often tripped over her own feet and dropped objects.

Social history: Danielle has a 5-month-old brother. Her mother, who is 31 years old, works part-time at the local library. Her father, 34, is a crane operator who has always been a poor reader. Danielle's mother has a Bachelor of Science degree, and her father received his high school equivalency diploma soon after Danielle was born. The family lives in a small apartment and is experiencing financial hardship. They have no immediate family or support system in the area, except for their local church and a few close friends.

Case Study 3

Mike is a 37-year-old, emaciated man referred to the community mental health agency after a short inpatient admittance intended to stabilize medications. He is experiencing chronic schizophrenia-depressive disorder.

Intake history: During the intake interview, Mike exhibited a disorderly appearance. His affect was flat and he appeared frightened. Mike had poor eye contact, his speech was loose and fragmented, and his insight was poor. He felt that he was "boxed in" and that people were against him. Recent and past memory was fair. He denied suicidal ideation.

Medical history: No history of major illnesses, except for double hernia surgery as an infant. Mike's psychiatric history spans approximately 12 years, with five voluntary admissions in the local hospital's inpatient unit.

Social history: Mike's educational background included completion of high school and 1 year of college. He has held several short-term jobs over the past 5 years, such as working in a coffee shop. He is presently unemployed, receiving state aid, and reports he has no desire to return to work. Mike states he spends his days sleeping, smoking, and drinking coffee. Mike's father was a salesman, and his mother was a housewife. Mike has one older and one younger sister. He reports a close uncle had a history of alcohol abuse.

References

Heruti, R., & Ohry, A. (1995). The rehabilitation team: A commentary. American Journal of Physical Medicine and Rehabilitation, 74, 466–468.

Keith, R. A. (1991). The comprehensive treatment team in rehabilitation. Archives of Physical Medicine and Rehabilitation, 72, 269–274.

Kemp, B., Brummel-Smith, K., & Ramsdell, J. (1990). Geriatric rehabilitation (p. 372). Austin, TX: Pro-ed.

Kouzes, J. M., & Posner, B. Z. (1987). The leadership challenge: How to get extraordinary things done in organizations (p. 213). San Francisco: Jossey-Bass.

Ling, C. (1996). Performance of a self-directed work team in a home health care agency. Journal of Nursing Administration, 26, 36.

Purtillo, R., & Haddad, A. (1996). Health professional and patient interaction (5th ed.) (p. 93). Philadelphia: W. B. Saunders, Co.

Suggested Readings

American Occupational Therapy Association. (1996). The occupational therapy manager (rev. ed.). Bethesda, MD: Author.

Castledine, G. (1996). Encouraging team collaboration in healthcare. British Journal of Nursing, 5, 14.

Fordyce, W. (1981). On interdisciplinary peers. Archives of Physical Medicine and Rehabilitation, 62, 51–53.

Gottlieb, L., & Rowat, K. (1987). The McGill model of nursing: A practice-derived model. Advances in Nursing Science, 9(4), 57–61.

Hoeman, S. (1996). Rehabilitation nursing: Process and application (2nd ed.). St. Louis: Mosby.

Jelles, F., Van Bennekom, C., & Lankhurst, G. (1995). The interdisciplinary team conference in rehabilitation medicine: A commentary. American Journal of Physical Medicine and Rehabilitation, 74, 464–465.

Lucci, J. (1980). Occupational therapy case studies (2nd ed.). Garden City, NJ: Medical Examination Publishing Company, Inc.

Maloney, F. (1987). Physical medicine and rehabilitation. Philadelphia: Hanley & Belfus.

McKeehan, K. (1981). Continuing care: A multidisciplinary approach to discharge planning. St Louis: Mosby.

Mears, P. (1994). Health care teams. Delray Beach, FL: St. Lucie Press.

Melvin, J. (1989). Status report on interdisciplinary medicine. Archives of Physical Medicine and Rehabilitation, 70, 273–276.

Purtillo, R. (1988). Ethical issues in teamwork: The context of rehabilitation. Archives of Physical Medicine and Rehabilitation, 69, 318–322.

Sladyk, K. (1997). Occupational therapy student primer: A guide to college success. Thorofare, NJ: Slack, Inc.

CHAPTER 3

Team Ethics in Rehabilitation

Dick Sobsey

Ethical dilemmas are common in rehabilitation. Occasionally, decisions must be made regarding life and death issues. More frequently, the consequences are subtler. The objectives of this chapter are to:

- Define ethics in rehabilitation
- Understand an ecological framework for categorizing ethics
- Recognize that ethics is subjective, based on social values, and cannot be based solely on logic or objectively verifiable information
- Recognize that multidisciplinary teamwork has its own set of ethical values and issues
- Identify and explore some of the current issues in rehabilitation ethics

Consider the following case study:

Case Study 1

William is an occupational therapist who likes working with clients with severe and chronic disabilities. After he described his clients' progress to Myrna, his agency administrator, she told him that their agency must shift program priorities to clients who have a greater probability of being restored to normal function. William argued that the health care system is ignoring those who need the most help, and he believes the agency has an ethical responsibility to serve these clients. Myrna, however, argued that the agency has an ethical responsibility to use limited program resources where they will do the greatest good for the most people.

Dilemmas like the one described in Case Study 1 are common in rehabilitation. Ethical decision making is an essential aspect of all human endeavors, but human services require particular attention to ethics. Rehabilitation requires even greater attention because team members often work closely with clients in situations that leave them vulnerable. For example, rehabilitation team members often work intensively with clients and their families during the early and often difficult stages of adjustment to disabilities acquired through stroke or spinal cord injuries (Trexler & Fordyce, 1996). In addition, rehabilitation professionals working as members of a team must balance ethical obligations to themselves, their teams, their respective disciplines, and society as a whole with their ethical responsibilities to their clients.

Until fairly recently, rehabilitation ethics were given little attention (Haas, 1993). In recent years, however, there has been considerable thought given to ethical issues and responsibilities in rehabilitation. As a result, there is significant consensus in many areas, and many guidelines and standards have been developed to assist team members from various disciplines. Nevertheless, it is important to point out that many ethical issues related to the practice of rehabilitation and multidisciplinary teamwork remain largely unexplored, whereas others remain the topic of great controversy and little consensus. This chapter presents some of the generally accepted guidelines and also explores some of the unresolved issues. While the information presented is based on considerable review of the literature, readers are reminded that the content is also strongly affected by the author's opinions. Because ethics are rooted in subjective values (e.g., what is good, bad, right, or wrong) rather than objective information, they are always subject to opinion. Logic can assist us in clarifying ethical issues, but it can never dictate the basic values on which ethics must be based.

Even though ethical values are subjective, it would be a mistake to think that these values are arbitrary or entirely determined within each

Case Study 2

Lois, whose 15-year-old son is recovering slowly from a traumatic brain injury, tells her son's physical therapist that she is so discouraged that she sometimes thinks about ending her son's suffering by smothering him. The physical therapist doesn't think Lois is serious, but she can't be sure. Reporting the statement to child protection authorities unnecessarily might cause more stress for the family and alienate the mother from the rehabilitation team. If Lois is serious about killing her son, however, failing to take action may be catastrophic.

individual. These values are largely socially and culturally determined. For example, citizens of the same country, members of a specific ethnic group, adherents to a particular religion, and practitioners of the same disciplines tend to share the same sets of values and codes of ethics. These ethical codes and guidelines are sometimes written down in laws, codes of conduct, charters, or other documents, but they are also shared informally through a variety of interpersonal interactions. While it is important for all members of a team to ascribe to similar or at least compatible ethical principles, each individual ultimately must make her or his own decisions and develop a personal set of ethics.

Often rehabilitation professionals must choose one moral obligation over another that conflicts with it or attempt to strike a delicate compromise between the two (Haas, 1993). In addition, changes in our social environment, technology, and professional practice continue to add new ethical dimensions and modify existing ethical responsibilities (Haas, 1993).

Ethics in Rehabilitation

Such dilemmas as the one discussed in Case Study 2 are not easily solved. Members of rehabilitation teams have many ethical responsibilities, and sometimes two or more responsibilities conflict with each other. Uncertainty and incomplete information often compound these conflicts. In this case, for example, the moral obligation to protect a child from danger conflicts with the moral obligation to preserve confidentiality. If the threat to the child were unambiguous, the duty of protection would clearly outweigh the protection of confidentiality. Because the threat is uncertain, however, the correct course of action remains unclear. Ultimately, the balance between the two ethical responsibilities depends on the perceived seriousness of the mother's statement. While ethical principles and guidelines can provide some assistance in such cases, they can never be expected to dictate the right decision. As Scott points out, those who expect guidelines to provide clear answers to difficult ethical questions are certain to be disappointed (Scott, 1998).

The relative recency of increased attention to ethical issues in rehabilitation may be due to several factors. First, because rehabilitation medicine is in itself relatively new, the currently emerging interest in ethical issues may signal maturity of the discipline. Second, as members of an emerging field, rehabilitation professionals may have chosen to focus on a few central issues (e.g., the recognition of rehabilitation medicine as a distinct field). Finally, rehabilitation professionals may have been content to be guided by more general medical or health care ethics (Haas, 1993). The current interest in rehabilitation ethics, however, has identified unique areas of focus for rehabilitation disciplines (Brillhart, 1995; Haas, 1995; Imrie, 1997; Lucke, 1998).

Garrett, Baillie, and Garrett (1998) provide the following definition:

> Ethics is that branch of philosophy that seeks to determine how human actions may be judged right or wrong. When the study of ethics is applied to a professional field, it becomes necessary to discuss not only basic ethical positions, but also the nature of the profession and the conditions under which that profession operates.

Therefore, rehabilitation ethics must be based on a general set of ethics that applies to all human conduct and must also incorporate values and procedures specifically related to the field of rehabilitation. In addition, the team approach to rehabilitation requires that specific attention be provided to the ethics of multidisciplinary teamwork. Although professionals and academics have devoted a great deal of attention to rehabilitation ethics in the 1980s and 1990s, the ethics of multidisciplinary teamwork remain largely ignored. At least in part, the lack of attention for multidisciplinary aspects of ethics has been a result of the major roles of discipline-based professional associations in addressing ethical issues. These professional associations have done a great deal of excellent work in developing guidelines and identifying issues. However, because these associations are based in specific disciplines (e.g., psychology, occupational therapy, nursing), they have given only cursory consideration to the ethics of multidisciplinary teamwork.

Ethical principles may be conceptualized and organized according to a number of different frameworks. For example, some ethicists categorize ethical principles as teleologic (i.e., based on the predictable consequences of an action) or deontologic (based on the duties of the individual) (Hansen, 1993). Rehabilitation ethics might also be categorized by the specific rehabilitation disciplines (e.g., nursing ethics, occupational therapy ethics, social work ethics). Although this approach would be useful for studying the history and development of rehabilitation ethics, it is not used in this chapter for three reasons. First, because every rehabilitation discipline has developed its own ethical guidelines, merely listing them all would take

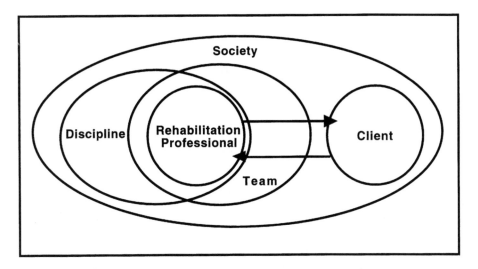

FIGURE 3.1. Ethical responsibilities. Interactions between the rehabilitation team member and client occur in the context of the team, the professional's specific discipline, and society as a whole.

up most of the chapter. Second, most of the ethical guidelines within each of the rehabilitation disciplines are similar to those of the other disciplines, therefore listing all of them would result in a great deal of repetition. Although the differences among the ethics developed by the various disciplines would be interesting to explore, that analysis goes beyond the scope of this chapter. Third, and most importantly, presenting ethical guidelines separately for each discipline would be inconsistent with the rehabilitation-team approach presented in this book. Therefore, this chapter presents a unified model of rehabilitation ethics. The ecological model of ethical responsibility is based on social contexts of moral responsibilities. In this model, ethical obligations are classified according to the context of the obligations.

As shown in Figure 3.1, a rehabilitation professional interacts with a client and has ethical responsibilities to that client. However, the rehabilitation professional also is acting as a member of a team and as a representative of a specific rehabilitation discipline. In addition, the professional, client, team, and discipline all exist within the context of larger society. Each of these social contexts for behavior has its own ethical domain. Therefore, ethical responsibility to clients must be balanced with ethical responsibilities to rehabilitation teams, each professional's specific discipline, society as a whole, and even with the professionals' moral obligations to themselves. Ethical behavior may be viewed as behavior that strikes the most appropriate balance of the duties among these various ethical domains.

Basic Principles of Ethics for Rehabilitation Teams

Table 3.1 presents basic principles of ethics for rehabilitation teams organized by domains of social context. These principles have been extrapo-
lated and blended from the ethical guidelines from a number of specific
rehabilitation disciplines.

Ethics of Self-Care

The identification of an ethical responsibility to one's own self may seem surprising to some. Others may even feel that such self-interest is inappropriate
or unethical. This is probably because many ethical problems have occurred
because individuals act in their own self-interest to the exclusion of the interest of others. As a result, the self-sacrificing professional who considers his or
her own interests last is often seen as more ethical than others. In fact, altruism—the ethical doctrine that the proper goal of behavior is for the general
good of society—is sometimes interpreted as contrary to any self-interest.

Recently, however, there has been greater recognition of the ethical
responsibility that rehabilitation professionals and other care providers
have to themselves. Psychologists have already given some recognition to
this ethical responsibility in their ethical guidelines, which state that psychologists must be aware that stress and other factors may impair their
ability to practice effectively (American Psychological Association, 1992).
Not surprisingly, research has demonstrated that psychologists believe that
they have an ethical responsibility to minimize stress and burnout in their
work. In addition, psychologists with strong belief in this ethical responsibility take more action to prevent burnout (Skorupa & Agresti, 1993).

While the ethics of self-care has received the greatest attention
among psychologists, it has also received growing attention in other rehabilitation disciplines, such as occupational therapy (Sweeney & Nichols,
1996) and nursing (Cameron, 1986). The American Nurses Association has
adopted an official policy that nurses have not only a right but an obligation to refuse assignments that put them in significant danger (American
Nurses Association, 1996).

This growing recognition is important for several reasons. First, reasonable attention to one's own needs is a legitimate and important concern. Second, because it is often necessary to balance the priorities given to
one's own interests with priorities given to the interests of others,
acknowledging and understanding self-interests is a necessary first step.
Third, rehabilitation professionals who sacrifice too much of their own
needs for others often become less effective in caring for others. Finally,
the rehabilitation professionals who do not properly care for themselves
set poor examples for their clients. Such poor examples are particularly
counterproductive when, as is often the case, client goals include developing enhanced self-care practices.

TABLE 3.1
Principle of Rehabilitation Ethics Organized by Domains of Social Context

---

Rehabilitation Professional Domain
Reasonable Self-Interest
1. Rehabilitation professionals will act on their own behalf to maintain reasonable levels of emotional and physical health.

Client Domain
Beneficence
1. Rehabilitation professionals will act to benefit their clients.
Nonmalfeasance
1. Rehabilitation professionals will take reasonable precautions to prevent harm to their clients.
2. Rehabilitation professionals will protect the privacy and confidentiality rights of their clients.
3. Rehabilitation professionals will refrain from all forms of sexual, physical, emotional, financial, and social exploitation of clients. They will avoid any relationships with clients, their families, or associates that might interfere with their professional judgment.
4. Rehabilitation professionals will identify the limits of their skills and expertise and seek supervision, or consultation when necessary, to protect clients from harm.
5. Rehabilitation professionals shall identify the limits of their skills and refer clients to other appropriate caregivers when necessary to ensure client safety.
Autonomy
1. Rehabilitation professionals will respect the rights of their clients to make their own decisions about therapy, including the right to refuse treatment.
2. Rehabilitation professionals will ensure that services are provided only if the client gives free and informed consent.
3. If engaging in research involving human subjects, rehabilitation professionals will ensure that all potential research participants are fully informed regarding potential risks and benefits. They must also ensure that potential research is free of coercion and undue influence while considering their decisions regarding consent.
Veracity or Truthfulness
1. Rehabilitation professionals shall provide information and education about therapeutic options (including potential benefits and risks) to ensure that clients can make properly informed decisions regarding consent.
Justice
1. Rehabilitation professionals will provide services in a manner equitable to all individuals.

Team Domain
Duties and Obligations
1. Rehabilitation professionals will assign service delivery to other professional, paraprofessional, or nonprofessional care providers only when adequate training and supervision are provided.
2. Rehabilitation professionals will ensure that those carrying out duties under their supervision do so in full accordance with professional ethics and the law.

continued

TABLE 3.1 *continued*

Veracity or Truthfulness
1. Rehabilitation professionals will disclose any potential conflicts of interest.
2. Rehabilitation professionals will share with team members information that assists the team in providing effective services.

Fidelity
1. Rehabilitation professionals will work toward common goals and objectives of the team.
2. Rehabilitation professionals will report barriers to team performance to the team and work with team members to eliminate such barriers.

Disciplinary Domain
Duties and Obligations
1. Rehabilitation professionals will be adequately trained and hold appropriate credentials to practice.
2. Rehabilitation professionals will use procedures and interventions that conform to the standards of their professional body.
3. Rehabilitation professionals will maintain competence through ongoing professional development and educational activities.
4. Rehabilitation professionals will perform all assessment and intervention based on current and accurate information.

Fidelity
1. Rehabilitation professionals will comply with the code of ethics for their specific rehabilitation disciplines.
2. Rehabilitation professionals will report any breaches of ethics to the appropriate authority.

Societal Domain
Justice
1. Rehabilitation professionals will carry out their professional duties in accordance with the laws of the society they inhabit.
2. Rehabilitation professionals will actively advocate for social conditions conducive to their clients' rehabilitation.
3. Rehabilitation professionals will ensure that services are available in an equitable manner.
4. Rehabilitation professionals will ensure that services are culturally sensitive or culturally neutral.

Note: Ethics may be classified in a number of ways. One method is by the focus of ethical responsibility. All members of the rehabilitation team have ethical responsibilities to (1) themselves, (2) their clients, (3) their teams, (4) their disciplines, and to (5) society as a whole.

The general principle of reasonable self-interest implies that every rehabilitation professional has an ethical responsibility to ensure that he or she is reasonably healthy, happy, and competent to meet professional standards. While competence may be considered a duty to the recipients of services or to the discipline itself, it may also be seen as the responsibility to oneself to ensure that one is mentally and physically prepared to practice.

Case Study 3

Erin, a caring and compassionate nurse, has been working overtime and coming in on her days off to help care for her patients. She is determined to provide the best care in spite of cutbacks and dwindling resources. Now, however, she is reaching the point of exhaustion. Her own health is deteriorating, and she is becoming short-tempered. She is starting to make mistakes, and some of them are serious ones. Her friends and coworkers have suggested that she take some time off, but Erin feels that she would be deserting her patients by doing so.

Meeting ethical responsibilities to one's self does not mean ignoring the needs of others; in fact, in the vast majority of cases, rehabilitation professionals who take good care of themselves are better able to provide high-quality care and treatment to others.

Ethical Responsibility to Clients

The area of ethics that has received the greatest attention among rehabilitation disciplines is ethical responsibility to clients. While there is considerable variation in official statements of ethical guidelines across disciplines and even within disciplines (because various professional bodies in the same discipline may issue their own guidelines), there is considerable consensus on basic ethical principles. These principles include altruism or beneficence, equality and dignity, freedom and autonomy, truthfulness or veracity, fairness or justice, privacy, and prudence (Kanny & Hansen, 1996).

Ethical Responsibility to Rehabilitation Teams

Rehabilitation professionals also have ethical responsibilities to their teams and to their respective disciplines. These responsibilities include fidelity, competence, performance, and truthfulness or veracity. Although the ethics of teaming is critical to successful application of multidisciplinary teamwork, few professionals and academics have written about it or discussed it.

Wachter (1976) appears to be among the first to point out the importance of interdisciplinary ethics. Around that time, a transdisciplinary model of teaming was being introduced to rehabilitation (Orelove & Sobsey, 1996). The transdisciplinary model mandates role sharing and role release, breaking down traditional boundaries among rehabilitation disciplines. It goes beyond coordinated service delivery to a unified approach that allows assessment and intervention traditionally directly provided by a member of a particular discipline to be provided by others. The model has been shown to be very valuable in delivering the services to individu-

Case Study 4

Mark is a speech pathologist working with young at-risk children in the schools. As part of a transdisciplinary team that stresses a consultative model, he trains parents and daycare workers to provide therapeutic intervention and provides them with supervision and support. Although he feels this model is ideal, he also feels that the model has been used as an excuse to eliminate jobs in speech pathology by allowing minimally trained nonprofessionals to do work traditionally reserved for trained therapists. As a result, he feels like his responsibilities to his team and clients conflict with his responsibilities to his discipline.

als who need assessment and intervention from many different disciplines outside hospital settings, but it has also required its own ethical guidelines. For example, most disciplines have established guidelines that ensure quality control by requiring services to be delivered directly by a trained and certified member of that discipline. In a transdisciplinary model, some of that control must be released, and quality assurance must be provided in some other manner.

While the transdisciplinary model is rarely mentioned directly in professional ethical guidelines, this model has been endorsed and guidelines for implementation have been developed by organizations such as the American Physical Therapy Association, the American Occupational Therapy Association, the American Speech-Language-Hearing Association, and the Association for Persons with Severe Handicaps (Orelove & Sobsey, 1996). These guidelines generally attempt to allow greater flexibility in who directly delivers services while ensuring quality control through cross-training (i.e., team members of different disciplines train each other), consultation, and supervision.

Teamwork also has its own ethical issues that must be addressed by rehabilitation teams (Purtilo, 1988; Purtilo & Meier, 1993). For example, the protection of privacy and confidentiality of a client may have special implications for team settings. When a client discloses information to one team member, can that team member assume that it can be shared with all other team members?

Ethical Responsibility to Rehabilitation Disciplines

Because professional associations that represent various professional disciplines have been the primary developers of ethical guidelines, they have naturally given close attention to the obligations of practitioners to their specific disciplines. Many of these obligations might also be considered obligations to oneself, to clients, to one's team, to society as a whole, or to all four. For example, exploitation of clients would primarily violate the ethical responsibility to clients, but it would also be likely to damage the reputation of the discipline and thus also violate an ethical obligation to the discipline.

Ethical Responsibility to Society as a Whole

Rehabilitation professionals have ethical responsibilities to society as a whole. The primary principles in this domain are justice and social responsibility. The most obvious implication of this principle is that rehabilitation professionals must practice within the relevant laws. It also appears to imply that rehabilitation professionals must not only work directly with their individual clients but must also advocate for conditions that optimize the potential rehabilitation of all clients. Noe (1997), for example, points to this implied duty in arguing that rehabilitation counselors must advocate for the elimination of discrimination against people with mental illness.

> Although advocacy and beneficence are not directly stated in the APA Ethical Principles of Psychologists; Principle F; Social Responsibility implies that psychologists have an ethical obligation for advocacy (p. 23).

Noe argues that discrimination presents such a great obstacle to the successful rehabilitation of people with mental illness that failure to address it is unethical. Scorzelli (1995) presents a similar ethical argument for rehabilitation professionals to advocate for program development to serve people with cerebral palsy in India. He suggests that service reform is so critical to successful rehabilitation that ignoring the need for advocacy dooms other efforts to failure.

Research Ethics

The protection of human participants in research has received more attention than most areas of rehabilitation ethics. This interest in research ethics developed after World War II, when the allied forces became aware that under the Nazi regime, physicians forced research subjects to undergo torturous procedures in the name of medical science. The Nuremberg code, which was first published as part of the *War Crimes Tribunal* transcript, was developed to protect research participants, especially those who might be vulnerable because of age, disability, or institutional residence (Elliott et al., 1997; Annas & Grodin, 1992). The major principles of the code were preserved in the World Medical Association's Declaration of Helsinki, which has been further amended several times and continues to be a major guidepost for researchers today (Elliott et al., 1997).

These basic principles also have been reflected in laws, guidelines of research funding agencies, and ethical codes of various professional organizations in rehabilitation (Gall et al., 1996). Some of the basic principles include:

- Agencies conducting research with human participants must have institutional review boards to protect the rights and safety of participants.
- Any potential risks to participants must be minimal and justified by potential benefits.
- Participants must consent before being involved in research.
- Participants must be informed and competent to consent.
- Participants must be free of undue influence to consent.
- Participants must be free to withdraw consent and discontinue participation at any time.
- Participants must be guaranteed that their rights of privacy and confidentiality are fully protected.
- Strict limits are placed on the use of deception.
- Special protection must be provided for captive subjects. Captive subjects are participants who are already in the care or control of the researcher or under the influence of the researcher. In most cases, this includes clients who might be involved in research conducted by the rehabilitation professionals who serve them.

The protection of human participants, particularly those who may be vulnerable to exploitation, must be of particular concern to members of rehabilitation teams. Historically, some of the worst ethical offenses have been committed against people with disabilities. One grim example has been chronicled by Gould, who described how retouched photos and false data were used to support the notion that developmental disabilities and psychiatric disorders were inherited (Gould, 1996). These pseudofindings were then used to justify the forced sterilization of thousands of people with developmental disabilities. In another disturbing example, researchers deliberately infected more than 700 people who had developmental disabilities with hepatitis virus so that they could study the effects of gamma globulin on the disease (Goldby, 1997). At another institution for people with developmental disabilities, 19 boys were deliberately fed radioactive calcium and iron in their oatmeal (Scripps Howard News Service, 1996). In yet another horrific example, the director of an institution referred a man with Down syndrome to be involuntarily sterilized to obtain samples of testicular tissue for his research project (Thomas, 1995). Every rehabilitation professional has a responsibility not only to refrain from such grossly unethical research, but also to prevent others from participating.

The primary focus of ethics in research has been the protection of human participants, but researchers also have other ethical responsibilities to society, their teams, and their disciplines. A few of these include ensuring the quality of research, acknowledgment of funding sources, and acknowledgment of those whose work or ideas contributed to the research (Gall et al., 1996).

Issues

Multidisciplinary teams must address a never-ending list of ethical questions. All of them are important. The ones that become important for a particular team or specific profession are generally those related to a decision that must be made or a problem that has arisen. The issues that are discussed in this chapter are only a few of many that must be addressed by rehabilitation teams around the world.

What Is Rehabilitation?

The definition of rehabilitation is continually evolving. Differing definitions reveal a central ethical issue. Most definitions focus on the restoring function. *Stedman's Medical Dictionary* (1990), for example, defines rehabilitation as "Restoration, following disease, illness or injury, of the ability to function in a normal or near normal manner." Similarly, the *Oxford English Dictionary* (1992) defines rehabilitation as "Restoration (of a disabled person, a criminal, etc.) to some degree of normal life by appropriate training." Such definitions raise important issues about the scope of rehabilitation and who might be expected to benefit from it. An individual born with a disability may not have experienced disease, illness, or injury and cannot be restored to a state that he or she never attained. In addition, some degenerative conditions make the restoration to an earlier level of function very unlikely. Equally important, an individual who experiences a permanent disability or who has attained a maximal level of restoration of physical function is beyond the scope of such narrow definitions of rehabilitation. While such technical distinctions may seem trivial, they underlie many issues about who is eligible for services. People with severe developmental disabilities, degenerative diseases, and conditions that make further improvement of physical function unlikely have often been considered poor candidates for rehabilitation and excluded from services because they are considered unlikely to benefit.

In addition, the expressed goal of achieving a "normal" life has been rejected by some potential candidates for rehabilitation. A striking example of this rejection occurred with large numbers of children who were born with phocomelia (very short limbs) as a result of the effects of the use of thalidomide during their mother's pregnancy. Rehabilitation professionals routinely attempted to teach these individuals to use artificial legs (Fletcher, 1980). Most of these individuals, however, rejected their prosthetic legs, developing less normal but more functional forms of mobility. Although artificial legs provided a more normal appearance, they provided poor mobility and precarious balance for individuals who had a high center of gravity and no arms to assist with balance or to catch them when they fell. Nevertheless, many therapists, physicians, and parents continued to insist that these children use their artificial legs because of their narrow focus on making the individual "normal" and their discomfort with the atypical methods of getting from place to place.

Increasingly, broader definitions of rehabilitation are being used. Wong and Neulicht, for example, present a definition of rehabilitation that adds empowerment to restoration as a central goal (1995). This and other broad definitions allow clients to determine their own rehabilitation goals and to focus on life satisfaction rather than normal motor function or even normal social function. This broader view of rehabilitation is consistent with the social trend toward acceptance of diversity and recognizes that social adjustment can be achieved in different ways for different individuals.

How Much Cultural Sensitivity Is Helpful?

Ann Fadiman's *The Spirit Catches You and You Fall Down* (1997) is a true story about a Hmong child named Lia with epilepsy, her family, and a California hospital. The health care team and the parents both want to do what is best for Lia, but tragically they are in conflict because of cultural differences. Lia suffers because of their conflict. One example of these cultural differences occurs when doctors tell her father through a translator that Lia is dying and will probably not last through the next day. Her father reacts by trying to run out of the hospital with his daughter, and the health care team views him as irrational and dangerous. They do not know that saying that Lia is dying is the same as saying that they are killing her in the Hmong culture. Eventually, when modern medical technology is no longer adequate, they send Lia home with her parents to die, but she survives for years on Hmong herbal medicines. It would be too simple to say her parents were right and the health care team was wrong. There are no real heroes or villains in this story. There are only good intentions failing because of poor communication and the inability to overcome cultural differences.

In an increasingly multicultural world, effective rehabilitation services must be culturally sensitive by responding to the cultural attitudes and beliefs of their clients. When they cannot be culturally sensitive, they must at least be culturally neutral by avoiding practices that offend the cultural attitudes and beliefs of their clients. It can be argued, however, that cultural sensitivity or neutrality can go too far. Some attitudes and beliefs may directly conflict with rehabilitation goals or the general welfare of clients. For example, a number of belief systems explain disability as a punishment for sin. In some cases, it is described as a punishment for sin in a previous life; in others, the disabled child is considered a punishment for a parent's sin.

These beliefs often create negative feelings within the family, threaten self-esteem, and reduce motivation for successful rehabilitation. If these difficulties can be resolved while maintaining cultural sensitivity, the problem may be easily solved. In many cases, however, successful rehabilitation may require the modification of these beliefs.

Assisted Suicide, Euthanasia, and Mercy Killing

In 1989, a 34-year-old man named Larry McAfee who had been left quadriplegic by a motorcycle accident contacted a lawyer. He wanted to go to court to demand that his respirator be shut off and that he be allowed to die. At the trial, McAfee testified, "Everyday when I wake up there is nothing to look forward to." Three weeks later, the Georgia judge granted permission for Larry McAfee to die, and McAfee's mother thanked him for doing so (Shapiro, 1993). Everyone was satisfied that it would be for the best. Larry McAfee was granted self-determination and personal autonomy, a victory some claimed for people with disabilities.

Advocates for the disability rights movement, however, were not cheering. They argued that this was not about free choice but rather a denial of choice. They argued that Larry McAfee wanted to die to escape from hospitals and nursing homes, not from paralysis. They believed that there is something wrong with a society that offers prevention programs to its nondisabled citizens who feel suicidal while it assists citizens with disabilities to kill themselves. They asked also whether only disability was seen as worse than death, when poverty, disgrace, loneliness, and all of life's other negative experiences are not seen as occasions for suicide. They argued that autonomy is an illusion in a health care system that drives people to suicide (Shapiro, 1993).

Who was right? In this case, it appeared to be the disability rights advocates. By the time McAfee got permission to die, he had been transferred to a better facility. With better care and treatment, McAfee no longer wanted to die. Instead of dying, he left the nursing home, got a job, and became a disability rights advocate. Interviewed some years later, McAfee said simply "If I ever have to return to an institution, then I prefer death, but never as long as we have it as good as this. My life is good now. I have hope" (Schindehette & Wescott, 1993).

The McAfee case points out some important issues for the rehabilitation team. The reality that a death wish may simply reflect a poor quality of care must not be forgotten, but it also raises questions about our own attitudes about significant disabilities. Bioethicists like Peter Singer and Joseph Fletcher have suggested that people with severe disabilities are not really "persons" and therefore killing them is not a serious offense (Shapiro, 1993). In a model of rehabilitation that empowers people with disabilities as equal partners, such beliefs cannot be simply ignored; they must be loudly refuted.

Ethics of Disability

Ultimately, the greatest issue in rehabilitation ethics may prove to be at the very root of our current ethical framework. Although rehabilitation ethics have done much to make professionals' responsibility to their clients a central focus, the terms and concepts have been generated by professionals, not clients. Some have suggested that we must start over, developing a new set of ethics that comes from clients, or at least with clients as equal partners (Asch, 1989). Perhaps the future will bring such a radical change.

Summary

This chapter described general unified ethical guidelines for rehabilitation professionals and presented some of the ethical issues that currently face the field. Ethics are based on socially determined values and will always be subject to individual understanding and opinion. No matter how sophisticated and refined our ethical guidelines, there will always be issues that require discussion.

References

American Nurses Association. (1996). Position statement: The right to accept or reject an assignment. Pulse, 33(1), 4–5, 11.

American Psychological Association (1992). Ethical principles for psychologists. American Psychologist, 47, 1597–1613.

Annas, G. J., & Grodin, M. A. (1992). The Nazi doctors and the Nuremberg code: Human rights in human experimentation (pp. xxii, 371). New York: Oxford University Press.

Asch, A. (1989). The meeting of disability and bioethics: A beginning rapprochement. In B. Duncan & D. E. Woods (Eds.), Ethical issues in disability and rehabilitation (pp. 85–89). Oakland, CA: World Institute on Disability.

Brillhart, B. A. (1995). Ethics in rehabilitation nursing. Rehabilitation Nursing, 20(1), 44–47.

Cameron, M. (1986). The moral and ethical component of nurse-burnout. Nursing Management, 17(4), 42B, 42D, 42E.

Elliott, D., Stern, J. E., & Institute for the Study of Applied and Professional Ethics. (1997). Research Ethics: A reader (pp. xii, 319). Hanover, NH: University Press of New England for the Institute for the Study of Applied and Professional Ethics at Dartmouth College.

Fadiman, A. (1997). The spirit catches you and you fall down. New York: Farrar, Strauss and Giroux.

Fletcher, I. (1980). Review of the treatment of thalidomide children with limb deficiency in Great Britain. Clinical Orthopaedics and Related Research, 148, 18–25.

Gall, M. B., Borg, W. R., & Gall, J. P. (1996). Educational research (6th ed.). White Plains, NY: Longman.

Garrett, T. M., Baillie, H. W., & Garrett, R. M. (1998). Health care ethics: Principles and practices (3rd ed.) (p. 1). Upper Saddle River, NJ: Prentice Hall.

Goldby, S. (1972). Experiments at the Willowbrook State School. In J. Katz (Ed.), Experimentation with human beings (pp. 1007–1010). New York: Russell Sage Foundation.

Gould, S.J. (1996). The mismeasure of man. New York: Norton.

Haas, J. F., MacKenzie, C. A. (1993). The role of ethics in rehabilitation medicine: Introduction to a series, American Journal of Physical Medicine & Rehabilitation, 72(1), 48–51.

Haas, J. F. (1995). Ethical issues in physical medicine and rehabilitation: Conclusion to a series. American Journal of Physical Medicine Rehabilitation, 74(Suppl. 1), S54–58.

Hansen, R. A. (1993). Ethics in occupational therapy. In H. L. Hopkins & H. D. Smith (Eds.), Willard and Spackman's Occupational Therapy (pp. 19–25). Philadelphia: J. B. Lippincott Company.

Imrie, R. (1997). Rethinking the relationships between disability, rehabilitation, and society. Disability and Rehabilitation, 19(7), 263–271.

Kanny, E., & Hansen, R. A. (1996). Core values and attitudes of occupational therapy practice. In American Occupational Therapy Association (Ed.), Occupational therapy code of ethics: Reference guide (pp. 6–8). Bethesda, MD: American Occupational Therapy Association.

Lucke, K. T. (1998). Ethical implications of caring in rehabilitation. Nursing Clinics of North America, 33(2), 253–264.

Noe, S. R. (1997). Discrimination against individuals with mental illness. Journal of Rehabilitation, 63, 20–27.

Orelove, F. P., & Sobsey, R. (1996). Educating children with multiple disabilities: A transdisciplinary approach (3rd ed.) (pp. xvi, 494). Baltimore: P. H. Brookes Publishing Co.

Oxford English dictionary (program, 2nd version) (1992). Oxford: Oxford University Press; Software.

Purtilo, R. B. (1988). Ethical issues in teamwork: The context of rehabilitation. Archives of Physical Medicine and Rehabilitation, 69(5), 318–322.

Purtilo, R. B., & Meier, R. H. D. (1993). Team challenges: Regulatory constraints and patient empowerment. American Journal of Physical Medicine and Rehabilitation, 72(5), 327–330.

Schindehette, S., & Wescott, G. (1993, January 18). Tube: Deciding not to die: A TV movie celebrates quadriplegic Larry McAfee's crusade to reclaim his life. People, 85.

Scorzelli, J. F. (1995). The development of educational and rehabilitation services for people with cerebral palsy in India. Journal of Rehabilitation, 61, 68–72.

Scott, P. A. (1998). Professional ethics: are we on the wrong track? Nursing Ethics, 5(6), 477–485.

Scripps Howard News Service. (1996, October 25). U.S. offers $4.8 million in radiation-test cases. The Dallas Morning News, p. 7A.

Shapiro, J. P. (1993). <u>No pity: People with disabilities forging a new civil rights movement</u>. New York: Times Books.

Skorupa, J., & Agresti, A. A. (1993). Ethical beliefs about burnout and continued professional practice. <u>Professional Psychology: Research and Practice, 24</u>(3), 281–285.

Stedman, T. L. (1990). <u>Stedman's medical dictionary, illustrated</u> (25th ed.) (xxxviii, 1784, [24] of plates). Baltimore: Williams & Wilkins.

Sweeney, G., & Nichols, K. (1996). Stress experiences of occupational therapists in mental health practice arenas: a review of the literature. <u>International Journal of Social Psychiatry, 42</u>(2), 132–140.

Thomas, D. (1995, July 2). Partial castrations were for research. <u>The Calgary Herald,</u> p. A11.

Trexler, L. E., & Fordyce, D. J. (1996). Psychological perspectives on rehabilitation: Contemporary assessment and intervention strategies. In R. L. Braddon (Ed.), <u>Physical medicine and rehabilitation</u> (pp. 66–81). Philadelphia: W. B. Saunders Company.

Wachter, M. D. (1976). Interdisciplinary teamwork. <u>Journal of Medical Ethics, 2</u>(2), 52–57.

Wong, H. D., & Neulicht, A. T. (1995). Ethics. In A. E. Del Orto & R. P. Marinelli (Eds.), <u>Encyclopedia of disability and rehabilitation</u> (pp. 305–309). New York: Simon & Schuster Macmillan.

Resources: Ethical Guidelines and Other Relevant Documents

American Association of Electrodiagnostic Medicine. (1994). Guidelines for ethical behavior relating to clinical practice issues in electrodiagnostic medicine. <u>Muscle & Nerve, 17</u>(8), 965–967.

American Fertility Society, Ethics Committee. (1994). Ethical considerations of assisted reproductive technologies. <u>Fertility & Sterility, 62</u>(5 Suppl. 1), 1S–125S.

American Medical Association. (1995). Ethical issues in managed care. Statement of principles. <u>Connecticut Medicine, 59</u>(5), 299.

American Nurses Association. (1995). American Nurses Association position statement on assisted suicide. <u>Trends in Health Care Law & Ethics, 10</u>(1–2), 124, 125–127.

American Nurses Association. (1996). Position statement. The right to accept or reject an assignment. <u>Pulse, 33</u>(1), 4–5, 11.

American Occupational Therapy Association. (1989). <u>Guidelines for occupational therapy services in the public schools</u> (2nd ed). Rockville, MD: Author.

American Occupational Therapy Association. (1994). Occupational therapy code of ethics. <u>American Journal of Occupational Therapy, 48</u>(11), 1037–1038.

American Physical Therapy Association. (1990). <u>Physical therapy practice in educational environments.</u> Alexandria, VA: Author.

American Physical Therapy Association. (1997). Standards of practice for physical therapy and the accompanying criteria. Physical Therapy, 77(1), 102–110.

American Psychological Association. (1992). Ethical principles of psychologists and code of conduct. American Psychologist, 47, 1597–1611.

American Rehabilitation Counseling Association, Commission on Rehabilitation Counseling Certification, National Rehabilitation Counseling Association. (1987). Code of professional ethics for rehabilitation counsellors. Journal of Applied Rehabilitation Counseling, 18(4), 26–31.

American Speech-Language-Hearing Association. (1992). Code of ethics. Issues in ethics. ASHA, 3(Suppl. 34), 1–21.

American Speech-Language-Hearing Association. (1988). Code of ethics of the American Speech-Language-Hearing Association 1988 (revised January 1, 1986). ASHA, 3(Suppl. 30), 47–50.

American Speech-Language-Hearing Association, Committee on Language Learning Disorders. (1991). A model for collaborative service delivery for students with language-learning disorders in the public schools. ASHA, 3(Suppl. 33), 44–50.

Australian Nursing Council. (1995). Code of ethics for nurses in Australia. The Australian Nursing Council, Inc., the Royal College of Nursing, Australia, and the Australian Nursing Foundation. Nursing Ethics, 2(1), 81–84.

Canadian Nurses Association. (1998). Code of ethics for registered nurses. Nursing Ethics, 5(1), 65–77.

United Nations General Assembly. (1948). Universal Declaration of Human Rights.

United Nations. (1991). Convention on the Rights of the Child. New York: Author.

World Medical Association. (1964). Declaration of Helsinki. Adopted by the 18th World Medical Assembly, Helsinki, Finland, June 1964 and amended by the 29th World Medical Assembly, Tokyo, Japan, October 1975; 35th World Medical Assembly, Venice, Italy, October 1983; and the 41st World Medical Assembly, Hong Kong, September 1989.

CHAPTER 4

Clinical Reasoning and Decision Making

Joy Higgs and Mark Jones

In the context of multidisciplinary rehabilitation, health professionals have key roles to play as autonomous primary health care professionals and as members of health care teams. In both cases, the importance of sound, effective clinical reasoning and decision making by the individual professional in collaboration with the team (including the client or patient) cannot be overstressed. The term *clinical reasoning* refers to the thinking and decision-making processes occurring during clinical practice. (In the literature, the term *clinical decision making* may be used interchangeably with *clinical reasoning*, or it may indicate a focus on the product [decisions] of the reasoning process, in particular the determination of diagnosis.) Clinical reasoning is directed toward enabling the clinician to take "wise" action, meaning taking the best-judged action in a specific context (Cervero, 1988; Harris, 1993).

In this chapter, we examine the nature of clinical reasoning and decision making and encourage readers to reflect on their own reasoning and decision-making skills. To serve the goal of self-directed and continuing education, we provide an overview of expertise in clinical reasoning and practice and discuss common errors in reasoning. In addition, the chapter explores the nature of multidisciplinary clinical decision making from several perspectives. This involves, first, discussion of the conceptual and practical differences between independent and collaborative decision making within the context of two interactive models of clinical practice and health care. Second, we consider implications of bringing together different models of clinical reasoning used by various disciplines in the management of individual client cases. Reflective exercises are interposed throughout the chapter to encourage readers to relate their current understanding of clinical reasoning to ideas espoused here and in recommended readings, and to promote a deeper individual understanding of this topic.

Nature of Clinical Reasoning and Decision Making

Definitions

Clinical reasoning has been defined as a process in which the clinician, interacting with the client and significant others (caregivers, health care team members), structures meaning, goals, and health management strategies based on clinical data, client choices, and professional judgment and knowledge (Higgs & Jones, in press, a). This process is centered on the client, the client's clinical problem(s), and the related environment. The major function of clinical reasoning is to enhance understanding (by clinician and client) of the clinical problem in order to provide the basis for sound health management. This model of clinical reasoning is explored further in the section "An Integrated, Client-Centered Model of Clinical Reasoning."

To compare this definition across the professions, consider the following images of clinical reasoning.

In *occupational therapy*, clinical reasoning "may be best described as the use of multiple reasoning strategies throughout the various phases of client management. Hypothetico-deductive modes of reasoning (including procedural reasoning as presented by Fleming [1991a]) are used when therapists think about client problems in terms of the disease and within the context of occupational performance. Interactive reasoning (Fleming, 1991b) involves developing an understanding of the naming of existing problems from the client's perspective. It employs processes of narrative thinking (Mattingly, 1991) and critical discourse with clients (Crepeau, 1991). Conditional reasoning (Fleming, 1991b) is a less definite process by which occupational therapists imagine the client in the future, and in so doing, imagine the therapy outcome and the therapeutic action required to achieve that outcome. Underpinning all these processes is a process of ethical reasoning and critical reflection"(Chapparo & Ranka, 1995).

In *physiotherapy*, "clinical reasoning refers to the thought processes associated with a clinician's examination and management of a client" (Jones et al., 1995). Modes of reasoning used in physiotherapy include hypothetico-deductive reasoning, pattern recognition, knowledge reasoning integration, and integrated models of reasoning involving client-centered and collaborative decision making (Edwards et al., 1998; Jones, 1992; Jones et al., in press).

In *nursing*, clinical reasoning can be defined as "the cognitive processes and strategies that nurses use to understand the significance of client data, to identify and diagnose actual or potential client problems, and to make clinical decisions to assist in problem resolution and to enhance the achievement of positive client outcomes" (Fonteyn, 1995).

In the *speech* and *hearing sciences,* clinical reasoning involves the application of relevant knowledge and skills to evaluation, diagnosis, and rehabilitation and is part of a larger clinical decision-making system involving interaction between clinician, client, task, and environment. It is a dynamic system that "acknowledges the natural complexity of the clinical situation, reminding us of the interactive character of these four components and of their influence on system output" (Doyle, 1995).

Reflective Exercise 1

What do you know about the topic of clinical reasoning? What does *clinical reasoning* mean to you? What are the key dimensions of your notion of clinical reasoning? Answer this question now to identify your current understanding of this topic. Then on completion of this chapter, review and revise your answer to this question, incorporating any additional concepts that you had previously not considered.

Context of Clinical Reasoning

Clinical reasoning is a complex process occurring within a multidimensional context. In clinical settings, clinicians frequently face ill-defined problems, goals that are complex, and outcomes that are difficult to predict clearly. Professional judgment and decision making within these ambiguous and uncertain health care situations are an inexact science (Kennedy, 1987) that require reflective practice and excellent skills in clinical reasoning (Schön, 1983). To interpret the way in which professionals cope with the uncertainties and challenges of clinical reasoning, we need to look beyond science. Harris (1993), for instance, presents the concept of professional practice as comprising a blend of art, craft, and technology.

The context in which clinical reasoning occurs plays an important role in the process of clinical reasoning, both in terms of the parties who are involved in the reasoning process and in terms of the many environmental factors that need to be taken into consideration. The context of clinical reasoning comprises a number of elements. These are outlined in Table 4.1.

Reflective Exercise 2

Consider each of the contexts in Figure 4.1. What values and beliefs do you bring to your clinical reasoning? How does your professional frame of reference (i.e., the way you define your profession and see your role, the rules and standards of professionalism that guide your actions) influence the clinical decisions you make and the way you involve others in clinical reasoning? Reflect on specific instances when your clients' personal frames of reference (their values, principles, goals, and context) have significantly influenced the process of clinical reasoning.

TABLE 4.1
Clinical Reasoning Contexts

Context	Features
The personal context of individual clients	The client's unique cultural, family, work, and socioeconomic frames of reference and state of physical and psychological health. The client's beliefs, values, expectations, and perceptions and needs in relation to clinical problems.
The unique multifaceted context of the client's clinical problem	Clinical problems frequently involve overlapping disabilities, clinical syndromes, and pain mechanisms as well as multiple physical, environmental, and psychosocial factors that contribute to the client's problem(s).
The specific context of health care for the client under consideration	This may be a mass-media health-promotion program, high-technology intensive-care hospital context, a multidisciplinary pain clinic, or a specific sports rehabilitation facility. Commonalities across settings include a focus on restoration of improved quality of life, and education directed toward prevention of future problems.
The wider health care environment	Factors influencing health include the environment, socioeconomic conditions (of client, nation, and global arena), cultural beliefs, and human cognition and behavior.
The knowledge explosion	An increasing body of scientific, technical, and professional knowledge. The need for self-directed professional updating.
The personal and professional framework of the clinician	The clinician's cultural, family, work, and socioeconomic frames of reference, and his or her beliefs, values, and attitudes. The ethical standards/requirements of the profession and the context of professionalism.
Multidisciplinary team work	A meeting ground for various professional cultures and modes of reasoning. The combination of individual professionals' frames of reference.
Rehabilitation	Restoration of function, enhanced understanding, and improved quality of life.

Source: Based on Higgs, J., & Jones, M. (1995). Clinical reasoning. In J. Higgs & M. Jones (Eds.), Clinical reasoning in the health professions. Oxford: Butterworth–Heinemann.

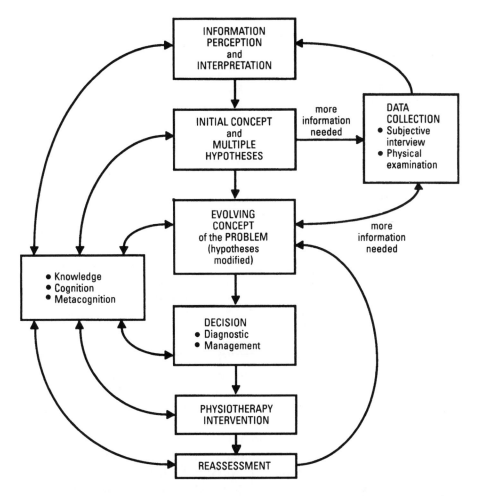

FIGURE 4.1. Hypothetico-deductive reasoning. (Reprinted with permission from Higgs, J., & Jones, M. [1995]. Clinical reasoning. In J. Higgs, & M. Jones [Eds.], <u>Clinical reasoning in the health professions</u> [p. 12]. Oxford: Butterworth–Heinemann.)

Models of Clinical Reasoning and Decision Making Used in Different Health Professions

The models that researchers and scholars use to interpret and explain clinical reasoning and decision making are influenced by the approaches used to generate these models. These approaches can be briefly described.

Process-oriented research emphasizes behaviors and cognition (particularly of the clinician). In this field, early research focused on attempting to analyze the behaviors (and steps) involved in problem solving and supported the notion of the generic nature and transferability of effective problem-solving skills (Grant, 1992). Later research based on cognitive psychology emphasized the nature of clinical reasoning and development of clinical reasoning expertise, and recognized the importance of the clinical knowledge base of the individual (Elstein et al., 1978). Recent developments in the cognitive tradition have included the use of propositional analysis (Patel & Groen, 1986; Schmidt et al., 1988).

Content (knowledge)-oriented research recognizes the interdependence of clinical reasoning and knowledge. The importance of knowledge in clinical reasoning is strongly demonstrated in the model of clinical reasoning expertise developed by Boshuizen and Schmidt (1992), in which expertise is linked to depth and organization of clinical knowledge initially acquired through formal professional schooling and later refined through reflective clinical practice.

For some time in nursing and occupational therapy, and more recently in physiotherapy, clinical reasoning research has questioned the domination of this field by positivistic research (i.e., reductionist, noncontextual quantitative analysis of discrete events). Recent qualitative research in the *interpretive* and *critical research* traditions has emphasized the importance of considering clinical reasoning as a process operating within the arena of human interactions. This research has explored the processes of reasoning practice in the allied health and nursing professions (particularly elements of collaboration and education, as discussed below) and has considered the nature of different forms of knowledge used in clinical reasoning. Higgs and Titchen (1995) provide a categorization of knowledge comprising *propositional knowledge* derived from theory or research (e.g., knowledge resulting from clinical trials and theories of professional practice), *professional craft knowledge* derived from professional experience (e.g., knowledge about wise action in dealing with people facing health crises), and *personal knowledge* derived from personal experience (e.g., knowledge of moral behavior and interpersonal interactions). They argue that the human sciences need a view of knowledge that accords validity to both propositional knowledge and nonpropositional or experience-based knowledge, that seeks both personal and public validation, and that recognizes that knowledge is a dynamic phenomenon.

Reflective Exercise 3

Consider the different forms of knowledge (propositional knowledge, professional craft knowledge, and personal knowledge) discussed above and reflect on the different forms of knowledge. How are these forms of knowledge valued—by you, by your colleagues, by your profession?

Various Clinical Reasoning Models

Various models have been used to interpret and explain the process of clinical reasoning. These include hypothetico-deductive reasoning (Elstein et al., 1978); pattern recognition (Barrows & Feltovich, 1987); knowledge reasoning integration (Schmidt et al., 1990); reasoning as a process of integrating knowledge, cognition, and metacognition (Higgs & Jones, 1995); and multimode reasoning (Fleming, 1991b).

Hypothetico-Deductive Reasoning

The hypothetico-deductive reasoning model of clinical reasoning arose from medical research (Barrows et al., 1978; Elstein et al., 1978) and has been identified as one approach used in physiotherapy (Jones, 1992), occupational therapy (i.e., "procedural reasoning" [Fleming, 1991b]), and nursing in diagnostic reasoning (Padrick et al., 1987). This reasoning approach involves the generation of diagnostic and nondiagnostic hypotheses based on clinical data and knowledge, and the testing of these hypotheses through further inquiry, physical testing, and ongoing management (see Figure 4.1).

Pattern Recognition

Pattern recognition or inductive reasoning is another interpretation of clinical reasoning. Groen and Patel (1985) ascertained that expert reasoning in nonproblematic situations resembles pattern recognition or direct automatic retrieval of information from a well-structured knowledge base. In problematic situations, however, experts consider and evaluate alternatives rather than using this rapid recognition approach (Elstein et al., 1990). Inductive reasoning has both strengths and weaknesses. Although it lacks certainty, inductive reasoning is fast and efficient and enables conclusions to be reached in the face of imprecise data and limited premises. By comparison, hypothetico-deductive reasoning is generally regarded as being a slower, more demanding, and more detailed process (Arocha et al., 1993). (For further discussion of pattern recognition, including explanations of the process, see Higgs & Jones [2000a].)

Knowledge-Reasoning Integration

Recent research in the health sciences has demonstrated that clinical reasoning is not a separate skill that can be developed independently of relevant professional knowledge and other clinical skills, such as investigative skills (Schmidt et al., 1990). Part of the process of professional education involves the acquisition of a body of knowledge that is specific to the profession in question (i.e., domain-specific knowledge). Increasing evidence supports the importance of domain-specific knowledge and an organized knowledge base in clinical problem-solving expertise (Elstein et al., 1990; Hassebrock et al., 1993; Patel et al., 1990; Schmidt et al., 1990). The interaction between such knowledge and skills in reasoning is central to clinical reasoning expertise.

Knowledge-reasoning integration is a central element of the stage theory of expertise development proposed by Boshuizen and Schmidt (1992). This model is based on the observation that developing reasoning expertise is largely the result of changes in knowledge structure. The student's progress to expert clinician is accompanied by a transition from knowledge organization dominated by biomedical knowledge, through encapsulation of knowledge into concept clusters with clinically relevant foci, to structuring of knowledge around *illness scripts* (consisting of the enabling conditions of the problem, the pathophysiologic processes occurring, and the consequences or signs and symptoms of the problem), and finally to *instantiated scripts* (actual detailed cases/specific instances). Patel and Kaufman (1995) critique this model, regarding it as idealized. They suggest that the key role played by basic sciences may be in facilitating explanation and coherent communication rather than in facilitating clinical reasoning itself.

Interpretive Models

Interpretive research into clinical reasoning has been conducted by Benner (1984) in nursing, by Crepeau (1991) and Fleming (1991a) in occupational therapy, and by Jensen et al. (1999) in physiotherapy. The clinical reasoning processes that such approaches describe focus on strategies that seek a deep understanding of the client's perspective and the influence of contextual factors, in addition to the more traditional "clinical" understanding of the client's condition.

In nursing, a number of studies (Agan, 1987; Pyles & Stern, 1983; Rew, 1990; Rew & Barrow, 1987) have emphasized the role of intuitive skills in clinical reasoning, linking intuitive knowledge to past experience with specific client cases. Fonteyn and Fisher (1992) have linked nurses' experience and associated intuition to the use of advanced reasoning strategies or heuristics. Such heuristics include pattern matching and listing items relevant to the working plan (Fonteyn & Grobe, 1993).

Interpretive models of clinical reasoning include the following:

- *Diagnostic reasoning* is that reasoning that aims to reveal the client's impairment(s), disability(ies), and handicap(s) and the underlying pathobiological mechanisms. While diagnostic reasoning is the most familiar reasoning strategy, in clinical practice it is combined with other strategies to establish client rapport and to educate and promote client self-efficacy and responsibility.
- *Interactive reasoning* occurs when dialogue in the form of social exchange is used deliberately to enhance or facilitate the assess-

ment/management process. This reasoning provides an effective means of better understanding the context in which the client's problem(s) exist while creating a relationship of interest and trust.

- *Narrative reasoning* involves the use of stories regarding past or present clients to further understand and manage a clinical situation. Such real-life scenarios bring credibility to the advice or explanation that they are used to support and can be strategically employed by practitioners to strengthen their message.
- *Collaborative reasoning* refers to shared decision making that ideally occurs between practitioner and client. Here the client's opinions, as well as information about the problem, are actively sought and used.
- *Predictive* or *conditional reasoning* is part of the practitioner's thinking directed to estimating client responses to treatment and likely outcomes of management, based on information obtained through the client interview, physical examination, and response to management.
- *Ethical/pragmatic reasoning* alludes to those less recognized but frequently made decisions regarding moral, political, and economic dilemmas that clinicians regularly confront, such as deciding how long to continue treatment.
- *Teaching as reasoning* occurs when practitioners consciously use advice, instruction, and guidance for the purpose of promoting change in the client's understanding, feelings, and behavior.

An Integrated, Client-Centered Model of Clinical Reasoning

Over a number of years, we have been developing an integrated, client-centered model of clinical reasoning. In 1995, we presented clinical reasoning as a process of reflective inquiry comprising three core elements: knowledge, cognition or thinking, and metacognition, which seeks to promote a deep and contextually relevant understanding of the clinical problem to provide a sound basis for clinical intervention (Higgs & Jones, 1995). These elements interact throughout the process of receiving, interpreting, processing, and using clinical information during decision making, clinical intervention, and reflection on actions and outcomes. This model is consistent with the findings of Alexander and Judy (1988) that domain-specific knowledge and skills in cognition (critical, creative, reflective, and logical/analytic thinking) and metacognition are essential for effective thinking and problem solving.

In our clinical reasoning model, the ongoing processing and reprocessing of data is presented as a series of clinical reasoning loops (Figure 4.2). Based on this deepening understanding, decisions are made concerning intervention, and actions are taken. The interaction between cognition, metacognition, and knowledge is illustrated in Figure 4.3. The process of reasoning

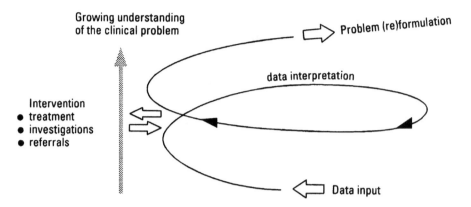

FIGURE 4.2. Clinical reasoning loop. (Reprinted with permission from Higgs, J., & Jones, M. [1995]. Clinical reasoning. In J. Higgs & M. Jones [Eds.] , Clinical reasoning in the health professions [p. 7]. Oxford: Butterworth–Heinemann. © Higgs and Jones, 1995.)

occurs within contextual parameters, including the client's and the clinician's frames of reference, the clinical case, and the clinical situation.

The model we have developed for the second edition of our clinical reasoning book (Higgs & Jones, 1999, b) builds on three core elements: (1) cognition or reflective inquiry; (2) a strong discipline-specific knowledge base; and (3) metacognition, which provides the integrative element between cognition and knowledge. We have expanded the interpersonal and contextual dimensions of the clinical reasoning model to give greater emphasis to:

- Mutual decision making, or the role of the client or patient in the decision-making process
- Contextual interaction, or the interactivity between the decision makers and the situation or environment of the reasoning process
- Task impact, or the influence of the nature of the clinical problem or task on the reasoning process

The importance of these three dimensions lies in the growing expectation by consumers that they play an active role in their own health care. The image of compliant, dependent clients is replaced by one of informed health care consumers who expect their needs and preferences to be listened to, who increasingly want to participate in decision making about their health, and who expect to take action to enhance their health.

The increasing reliance of health care systems on "user-pays" funding strategies means that consumers are purchasing (rather than "receiving") health care, and as a result, their expectations of service, quality, and own-

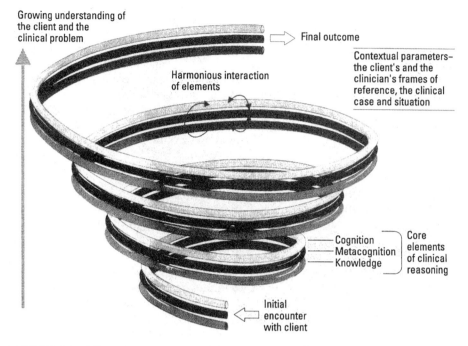

Growing understanding of
the client and the
clinical problem

Final outcome

Harmonious interaction
of elements

Contextual parameters—
the client's and the
clinician's frames of
reference, the clinical
case and situation

Cognition
Metacognition
Knowledge

Core
elements
of clinical
reasoning

Initial
encounter
with client

FIGURE 4.3. Clinical reasoning model. (Reprinted with permission from Higgs, J., & Jones, M. [1995]. Clinical reasoning. In J. Higgs & M. Jones [Eds.], <u>Clinical reasoning in the health professions</u> [p. 6]. Oxford: Butterworth–Heinemann. © Higgs and Jones, 1995.)

ership of health programs are increasing. Similarly, caregivers need and wish to play a greater role in health management and decision making. The self-help and user-pays context also highlights the need to pay greater attention to the client's environment. This includes the physical home and work environment, clients' personal circumstances (e.g., culture, family, finances), and their access to health care. Access involves considerations such as location of health care facilities, transportation options, language and cultural factors, and economic provisions for health care.

These situational factors also interact with the nature of the clinical problem or task facing the health care team and the client (and caregivers). Clinical problems facing clients and health professionals can be difficult, changeable, uncertain, and multidimensional. They involve human and nonhuman elements. They are affected by local and global contexts and occur in the context of uncertainty, changeability, and the indeterminate knowledge base of the health sciences.

In our model, the process of clinical reasoning is represented by an upward and outward spiral (see Figure 4.3.) This image is intended to demonstrate clinical reasoning as both a cyclical and a developing process. The process is centered on the client and the client's clinical problem(s) and the related environment. The major function of clinical reasoning is to enhance understanding (by clinician and client) of the clinical problem to provide the basis for sound health management. Greater focus on evaluating and addressing these factors is warranted with the increasing evidence that the meaning that clients give to their problems—including their understanding and their feelings regarding their problems—can significantly influence their levels of pain tolerance, disability, and eventual outcome (Borkan et al., 1991; Feuerstein & Beattie, 1995; Malt & Olafson, 1995).

Clinical reasoning effectiveness relies on the clinician's reasoning proficiency and the client's capacity and willingness to participate in clinical decision making. The quality of reasoning can be represented by parameters such as the speed of decision making, the depth of understanding of the clinical problem that is achieved, involvement of the client in goal setting and management decisions, and the validity and relevance of the management approach adopted. These outcomes are influenced by the abilities and performance of the health professionals participating in the rehabilitation team (e.g., their knowledge base, familiarity and experience with this type of case, reasoning skills), client factors (e.g., clients' needs, communication skills, circumstances, choices), and environmental factors (e.g., institutional expectations, profession-specific frameworks of operation, complexity of the case).

During the reasoning process, the core elements of the nature of the task—knowledge, cognition, and metacognition—combine in a process of decision making and interaction between the reasoner(s) and their context. Cognitive skills (such as analysis, synthesis, and evaluation of data collected) are used to process clinical data against the clinician's existing knowledge base in consideration of the client's needs and the clinical problem. At the same time, metacognition is used by the clinician to monitor thinking processes, conclusions, and knowledge adequacy; to detect links or inconsistencies between clinical data and existing clinical patterns or expectations based on prior learning; to reflect on the soundness (accuracy, reliability, validity) of observations and conclusions; and to critique the reasoning process itself (for logic, scope, client relevance, efficiency, creativity, etc.). Clinical reasoning involves the clinician's interaction with the client and other team members, each decision or action producing a clearer picture of the clinical problem and context influences or targets, which in turn generates further information and questions in the continuing process of data interpretation and mutual decision making.

Many human problems have multiple interpretations and solutions. The key to effective and accountable clinical practice is for the clinician's (and team's) understanding of the problem to be substantial so as to avoid potential harmful or ineffective intervention outcomes, and for the clinical management to be justifiable in terms of sound arguments based on the propositional, professional, and personal knowledge of the clinician and (as appropriate) the personal knowledge of the client.

Reflective Exercise 4

How do you reason? Consider the various models of clinical reasoning and decision making discussed above and reflect on the strategies and modes of reasoning you use. Do your strategies differ in different contexts, and if so, what factors (e.g., resources, client preferences, culture, competencies) influence these strategies? Consider your knowledge base (including theoretical, research, and experience-based knowledge) and ask yourself if there are some areas of your knowledge base that you need or would like to improve?

Expertise in Clinical Reasoning

The attainment of clinical reasoning and clinical practice expertise is a target of clinicians and an expectation of health care consumers. What is expertise and how is it developed?

Glaser and Chi (1988) have identified seven characteristics of experts:

1. Experts excel mainly in their own domains.
2. Experts perceive large meaningful patterns in their domain.
3. Experts are fast: they are faster than novices at performing the skills of their domain, and they quickly solve problems with little error.
4. Experts have superior short-term and long-term memory.
5. Experts see and represent a problem in their domain at a deeper (more principled) level than novices; novices tend to represent a problem at a superficial level.
6. Experts spend a great deal of time analyzing a problem qualitatively.
7. Experts have strong self-monitoring skills.

In addition to these generic skills of experts, which are applicable to clinical reasoning expertise, there are particular characteristics of experts that are pertinent to the health professions. We propose that clinical expertise, of which clinical reasoning is a critical component, can be viewed as a continuum along multiple dimensions. These dimensions include clinical outcomes; attributes such as professional judgment, technical clinical skills, communication, and interpersonal skills (to involve the client and others in decision making and to consider the client's perspectives); a sound knowledge base; and cognitive and metacognitive proficiency. A number of writers identify the importance of an expert's affective disposition to think in this reflective manner. Affective dispositions that skilled clinical thinkers must have include inquisitiveness, self-confidence, open-mindedness, flexibility, honesty, diligence, reasonableness, empathy, and humility (Brookfield, 1987; Ennis, 1987; Fonteyn & Ritter, 2000; Jensen et al., 1999). We have identified the following additional characteristics (see Higgs & Jones [2000b] for further discussion):

1. Experts value the participation of relevant others (clients, caregivers, team members) in the decision-making process.
2. Experts use high levels of metacognition in their reasoning.
3. Experts recognize the value of different forms of knowledge in their reasoning and use this knowledge critically.
4. Experts are client-centered.
5. Experts share their expertise to help develop expertise in others.
6. Experts are able to communicate their reasoning well and in a manner appropriate to their audience.
7. Experts have appropriate affective dispositions (e.g., inquisitiveness) to think in a reflective manner.

Skills of reasoning that contribute to the development of expertise include critical thinking skills, professional judgment, metacognition, and interpersonal skills. Fonteyn (1998) provides details of a "Thinking in Practice" study, which identified 12 strategies that nurses use in practice: (1) recognizing a pattern, (2) setting priorities, (3) searching for information, (4) generating hypotheses, (5) making predictions, (6) forming relationships, (7) stating a proposition, (8) asserting a practice rule, (9) making choices, (10) judging the value, (11) drawing conclusions, and (12) providing explanations. Each of these strategies forms a valuable element of clinical reasoning. Students learning to perform clinical reasoning need to practice each skill and gain feedback on the effectiveness of their performance from peers and tutors within the overall process of clinical reasoning.

In addition to developing thinking strategies, students need to develop a sound knowledge base. Carnevali (1995) argues that enhancing clinical reasoning is a personal process. It is each clinician's responsibility to develop expertise in the following aspects of reasoning expertise:

- Understanding what is currently known of memory systems and the diagnostic reasoning processes used
- Systematically storing one's theoretic and clinical knowledge base in long-term memory to facilitate its access for clinical judgment and decision-making activities
- Building a growing body of clinical experiences involving a variety of clinical phenomena, situations, and treatments, and storing them for ease of retrieval
- Gaining expertise in discipline-specific data acquisition and the use of one's cognitive processes in varying clinical situations and care settings (p. 180)

Reflective Exercise 5

What characteristics of experts do you exhibit? Which areas of expertise do you most need to develop now and in the future? How are your clinical reasoning skills developing? Reflect on your clinical education experiences with your peers. Do you demonstrate any of the following types of professional judgment that Fish and Coles (1998) present as a continuum:

- *Intuitive judgment* (i.e., unreflective, reactive)
- *Strategic judgment* (i.e., reflection only after the event, if at all)
- *Reflective judgment* (i.e., reflection on actions both during and after events, taking an evaluative stance and thinking critically)
- *Deliberative judgment* (i.e., deliberation on ends and means, being disposed to being critical and taking nothing for granted, breaking out of habitual ways of seeing, questioning the accepted)

If you want to read further on this topic, refer to Carnevali (1995) and follow her exercises to enhance your reasoning skills; and to Fonteyn (1998), Chapter 27, which refers to the California Critical Thinking Skills Test. This test "provides an excellent measure of all 12 of the dominant thinking strategies" used by nurses.

Clinical Reasoning Errors

A critical element of learning to be a good clinical reasoner is understanding and avoiding errors in reasoning. Errors of reasoning may occur at any stage of the clinical reasoning process, including errors of perception, inquiry, interpretation, synthesis, planning, and reflection (Jones, 1992). Scott (2000) highlights three critical causes of clinical reasoning errors:

1. Faulty elicitation or perception of clinical cues
2. Inadequate knowledge (e.g., about a clinical condition)
3. Misapplication of knowledge to a specific problem

Reasoning errors don't only stem from incomplete propositional knowledge. For example, faulty perception or elicitation of cues may be related to inadequate knowledge (both experimental and experienced based) of the relevant cues and underdeveloped craft knowledge in recognizing those cues. Similarly, misapplication of known facts to a specific problem relates to incorrect use of heuristics, an example of poor procedural knowledge.

Common types of clinical reasoning errors are described by Watts (1995) as follows:

Vagueness. The purpose of evaluation or treatment is unclear, and there is insufficient information to judge wisdom of decisions.

Narrowness. Familiar approaches that seem effective are used without consideration of alternative methods.

Rigidity. Standardized regimens of evaluation and treatment are used routinely with little consideration of important differences in individual client needs and response. Treatment reactions are not monitored to detect unexpected results.

Irrationality. Choices are based on convenience, habit, subjective impressions, and the word of people advocating specific techniques, rather than on sound evidence.

Wastefulness. Investigations are extensive, but their results have little influence on treatment selection. Costly treatment techniques are used without considering whether more economical methods might be equally effective.

Insensitivity. Clients' and families' personal values and psychosocial concerns are ignored, and physical performance enhancement is given higher priority than enhanced quality of life.

Mystery. The clinician's process of decision making cannot be explained in terms clients and colleagues can understand, and so others cannot question and contribute to this process.

Similarly, Scott (2000) identifies a number of common reasoning errors:

Forming the wrong initial concept of the problem (framing error). If students fail to attend to or correctly interpret initial or critical cues, they can form incorrect initial concepts of the clinical problem. This can result in incorrect or inadequate diagnostic or management decisions being made, much time wasted in pursuing incorrect lines of inquiry, and incorrect (e.g., harmful, wasteful, or useless) treatments. Time spent in carefully checking and interpreting cues, questioning the validity of the emerging picture of the clinical problem, and clarifying client responses rather than assuming can help avoid this error.

Failure to generate plausible hypotheses and adequately test them. Students (or clinicians) can miss cues, misdiagnose, or fail to take sufficient information into consideration, and as a result, they can fail to generate sound diagnostic or management hypotheses. This problem is further compounded if the problem is not detected or the process of testing hypotheses is also erroneous (e.g., clinicians may seek to confirm inadequate or erroneous hypotheses or may test hypotheses insufficiently). Attending to both supporting and negating evidence and disproving hypotheses—rather than assuming that evidence for one hypothesis implies that competing hypotheses are not valid—will assist in avoiding this error.

Inadequate testing and premature acceptance of hypotheses. Problems can arise when students/clinicians prematurely accept hypotheses (e.g., they may adopt favored, common, obvious hypotheses) and then during the testing process fail to detect that an error in reasoning has occurred because they are expecting the hypothesis to be confirmed. Critical checking of reasoning and test results is important to prevent this problem.

It is an important challenge for students and teachers alike to avoid the problem of clinical reasoning errors during clinical practice. Critical self-evaluation by the student and constructive feedback by the tutor are essential to avoid the problem of errors becoming a habit, which could go undetected for some time and result in ineffective or hazardous clinical intervention.

Reflective Exercise 6

From your past experience, can you remember specific instances in which you committed any of the above errors? How was the error detected—by you or others? What consequences arose?

In your future clinical practice, take time out to reflect on your clinical reasoning and seek any evidence of errors in your reasoning and decision making. Look out for the following errors:

- Neglecting important information
- Misinterpreting information/making assumptions
- Basing decisions on insufficient evidence
- Focusing too much on favorite or obvious hypotheses
- Missing contraindications or precautions
- Missing serious pathology cue detection and linkage to hypotheses
- Misdiagnosing
- Taking unwarranted action
- Failing to monitor your own reasoning (metacognition)
- Failing to detect inconsistencies
- Reaching firm conclusions prematurely
- Using recipes, not reasoning
- Failing to involve the client in decision making

Multidisciplinary Clinical Decision Making

Clinical decision making can rarely be considered an individual activity or an individual responsibility. In the rehabilitation context, we are commonly working with alert clients who can and generally want to participate in the decision-making process, particularly management planning. We are encouraging and educating clients toward this goal. The wider rehabilitation team includes professional colleagues, community agencies and workers, family, caregivers, and relevant others. The following discussion explores several key dimensions of multidisciplinary clinical reasoning and decision making.

A Social Ecology Model of Health
and the Interactional Professional

To deal effectively with the changing health care context and the changing expectations of individual health professionals and health care teams, we need to rethink the way that health systems operate. One way of reconceptualizing health care is via a social ecology model for health care participation and provision (Higgs et al., 1999). In this framework, health professionals no longer operate in a stable comprehensive health care system. Rather, they are faced with an unprecedented dynamic of change and a growing emphasis on the wider social responsibility: social relevance. To work effectively as team members in this context, health professionals need to work interactively in clinical decision making and in the provision of health care. In addition, health professionals need to be aware of health care in the greater context of life and of their obligation and responsibility to help create and be informed by a more social ecological model of health care. This requires them to be proactive as well as reactive to changes in health care.

The practice in interaction is also the focus of a new model for the beginning practitioner, called "the interactional professional" (Higgs & Hunt, 1999). This model argues the need for today's health professionals to be effective in interacting with the immediate and larger work environment, with key players in that context and with situational elements pertinent to the client and case/task under consideration. Interactional health professionals seek and value the input of others—particularly clients, caregivers, and other health care team members—in the reasoning and decision-making processes in order to achieve the goal of providing quality care that is appropriate and acceptable (to the client).

In both of these models, the role for the health care consumer is radically different in many respects to the dependent client role of traditional health care. Consumers of health care are becoming increasingly well informed about their health and about health care services. Terms such as *self-help* and *holistic health care* are central to today's health care, and the goal of achieving effective participation by consumers in their health care is widespread, requiring health professionals to involve their clients in clinical decision making whenever possible. Increasingly, clients' choices, rights, and responsibilities in relation to their health are changing. Payton et al. (1990) advocate client involvement in decision making concerning the management of the client's health and well-being. They argue that this process of client participation is based on recognizing the worth of individuals and their capacity for self-determination. Using understanding of their clients' rights and responsibilities, clinicians need to develop their own guidelines for involving the client in reasoning and decision making. Mutual decision making requires not only a sharing of ownership of decisions but also the development of skills in negotiating and explaining so as to facilitate effective two-way communication.

Scenario 1

You have been asked to participate in a debate. You are to comment on this statement: "Professional education in (your health profession) should prepare graduates to work in a global context (e.g., in different international settings and in a professional context that is influenced by international events, technology, and knowledge)." Choose to defend or oppose this position. What are the 5 main arguments you would present to argue your case?

Scenario 2

It is your turn to present an in-service education session to your peers. The topic negotiated is "What type of beginning practitioner does our profession need?" In preparing this talk, consider in particular: What clinical reasoning and decision-making competencies does this new graduate need (and why)? What interpersonal skills and performance should the profession, colleagues, clients, and caregivers be able to expect of the new graduate, and what other key characteristics should the beginning practitioner be able to demonstrate?

A Meeting of Professional Cultures and Modes of Decision Making

Although many elements of professionalism (including duty of care, quality health care goals, client-centered care, accountability) extend across the health professions, each profession has special features that define its professional culture. This distinctiveness of the professions arises from two processes: professionalization and professional socialization (Cant & Higgs, 1999).

During *professionalization,* occupations are transformed into professions. This goal has been a strong aspiration of many of the health disciplines given the status, legitimization, and authority that professional recognition brings. However, in terms of multidisciplinary teamwork in rehabilitation and other settings, the price paid for professionalization is separatism, which occurs in conjunction with the development of distinctive professional cultures.

During *professional socialization,* individuals are inducted into the professional culture. From the team perspective, this has both advantages and disadvantages. The advantages are that professional socialization results in the acquisition of behaviors and values of professionalism and an understanding of the roles of different team members. This provides the basis for a common culture and recognition of the complementary contributions effective health care team members can make. Similarly, within their discipline, individuals acquire the technical skills and knowledge that enable them to contribute their disciplinary expertise to the team. However, professional socialization can also engender notions and practices of territoriality and individualism rather than collegiality.

Other factors that influence the creation of effective multidisciplinary and multicultural rehabilitation settings include the culture or ethos of the rehabilitation unit (e.g., encouragement of teamwork, equity, and resource sharing), financial considerations (e.g., rewards for quality or efficiency measures such as output), community expectations (e.g., for client-centeredness and empowerment), staffing levels and equity across professions, and physical environment factors (e.g., accessibility, isolation).

To create effective multidisciplinary rehabilitation teams, individuals, leaders, and groups need to develop strategies to promote collaborative clinical reasoning and decision making. Factors that could promote this outcome include (1) the practice and ability of individuals to articulate their reasoning, and (2) the use of team decision-making strategies in the rehabilitation unit, such as negotiation and practices (e.g., case meetings) that require communication and cooperation in decision making. Successful decision making also requires the desire of all participants to make the team paramount, rather than individuals.

Scenario 3

A new rehabilitation unit has been established. The eight health professionals appointed to the unit each have a specific role to play in establishing the unit. Your role is to prepare a paper to promote discussion on how to establish effective team decision making. How will you go about this task?

Conclusion

As individual health professionals and as members of multidisciplinary rehabilitation teams, nurses, physiotherapists, speech and hearing therapists, occupational therapists, and other health professionals need to acquire and demonstrate effective clinical reasoning and decision making. In this chapter, we have explored many elements of the nature and practice of clinical reasoning. We have stressed the importance of critical reflection in reasoning; metacognition and ongoing self-evaluation; the development and use of rich, sound, and well-organized knowledge bases comprising domain-specific and relevant generic knowledge; and good reasoning skills. In addition, the importance of the patient's role in the decision-making process has been emphasized. Readers are encouraged to reflect on the material and learning activities presented and to expand their own reasoning awareness and competence.

References

Agan, R. (1987). Intuitive knowing as a dimension of nursing. <u>Advances in Nursing Science, 10,</u> 63–70.

Alexander, P. A., & Judy, J. E. (1988). The interaction of domain-specific and strategic knowledge in academic performance. Review of Educational Research, 58, 375–404.

Arocha, J. F., Patel, V. L., & Patel, Y. C. (1993). Hypothesis generation and the coordination of theory and evidence in novice diagnostic reasoning. Medical Decision Making, 13, 198–211.

Barrows, H. S., Feightner, J. W., Neufield V. R., & Norman G. R. (1978). An analysis of the clinical methods of medical students and physicians: Report to the Province of Ontario Department of Health. Hamilton, ON: McMaster University.

Barrows, H. S., & Feltovich, P. J. (1987). The clinical reasoning process. Medical Education, 21, 86–91.

Benner, P. (1984). From novice to expert: Excellence and power in clinical nursing practice. London: Addison-Wesley.

Borkan, J. M., Quirk, M., & Sullivan, M. (1991). Finding meaning after the fall: Injury narratives from elderly hip fracture clients. Social Science and Medicine, 33, 947–957.

Boshuizen, H. P. A., & Schmidt, H. G. (1992). On the role of biomedical knowledge in clinical reasoning by experts, intermediates and novices. Cognitive Science, 16, 153–184.

Brookfield, S. D. (1987). Developing critical thinkers. San Francisco: Jossey-Bass Publishers.

Cant, R., & Higgs, J. (1999). Professional socialisation. In J. Higgs & M. Jones (Eds.), Educating beginning practitioners (pp. 46–51). Oxford: Butterworth–Heinemann.

Carnevali, D. (1995). Self-monitoring of clinical reasoning. In J. Higgs & M. Jones (Eds.), Clinical reasoning in the health professions (pp. 179–190). Oxford: Butterworth–Heinemann.

Cervero, R. M. (1988). Effective continuing education for professionals. San Francisco: Jossey-Bass.

Chapparo, C., & Ranka, J. (1995). Clinical reasoning in occupational therapy. In J. Higgs & M. Jones (Eds.), Clinical reasoning in the health professions (pp. 88–100). Oxford: Butterworth–Heinemann.

Crepeau, E. B. (1991). Achieving intersubjective understanding: Examples from an occupational therapy treatment session. American Journal of Occupational Therapy, 45, 1016–1025.

Doyle, J. (1995). Teaching clinical reasoning to speech and hearing students. In J. Higgs & M. Jones (Eds.), Clinical reasoning in the health professions (pp. 224–234). Oxford: Butterworth–Heinemann.

Edwards, I. C., Jones, M. A., Carr, J., & Jensen, G. M. (1998). Clinical reasoning in three different fields of physiotherapy: A qualitative study. Proceedings of the Fifth International Congress of the Australian Physiotherapy Association, 298–300.

Elstein, A. S., Shulman, L. S., & Sprafka, S. A. (1978). Medical problem solving: An analysis of clinical reasoning. Cambridge, MA: Harvard University Press.

Elstein, A. S., Shulman, L. S., & Sprafka, S. A. (1990). Medical problem solving: A ten-year retrospective. Evaluation and the Health Professions, 13, 5–36.

Ennis, R. H. (1987). A taxonomy of critical thinking dispositions and abilities. In

J. B. Baron & R. J. Sternberg (Eds.), <u>Teaching thinking skills: Theory and practice</u> (pp. 9–26). New York: W. H. Freeman and Company.

Feuerstein, M., & Beattie, P. (1995). Biobehavioral factors affecting pain and disability in low back pain: Mechanisms and assessment. <u>Physical Therapy, 75,</u> 267–280.

Fish, D., & Coles, C. (1998), Developing professional judgement. In D. Fish & C. Coles (Eds.), <u>Developing professional judgement in health care: Learning through the critical appreciation of practice</u> (pp. 289–307). Oxford: Butterworth–Heinemann.

Fleming, M. H. (1991a). Clinical reasoning in medicine compared with clinical reasoning in occupational therapy. <u>American Journal of Occupational Therapy, 45,</u> 988–996.

Fleming, M. H. (1991b). The therapist with the three track mind. <u>American Journal of Occupational Therapy, 45,</u> 1007–1014.

Fonteyn, M. (1995). Clinical reasoning in nursing. In J. Higgs & M. Jones (Eds.), <u>Clinical reasoning in the health professions</u> (pp. 60–71). Oxford: Butterworth–Heinemann.

Fonteyn, M. E. (1998). <u>Thinking strategies for nursing practice.</u> Philadelphia: Lippincott.

Fonteyn, M., & Fisher, S. (1992, October). <u>The study of expert nurses in practice.</u> Paper presented at Transformation Through Unity: Decision-Making and Informatics in Nursing, University of Oregon Health Science Center, Portland, Oregon.

Fonteyn, M., & Grobe, S. (1993). Expert critical care nurses' clinical reasoning under uncertainty: Representation, structure and process. In M. Frisse (Ed.), <u>Sixteenth annual symposium on computer applications in medical care</u> (pp. 405–409). New York: McGraw-Hill.

Fonteyn, M., & Ritter, B. (2000). Clinical reasoning in nursing. In J. Higgs & M. Jones (Eds.), <u>Clinical reasoning in the health professions</u> (2nd ed.) (pp. 107–116). Oxford: Butterworth–Heinemann.

Glaser, R., & Chi, M. T. H. (1988). Overview. In M. T. H. Chi, R. Glaser, & M. J. Farr (Eds.), <u>The nature of expertise</u> (pp. xvi-xxviii). Hillsdale, NJ: Lawrence Erlbaum Associates.

Grant, R. (1992). Obsolescence or lifelong education: Choices and challenges. <u>Physiotherapy, 78,</u> 167–171.

Groen, G. J., & Patel, V. L. (1985). Medical problem-solving: Some questionable assumptions. <u>Medical Education, 19,</u> 95–100.

Harris, I. B. (1993). New expectations for professional competence. In L. Curry & J. Wergin (Eds.), <u>Educating professionals: Responding to new expectations for competence and accountability</u> (pp. 17–52). San Francisco: Jossey-Bass.

Hassebrock, F., Johnson, P. E., Bullemer, P., Fox, P. W., & Moller, J. H. (1993). When less is more: Representation and selective memory in expert problem solving. <u>American Journal of Psychology, 106,</u> 155–189.

Higgs, C., Neubauer, D., & Higgs, J. (1999). The changing health care context: Globilization and social ecology. In J. Higgs & H. Edwards (Eds.), <u>Educating beginning practitioners</u> (pp. 30–37). Oxford: Butterworth–Heinemann.

Higgs, J., & Hunt, A. (1999). Rethinking the beginning practitioner: "the interactional professional." In J. Higgs & H. Edwards (Eds.), <u>Educating beginning practitioners</u> (pp. 10–18). Oxford: Butterworth–Heinemann.

Higgs, J., & Jones, M. (1995). Clinical reasoning. In J. Higgs & M. Jones (Eds.), <u>Clinical reasoning in the health professions</u> (pp. 3–23). Oxford: Butterworth–Heinemann.

Higgs, J., & Jones, M. (2000a). Clinical reasoning in the health professions. In Higgs, J., & Jones, M. (Eds.), <u>Clinical reasoning in the health professions</u> (2nd ed.) (pp. 3–14). Oxford: Butterworth–Heinemann.

Higgs, J., & Jones, M. (Eds.), (2000b). <u>Clinical reasoning in the health professions</u> (2nd ed). Oxford: Butterworth–Heinemann.

Higgs, J., & Titchen, A. (1995). Propositional, professional and personal knowledge in clinical reasoning. In J. Higgs & M. Jones (Eds.), <u>Clinical reasoning in the health professions</u> (pp. 129–146). Oxford: Butterworth–Heinemann.

Jensen, G. M., Gwyer, J., Shepard, K. F., & Hack, L. M. (1999). <u>Expertise in physical therapy practice.</u> Boston: Butterworth–Heinemann.

Jones, M. A. (1992). Clinical reasoning in manual therapy. <u>Physical Therapy, 72,</u> 875–884.

Jones, M., Jensen, G., & Edwards, I. (2000). Clinical reasoning in physiotherapy. In J. Higgs & M. Jones, (Eds.), <u>Clinical reasoning in the health professions</u> (2nd ed.) (pp. 117–127). Oxford: Butterworth–Heinemann.

Jones, M., Jensen, G., & Rothstein, J. (1995). Clinical reasoning in physiotherapy. In J. Higgs & M. Jones (Eds.), <u>Clinical reasoning in the health professions</u> (pp. 72–87). Oxford: Butterworth–Heinemann.

Kennedy, M. (1987). Inexact sciences: Professional education and the development of expertise. <u>Review of Research in Education, 14,</u> 133–168.

Malt, U. F., & Olafson, O. M. (1995). Psychological appraisal and emotional response to physical injury: A clinical, phenomenological study of 109 adults. <u>Psychiatric Medicine, 10,</u> 117–134.

Mattingly, C. (1991). The narrative nature of clinical reasoning. <u>American Journal of Occupational Therapy, 45,</u> 998–1005.

Padrick, K., Tanner, C., Putzier, D., & Westfall, U. (1987). Hypothesis evaluation: A component of diagnostic reasoning. In A. McClane (Ed.), <u>Classification of nursing diagnosis: Proceedings of the Seventh Conference</u> (pp. 299–305). Toronto: C.V. Mosby.

Patel, V. L., & Groen, G. J. (1986). Knowledge-based solution strategies in medical reasoning. <u>Cognitive Science, 10,</u> 91–116.

Patel, V. L., Groen, G. J., & Arocha, J. F. (1990). Medical expertise as a function of task difficulty. <u>Memory and Cognition, 18,</u> 394–406.

Patel, V. L., & Kaufman, D. R. (1995). Clinical reasoning and biomedical knowledge: Implications for teaching. In J. Higgs & M. Jones (Eds.), <u>Clinical reasoning in the health professions</u> (pp. 117–128). Oxford: Butterworth–Heinemann.

Payton, O. D., Nelson, C. E., & Ozer, M. N. (1990). <u>Client participation in program planning: A manual for therapists.</u> Philadelphia: F. A. Davis.

Pyles, S., & Stern, P. (1983). Discovery of nursing gestalt in critical care nursing: The importance of the grey gorilla syndrome. <u>Image: The Journal of Nursing Scholarship, 15,</u> 51–57.

Rew, L. (1990). Intuition in critical care nursing practice. <u>Dimensions of Critical Care Nursing, 9,</u> 30–37.

Rew, L., & Barrow, E. (1987). Intuition: A neglected hallmark of nursing knowledge. <u>Advances in Nursing Science, 10,</u> 49–62.

Schmidt, H., Boshuizen, H. P. A., & Hobus, P. P. M. (1988). Transitory stages in the development of medical expertise: The "intermediate effect" in clinical case representation studies. In V. L. Patel & G. J. Groen (Eds.), <u>Proceedings of the tenth annual conference of the Cognitive Science Society</u> (pp. 139–145). Hillsdale, NJ: Lawrence Erlbaum Associates.

Schmidt, H. G., Norman, G. R., & Boshuizen, H. P. A. (1990). A cognitive perspective on medical expertise: Theory and implications. <u>Academic Medicine, 65,</u> 611–621.

Schön, D. A. (1983). <u>The reflective practitioner: How professionals think in action.</u> London: Temple Smith.

Scott, I. (2000). Teaching clinical reasoning: A case-based approach. In J. Higgs & M. Jones (Eds.), <u>Clinical reasoning in the health professions</u> (2nd ed.) (pp. 290–297). Oxford: Butterworth–Heinemann.

Watts, N. (1995). Teaching clinical decision analysis in physiotherapy. In J. Higgs & M. Jones (Eds.), <u>Clinical reasoning in the health professions</u> (pp. 179–190). Oxford: Butterworth–Heinemann.

Suggested Readings

Chapparo, C., & Ranka, J. (2000). Clinical reasoning in occupational therapy. In J. Higgs & M. Jones (Eds.), <u>Clinical reasoning in the health professions</u> (2nd ed.) (pp. 128–137). Oxford: Butterworth–Heinemann.

Elstein, A., & Schwartz, A. (2000). Clinical reasoning in medicine. In J. Higgs & M. Jones (Eds.), <u>Clinical reasoning in the health professions</u> (2nd ed.) (pp. 95–106). Oxford: Butterworth–Heinemann.

Fleming, M., & Mattingly, C., (2000). Action and narrative: Two dynamics of clinical reasoning. In J. Higgs & M. Jones, (Eds.), <u>Clinical reasoning in the health professions</u> (2nd ed.) (pp. 54–61). Oxford: Butterworth–Heinemann.

Fonteyn, M., & Ritter, B. J. (2000). Clinical reasoning in nursing. In J. Higgs & M. Jones (Eds.), <u>Clinical reasoning in the health professions</u> (2nd ed.) (pp. 107–116). Oxford: Butterworth–Heinemann.

Higgs, J., & Jones, M. (Eds.), (2000). <u>Clinical reasoning in the health professions</u> (2nd ed.) Oxford: Butterworth–Heinemann.

Jones, M., Jensen, G., & Edwards, I. (2000). Clinical reasoning in physiotherapy. In J. Higgs & M. Jones, (Eds.), <u>Clinical reasoning in the health professions</u> (2nd ed.) (pp. 117–127). Oxford: Butterworth–Heinemann.

Perry, A. (Ed.), (1997). <u>Nursing: A knowledge base for practice,</u> London: Arnold.

CHAPTER 5

Case Management

Donna L. Smith

The need for integration of health and human services is not new. However, in recent decades, the number of people with chronic and complex conditions has grown, the number of service providers has increased, funding arrangements have become more diverse, and costs have become an increasing concern. In the 1990s, the health and human service systems in most Western countries were restructured, often with the declared goal of improving the integration of services. In the new millennium, achieving integrated, client-centered services will remain an important, if elusive, goal.

Case management is a process that has been used since the 1970s to improve the integration of services. In this chapter, the origins of case management are described, and the terminology used to describe it is introduced. Many different definitions of case management have been proposed, and terminology traditionally used in this field is now dated. A working definition of case management is presented, and some of the organizational arrangements and delivery models for case management services are discussed.

Various goals can be achieved through case management. The goals and priorities for case management have a bearing on the role of a case manager. The goals of organizations within which case management services are provided can sometimes be in conflict with professional goals.

The case management process and the role of a case manager are discussed in terms of core activities. These are illustrated through two case studies, one in the primary health care setting and the other spanning tertiary care, rehabilitation settings, and the community. The case studies highlight the need for service integration within and between disciplines, departments, programs, agencies, and regions.

As demonstrated by the case studies, the case manager's role is complex, requiring expert knowledge of the client group and the applicable service delivery systems as the basis for discretionary decision making. For this reason, many authorities agree that professional preparation in a health or human service discipline, combined with experience in working with the client group, should be the minimum qualifications for the case management role.

Experts believe that case management can "add value" by improving the continuity and outcomes of care. There is a growing research literature about case management and its outcomes, and some highlights are presented. The importance of evidence-based practice in this evolving field is emphasized.

Professionals trained in health or human service disciplines learn foundational skills for case management while obtaining their undergraduate degrees. Whether entering the work force for the first time or redirecting their careers, they can expect to have opportunities to practice as case managers. Interdisciplinary continuing education for case management practice will increasingly become available to assist them in preparing for the challenges of existing or future roles.

Origins of Case Management

The process that came to be called *case management* arose within the professional cultures of social work, nursing, and medicine more than a century ago as visiting nurses, community social workers, and "family doctors" did their best to respond to the needs of vulnerable people who needed help. Only the very wealthy could afford health services, and the limited services available to other members of society were provided by individual professionals or charitable organizations operating independently of each other. Industrialization and urbanization caused social problems to multiply. The need for more encompassing health and social programs was recognized in the aftermath of the First World War, the Great Depression, and the Second World War. Over several decades, a patchwork of programs developed.

In the 1970s, the term *case management* began to appear in the professional literature. Many long-term residents of mental hospitals were discharged to the community, and an increasing number of older people began to seek health and social support services. At the same time, the systems for delivering health and human services were becoming more complex, and new health disciplines were emerging. New program models were developed, with services being delivered in more locations and under a wider variety of organizational auspices and funding arrangements. As this happened, the need to coordinate services extended beyond vulnerable populations to many other client groups, particularly those with multiple chronic conditions and complex health and social needs. Many different ways of funding and paying for services evolved, adding additional complexity to the processes of accessing, providing, and coordinating services. These factors accelerated the development and formalization of case management.

As new technologies made it possible to prolong the lives of people with severe disabilities, injuries, and chronic illnesses, the costs of providing ongoing services to these client populations began to increase significantly. Workers' Compensation programs and other disability programs offered by insurance companies in the for-profit sector recognized the need to control costs by limiting access to expensive services and by coordinating and monitoring ongoing services to assure their appropriateness and quality. As health costs rose in publicly funded systems such as Medicare and Medicaid in the United States, the National Health Service in the United Kingdom, and in services insured under the provisions of the Canada Health Act in Canada, the goals of achieving efficiency and cost reduction became widely accepted.

The success of case management in the community had demonstrated that a coordinated approach to targeting at-risk populations, identifying their needs, and then providing and monitoring the services of all providers could result in greater quality and efficiency. Unnecessary costs could be avoided by reducing or eliminating duplication of services and by preventing mistakes resulting from poor coordination and communication. It had also been demonstrated that proactive intervention to identify needs and provide low-cost services could often reduce the need for high-cost tertiary services or improve their utilization.

Case Management Terminology and Definition

At the end of the twentieth century, it is obvious that clients or patients do not want to be thought of as "cases" to be "managed" (Everett & Nelson, 1992). The term *case management* continues to be used and facilitates access to much of the formal professional literature. However, other terms—such as *care management, care coordination,* and *service coordination*—have been introduced in recent years and are generally more acceptable to client groups. Case management models have been described in terms of disease entities and settings, the educational background of case managers, or the characteristics of the organization or system in which case management is provided (More & Mandell, 1997; Roberts-DeGenarro, 1987, 1993).

Traditionally, health and human service systems have been organized around the priorities and schedules of professionals or the organizations that provide or pay for services. When confronted with a need or problem, clients and their families often have to engage in what the organizational theorist Charles Perrow (1970) has called "unanalyzable search procedures." These are required when a "nonroutine" problem is encountered and a person has no prior experience or no readily available guidance as to how it can be solved. Clients and their families must often use a process of trial and error to discover what services are available and how to locate and pay for them. Viewed from the client's perspective, it is confusing, time consuming, inconvenient, anxiety provoking, and costly to engage in this process without the necessary information, support, and assistance. The knowledge base and experience that professionals bring to their work equips them for the discretionary decision making needed to engage in an unanalyzable search on behalf of their clients. Case management can be thought of as a process in which the case manager engages in search behavior to obtain needed services or resources with, or on behalf of, a client or family.

As discussed earlier, the need for case management services and the potential value that they can add to clients' well-being and system efficiency has now been recognized. In the years to come, there will be many opportunities for professionals in health and human service disciplines to practice as case managers. Codes of ethics and other professional values will lead professionally prepared case managers to seek ways of reconciling the requirements for client-centered, values-based practice with the financial goals of their employers. Financial accountability and cost avoidance can often be achieved as a by-product of quality-driven, client-centered case management practice (Koska, 1990; Smith & Smith, 1999). This view informs the working definition of case management presented in this chapter. Case management is defined as a process and a professional service to achieve client-centered service integration by facilitating access to services and through assessment, planning, coordination, delivery, and monitoring to assure that they are appropriate and accountable.

Organizational Arrangements and Delivery Models

Case management is sometimes described in terms of the setting or client group being served. In a book regarded as a classic in the case management literature, Applebaum and Austin (1990) explained how case management programs for long-term-care clients were tested in more than 15 federally funded demonstration projects in the United States between 1973 and 1985. They identified intensity, breadth, and duration as features that distinguished long-term-care case management from coordination of services within existing programs. *Intensity* refers to the amount of time the case manager spends with clients, *breadth* refers to the utilization of a broad span of services, and *duration* refers to the amount of time the case manager is involved with the client. These dimensions remain relevant in explaining the difference between case management for people who need a variety of services over an extended period of time and those people who receive services focused around a single and relatively straightforward episode of care in a hospital or health agency.

Case management can also be described in terms of where the case manager is based or employed. The term *internal case management* (More & Mandell, 1997) describes the work case managers do within acute care hospitals and some other institutions to limit variance from expected lengths of stay, outcomes, and costs. A feature of this approach is usually multidisciplinary "critical pathways" or "care maps" developed around the events expected during the hospital stay for various diagnostic-related groups (DRGs) of patients. Case management based in rehabilitation and subacute care facilities as well as in home care programs can also be considered forms of internal case management, in which the case manager is employed by a health care facility or network. In contrast, *external case managers* may work directly for insurance companies or managed care organizations, or may be employed by private case management companies. They may also be self-employed, working directly for clients.

Case management within primary and community care settings has been described as "beyond the walls" by Cohen and Cesta (1997), in contrast to that provided "within the walls" of hospitals or other institutional care settings. Beyond-the-walls case management clearly has features in common with the long-term-care case management models that were described by Applebaum and Austin (1990). They discussed some of the advantages and disadvantages of delivering case management services from a freestanding agency, a special unit in a planning agency, a special unit in an information and referral agency, a special unit in a provider agency, and a special unit in a hospital.

Much of the literature about case management has focused on its value in the long-term care of older people (Austin, 1983, 1992; Shapiro, 1995). But people with mental health problems and a number of other conditions may also have a need for ongoing services. In fact, for people of any age who have multiple health or social problems, the distinction between acute and long-term care is often meaningless because they require a variety of acute, continuing care, and social support services over long periods of time, or from time to time, for the rest of their lives. For these people, the value added by case management is in the continuity of attention they receive from a case manager who collaborates with them to plan and coordinate the various transitions they must make within and between service providers, programs, locations, and systems.

Goals of Case Management

In recent decades, it has become clear that difficulty in accessing services and problems caused by fragmentation and discontinuity in care are no longer restricted to the vulnerable members of society. People of all social classes are living longer and have more chronic illnesses and greater needs for multiple services. Health and human service systems continue to increase in complexity and cost. The need for understandable and convenient access to services and for continuity and integration of services is now widely recognized. Calls for seamless, integrated, and cost-effective systems have driven initiatives to reform and restructure the way that health and human services are delivered in Western countries.

One effect of this has been that case management strategies, originally designed for and implemented in the community, have been adopted and modified to meet the needs of the acute case and hospital sector. In the 1980s and 1990s, programs for prospective hospital reimbursement based on norms developed for various DRGs were introduced in the United States. Health maintenance organizations (HMOs) proliferated, creating incentives for the use of screening, gatekeeping, and coordinating mechanisms. Therefore, in the last decade there has been an "explosion" of literature about the application and benefits of case management in acute care and HMOs (McClelland, 1996). Exposure to this literature without an awareness of the origins and history of case management might lead thoughtful professionals to conclude that it is nothing more than the most recent management fad. For example, the community origins of case management are overlooked in a recent textbook of nursing administration in which an author explained that "case management began in 1980 at the New England Medical Center as a model that maintained quality while streamlining costs," and that "the system originated because of the DRG restrictions on length of stay patients were permitted, and the amount of care allotted during the stay" (Komplin, 1995). The growing use of case management for this purpose has resulted in role conflict and ethical dilemmas for professionals who are case managers (Erlen & Mellors, 1998; Gordon & McCall, 1998; Heater, 1998; Koska, 1990; McClelland et al., 1996; Mohr & Mahon, 1998).

This overview of the origins and development of case management illustrates that case management can be used to achieve a variety of goals. Case management has been described as a "creature of its environment, tuned to the specific needs of its host system," and definitions of case management are often "derived from the nature and needs of the system whose component parts it will be coordinating and integrating" (Beatrice, 1981). Today, case management services are still provided by some organizations to advocate for vulnerable populations and to assist them in gaining access to needed services. The frail elderly and people with mental health needs for whom case management services were originally developed have a continuing need for service. However, other populations— including abused women, children, or elders; people with acquired immunodeficiency syndrome (AIDS); people with problems of substance abuse; people affected by poverty; and people with disabilities, including those resulting from accidents and brain injury—have now been identified as needing case management services.

As the goals of controlling access to high-cost services (often called *gatekeeping*) and managing the utilization of services by clients with complex, multiple needs have gained prominence, some authorities have made a sharp distinction between *system-centered* and *client-centered* case management. System-centered case management serves a rationing and priority-setting function in common with utilization and benefits management. Client-centered case management focuses on advocating for clients and coordinating their services within a fragmented delivery system (Kane, 1992). Standards adopted by the National Association of Social Workers (1992) in the United States acknowledge the potential for role conflict that is inherent in these differing perspectives. The standards advocate that professionals not only put the client's needs first, but also be able to justify how resources are spent on behalf of the client. As McClelland et al. (1996) pointed out, a public policy environment based on a "leaner and meaner" philosophy has made it unfashionable to express concern about the adequacy of funding for social, health, and mental health services, but this issue remains fundamental because "society cannot cost contain or 'case manage' its way around, or out of, a central value and social policy dilemma."

Case Management Process: What Do Case Managers Do?

Case managers use their knowledge and skills to identify and assess individuals and groups who are at risk for complex health and social problems and to facilitate their access to services. Working in collaboration with the client and family, and often within an interdisciplinary team environment, they set goals and develop service plans through which these goals can be achieved. The case manager arranges for appropriate services and sometimes provides direct services. By monitoring the adequacy, quality, and appropriateness of services and by arranging for reassessment as the client's needs or condition changes, the case manager can determine whether changes to the service plan are necessary. These activities of targeting, assessment, care planning, implementation, monitoring, and reassessment have been called the *core activities* of case management (Smith & Smith, 1998).

Coordinating Assessment and Access to Services

Identifying at-risk clients and facilitating their access to services are complex processes. The amount of professional expertise and coordination required depends on the complexity of the client's needs. It also depends on the number of care providers, service locations, and funding mechanisms involved. For example, it is relatively straightforward and uncomplicated to facilitate access to services for an individual with a single health problem that has already been identified or diagnosed and that can be dealt with by one professional service in one location. An elderly patient with diabetes whose condition is stable may be referred to a foot care clinic. His regular attendance at the clinic provides an opportunity for health monitoring and regular reassessment with a health promotion focus. Similarly, groups of otherwise healthy adults whose lower back pain has been appropriately assessed can receive coaching and supervision from a physiotherapist in a group exercise program offered from a gymnasium in a hospital or school. However, as the number of different caregivers, services, programs, locations, and funding mechanisms increases, facilitating access to services becomes more challenging. This is illustrated in the case study that follows.

Case Study 1

Mrs. McNeil was an 85-year-old woman who had lived alone in her own home since being widowed 5 years ago. Although she had diabetes and hypertension, she was in good physical and mental health and had a circle of friends her own age. She was unable to hear without a hearing aid. She did not drive, but walked downtown every day and met people she knew in the stores, post office, or coffee shop. The northern community in which she lived had a population of about 2,500. Her only child, Sandra, lived 225 miles away in the provincial capital of Overton, but telephoned every evening for a chat.

One evening Mrs. McNeil told her daughter: "I didn't want to mention this to you, but I can feel a lump in my breast under my arm. At first I ignored it, but it started to hurt, so I went to see Dr. Todd. He said I needed a CAT scan and that he would book one for me in Snow City. I just thought you should know."

Fortunately, Sandra was a nurse who worked with frail older people, and she understood the way the health system was organized. She began to think about how the diagnostic process and possible treatment might unfold for her mother. Although Snow City was only 125 miles from where Mrs. McNeil lived, it was almost 400 miles from Overton where Sandra lived and worked. It might have been possible for Mrs. McNeil to arrange to have someone from her home town drive her to Snow City for the CAT scan. However, she knew no one there, and if follow-up treatment or hospitalization were necessary, she would have been alone in an unfamiliar hospital and city without support from family or friends. Mrs. McNeil had confidence in Dr. Todd, her general practitioner, and Sandra felt that he had been attentive and vigilant with regard to her mother's care. However, when Sandra telephoned his office the next day, he did not return her call, but rather had his office nurse relay the message that because Mrs. McNeil was competent to make her own decisions, he would not discuss her care with anyone else, including her daughter.

Two days later Mrs. McNeil had not had any further communication from Dr. Todd's office regarding the scheduling of the CAT scan or other diagnostic procedures, and the lump under her arm continued to be painful. "What if this is cancer, Sandra?" she asked. "Won't I have to have an operation?" At this point Sandra told her mother, "I'll drive up tomorrow, and we'll decide how to sort this out."

Before leaving, Sandra communicated with her own general practitioner, Dr. Singh, to explain the situation and ask if he would see her mother. Dr. Singh said that he would be happy to do so and remarked, "I think we should start with a mammogram." Mrs. McNeil was relieved that she could be seen by Dr. Singh in Overton without delay. She was able to arrange for snow shoveling and housesitting on short notice, and the next day she and Sandra were on their way back to Overton.

Sandra called Dr. Singh's office to confirm the tentative appointment she had made for her mother and said to the office nurse, "Dr. Singh mentioned that my mother would probably need a mammogram. Could we have that done before our appointment with him?" After a few moments the office nurse came back on the line to say that an appointment for a mammogram had been confirmed for 3:30 p.m., an hour before the appointment with Dr. Singh.

The mammogram was completed and Mrs. McNeil was given her film to take to her appointment with Dr. Singh. Sandra drove her mother to both of these appointments. After examining Mrs. McNeil and looking at the mammogram, Dr. Singh said, "Mrs. McNeil, it looks to me as if this is a cyst. We want to be sure, though, so I'll book you for an ultrasound."

The ultrasound was booked 2 days later in a facility in downtown Overton. Sandra was able to trade shifts with a coworker, so she was free in the morning to take her mother to this appointment. When they arrived, the technician was unable to locate the mammogram film, which was to have been sent by courier from Dr. Singh's office. "We'll call them to get it sent and rebook you for another appointment," the technician told them. Although annoyed by this inconvenience, Sandra realized that there was no alternative and agreed to return with her mother in a few days' time.

By the time the ultrasound had been completed, the lump had become less painful. Dr. Singh telephoned to report that the ultrasound examination confirmed that the lump was a cyst. He said that as long as the discomfort continued to decrease and no other symptoms appeared, there was no need for Mrs. McNeil to return for a follow-up visit to his office. Mrs. McNeil and Sandra were relieved to have Dr. Singh's original diagnosis confirmed. Mrs. McNeil remained in Overton until the next time Sandra had a few days off, when they drove back to her home.

When there are no formal mechanisms for integrating services, family members must often act as informal case managers (Dring, 1989; Lamb & Stempel, 1994). Fortunately, in this case, Sandra was a nurse who worked with the elderly, so she had expert knowledge of the client group (the frail elderly) to which her mother belonged. As a health professional she also had "insider knowledge" of how the health system operated. She was therefore well equipped to act as the informal case manager for her mother.

Case managers apply their knowledge of client groups and service systems to anticipate the needs of clients, to collaborate with them to set mutually agreed-on goals, and to take their individual choices and preferences into account. In her encounters with the health system, Mrs. McNeil preferred to be near her daughter, and her daughter wanted to do all that she could to support her mother and help her maintain her independence. The goals of maintaining this system of support, and with it Mrs. McNeil's independence and self-confidence, would be uppermost in the mind of an expert case manager working with older people.

Another goal is to arrange for appropriate services in a manner that does not cause inconvenience or difficulty for the client and family or unnecessary costs to the system. In this case, Sandra was able to arrange by telephone to have the mammogram scheduled before the visit to the physician. Had this not been done, two visits to the physician would have probably been necessary to confirm the diagnosis. In addition, a mammogram was a more appropriate and less costly diagnostic procedure than the CAT scan originally suggested by Mrs. McNeil's physician. However, if Sandra had not been able to take time away from work to assist her mother, arranging for transportation to the necessary diagnostic and physician visits would have been a complicated and anxiety-provoking matter. An expert case manager involved in this situation would have assessed Mrs. McNeil's need for assistance and the capacity of her family or friends to assist her. If such informal assistance was not available or appropriate, the case manager would have arranged the necessary transportation, accommodation, and perhaps support from a volunteer or a paid assistant.

On the surface, this case may appear to be about the simple task of scheduling a diagnostic examination. However, it involved several different services located in different places and provided by different professionals. Even if the obvious difficulties of transportation to the diagnostic facilities in Snow City could have been overcome, the situation could have become very complicated for Mrs. McNeil and her daughter if the results of the scan had suggested a need for immediate treatment. Although self-reliant and independent in her own environment, Mrs. McNeil could quickly have become unable to communicate if her hearing aid had been misplaced during the diagnostic examination or surgery. Although Sandra was attentive and willing to assist her mother, it would have been very difficult and expensive for her to do so if treatment or surgery for her mother had been initiated in Snow City. In this case, coordination of services, although important, would not have been sufficient to achieve optimal health outcomes. Expert knowledge of both the client group and the service system was required to carry out an appropriate assessment and to plan for the necessary diagnostic services within a broader framework of long-term health goals.

Not all clients need case management services. Case managers must often determine which clients receive service and in what priority. Access to services is coordinated through the use of mechanisms such as targeting, screening, assessment, and prioritization of client's needs and requests. After determining which clients need services and which of the available services are most appropriate to meet the client's needs, the case manager refers or admits clients to these services.

Inevitably, certain values are built into the eligibility criteria and decision rules that are used to "triage" potential clients. Agencies or professionals whose mandate emphasizes or includes advocacy may give priority to those clients who have the greatest immediate need, who are the most vulnerable, or whose situation will worsen in the immediate future if services are not provided. There are usually many frail older people who have been assessed and placed on a waiting list for admission to continuing care services. If someone on the wait list is being abused by the family member with whom she or he is currently living, this person might receive priority for admission over someone who is in the hospital waiting to be discharged to a continuing care center. If the primary goal of coordinating access is to provide gatekeeping and cost control for an organization, system, or profession, the eligibility criteria and decision rules may reflect an approach that is sometimes described as "cherry picking" to select clients who are most likely to be able to pay or whose care is most straightforward and therefore costs the least to provide.

Uncertainty about how to access or obtain services can discourage people from behaving proactively to prevent or manage their health or social problems. When faced with a crisis, they often turn to the most visible or familiar services. In the health system, these have tended to be doctor's offices and emergency departments, which are among the most expensive of health and human services and which are often unequipped to deal with social or "low-tech" health problems. Although it is common to hear politicians, and some professionals, state that the public misuses or abuses emergency services, more appropriate alternatives that have the confidence of the public and that are convenient to use have been slow to develop.

The concept of a "single point of entry" or "one window" to services has been advocated and demonstrated to be an effective way of providing information, screening, coordinated assessment, and service planning for client groups such as the frail elderly and people with mental illness before they are faced with a crisis. "One-stop shopping" was developed in the business world to respond to consumers' needs for greater convenience and to help them save time. For example, at one time guests in a hotel had to call a different telephone number for each service they might require, such as housekeeping, room service, billing information, parking, and so on. Now it is usually possible to obtain any service by dialing one central number. Within the health and human service systems, "help lines" and telephone information referral services provide one way of simplifying search processes for clients and their families. When monitored by individuals with the appropriate knowledge and intervention skills, such services are often sufficient to enable many clients and families to meet their needs without further assistance. In other instances, the worker receiving the call is able to determine that the urgency or seriousness in the caller's situation requires follow-up by means of a visit by a worker or through arranging an appointment. This approach to screening, targeting, and initial service integration has proven to be efficacious and cost effective with certain client groups.

Another way to integrate services is to locate them in one place. Most professionals and many clients are now familiar with mechanisms such as intake or preadmission clinics. These have worked well for client groups whose health problem and treatment have already been identified. However, individuals with multiple needs or chronic illnesses or who are at risk for various reasons are not well served by traditionally organized services. The Community Health Center Model (Church & Lawrence, 1999) is one in which integrated, interdisciplinary health and human services are provided in one location so that people can receive primary health care in or near their own communities. This model has been shown to be both cost effective and popular with consumers, but its potential to interfere with the exclusive gatekeeping role of general practitioners and the economic incentives within the fee-for-service system of remunerating some professionals has delayed its widespread implementation. It can be expected that efforts to improve quality, customer satisfaction, and cost effectiveness in health and human service systems will result in new forms of providing service that focus on removing barriers and eliminating inconvenience duplication, omissions, and mistakes that have traditionally made it difficult for people to find and obtain the services they need.

Coordinating the Planning, Delivery, and Monitoring of Services

Once the assessment process is complete and initial goals and a service plan have been agreed on, clients with multiple needs, risk factors, or chronic conditions will require ongoing services. Arranging for and coordinating these services is important, both to clients' well-being and to the achievement of health outcomes. There are varying degrees of complexity involved in the mobilization and coordination of services.

Coordinating services provided by one professional group is the most common and least complex type of case management. Required in many settings, it is affected by variables such as work schedules, professional specialization, and professional culture. For example, in a rehabilitation services department, physiotherapists may be assisted by aides who are delegated to carry out certain treatments. Even if the same physiotherapist remains responsible for the client on successive visits, it is necessary for the therapist to communicate closely with the aide. If for any reason the same physiotherapist is not available throughout the client's attendance, additional coordination is necessary.

As the number of professional groups or departments providing service increases, so do the problems of communication and coordination. In general, services provided by many departments in one location, such as an acute care hospital, are easier to coordinate than those provided in different locations.

Complexity is increased if the funding for services comes from more than one organization or plan. The most complex situations are those in which the client has multiple health and social problems of a chronic nature. Such clients often need services from several different agencies and professionals simultaneously, or in sequence, and they may be eligible for funding support from more than one source. The next case study presents a prototypical situation that illustrates this complexity.

Case Study 2

Cheryl was 19 years of age, and she had finished her first year of university with top marks. She was active in a number of sports and especially loved running with her dog. She was attractive and had a fun-filled social life that included a steady boyfriend. Suddenly all this changed.

While traveling through the mountains in another province, she was involved in a serious car accident. Unconscious, she was taken by ambulance to the nearest hospital. Her parents were contacted and immediately set out to be with her. Fortunately, both were professionals and able to arrange for time away from their work. For several days it was uncertain whether Cheryl would survive. She received excellent care from a multidisciplinary team of intensive care specialists.

As Cheryl's condition began to stabilize, her parents were told that she could be moved back to her home city, Edgerton. Much to their surprise, they were told it would be up to them to arrange for the air ambulance and the recovery of costs from their provincial health plan. They found this very stressful but were able to do what was necessary to make the arrangements.

Staff who had been caring for Cheryl in the intensive care unit (ICU) communicated with staff in the ICU in Edgerton to arrange for Cheryl's transfer. However, when she arrived it was clear that this communication had not been entirely successful. The staff of the receiving unit had not appreciated the severity of Cheryl's condition, which was too unstable for her to be cared for in the location they had prepared.

There were some stressful hours as arrangements were made to move other patients to make room for Cheryl in the main ICU. At this time, about a week after her accident, she was still unconscious and breathing with the assistance of a ventilator. She had several broken bones and flesh wounds, and her neurologic signs were unstable. Her parents were told that it was uncertain when, or to what extent, she would regain consciousness and that if she did, it was unlikely that she would be able to walk again. Supported by family and friends, they maintained a vigil at Cheryl's bedside, speaking to her, touching her, and assisting with her care. As her physical condition improved, she showed some signs of responding to them. She had been transferred to a step-down unit, and after she had begun to breathe on her own, the ventilator was removed. She was then transferred to the neurologic ward within the same hospital.

As these transfers occurred, some of the same doctors remained involved with Cheryl's care. However, with the transfer from the ICU environment of the ward, a different group of physicians and medical house staff was involved. It seemed that they rarely talked to one another, and each offered a different viewpoint as to Cheryl's prognosis. The nursing staff on the various units was accustomed to arranging the transfer of patients from one unit to the other, and the respiratory therapists, physiotherapists, dietician, and clinical pharmacist who were participating in Cheryl's care remained the same except for the occasions when one or the other might need to be replaced due to illness or vacation. Although they had received some conflicting information about Cheryl's prognosis from the various professionals involved, Cheryl's parents remained generally satisfied with her care as these transfers occurred within the acute hospital environment.

Approximately 6 weeks after her accident, Cheryl regained consciousness. Her parents were then advised that she would need to be transferred to a rehabilitation program. Two programs were available for people who had suffered traumatic brain injury, one in Edgerton and one in a smaller center about 100 miles away. Cheryl's parents expressed a preference for the local program, feeling that this would enable Cheryl to see her family and friends, as well as her dog. They were told that there was a long waiting list in that program, that it was now urgent to discharge Cheryl from the hospital to make room for other patients, and that the out-of-town program was more suitable for Cheryl's needs. They felt they had little choice but to accept the transfer.

The rehabilitation program was located in renovated space in a provincial mental hospital. Cheryl's rehabilitation program consisted of physio-, occupational, and speech therapy. Having been an athlete and a runner before her accident, Cheryl embraced her physiotherapy program. She was aware that she needed help to improve her speech and participated willingly in her speech therapy program. However, when asked to do crafts (ceramics) in her occupational therapy program, she rebelled and was dismissed from the program. She had formed a good relationship with her physiotherapist, who eventually facilitated a relationship with an occupational therapist who was based in the town and not at the hospital. This enabled Cheryl to resume an occupational therapy program that was tailored more to her own interests and preferences.

Cheryl felt lonely and isolated. During her free time, she rode the exercise bike for hours on end. She continued to read and occasionally wrote letters. Her parents visited every week and sometimes more frequently. They attempted to bring her dog, but he traveled poorly, and this had to be discontinued. Although her friends had visited her frequently when she was in the acute care hospital, she now lost touch with them. Most of the other patients in the program were elderly, so she had limited age-appropriate companionship.

After approximately 5 months, Cheryl was discharged home. Her parents were told that she needed ongoing outpatient rehabilitation, but that patients from out of town were put on a waiting list behind those from the local inpatient rehabilitation program. Feeling that it was essential that Cheryl's therapy continue without interruption, her parents arranged to pay for her therapy privately. Then, because she was already in a program, she had even less priority on the waiting list for the publicly funded program.

Four years after her accident, Cheryl became independent in her activities of daily living. She had a contracture in one hand, and although she was still an attractive young person, her face had a "frozen" expression. She spoke in a monotone, but expressed herself quite well in short sentences. She recalled her experiences in the rehabilitation hospitals as an unhappy time that she would like to forget. She felt that her recovery was due to her physiotherapist, who "treated me like a real person" and "really enjoyed her job."

Cheryl resumed her university studies, working hard to succeed in one course per semester. She ran regularly with her dog. She still had limited social contact with people her own age, but her relationship with her parents remained close and supportive, although there was some conflict because she pressed them to allow her to resume driving. Her parents said that they were glad that their incomes and educational background allowed them to support Cheryl as they had and as they continued to do. Although she was not receiving any services at present, they recognized that she would need various sorts of ongoing social, vocational, and rehabilitation support. They expressed the wish to "just be her parents" again.

This case study illustrates a situation in which a family had no professional case management support in the complex journey between hospitals in two different provinces, and services were provided by a number of different professional groups in more than one location over a significant period of time. Initially, the coordination of care within individual professional disciplines and individual hospital units was adequate, although the information provided to the family was often contradictory. However, as the goal of care shifted from life support and discharge from the acute care hospital to that of supporting resumption of the life activities and developmental tasks of a young adult, there were obvious failures in service coordination and long-range client and family-centered planning.

It is clear that this family would have benefited from the expertise and support of an expert case manager who would have assisted them in spanning the boundaries between professional services, programs, and locations during the immediate aftermath of Cheryl's traumatic brain injury. As advocated by Cioschi and Goodman (1994) and reinforced by other authors (e.g., Brooks et al., 1986; Dring, 1989; Gilbert & Counsell, 1995; Smith, 1998), the complexity of this and similar chronic conditions suggests the need for a lifetime case management model.

For effectiveness in such a model, case managers must be able to advocate as care-delivery-team members and settings change for their clients. Care maps or models—which identify the barriers separating settings and services and the strategies for navigating the system to find the most commonly needed services—facilitate more integrated, client-centered service (Nikolaj & Boon, 1998; Raiwet et al., 1997). Case managers within such a model would assess and build on the strengths of both the client and the informal support system, with a view to supporting the long-range physical, social, vocational, and health requirements of each. Without such expert support, the potential for burnout among informal caregivers is high, and the resulting health and social costs are prohibitive (Smith, 1998).

Preparation, Research, and Professional Opportunities in Case Management

Case managers require expert knowledge of the client group, as well as of the service systems and sources of funds needed by the client groups they serve. As mentioned earlier in this chapter, a majority of the professional literature about case management has originated from the professions of social work and nursing. However, in recent years, other professions have developed an interest and expertise in case management, and this has now been reflected in the literature of the rehabilitation professions ("A Brief Look," 1994; Carswell-Opzoomer, 1990; Cook, 1995; Dyck, 1996; Krupa & Clark, 1995; Nelson, 1993). A high level of discretionary decision making is required of case managers as they apply their expert knowledge to collaborate with the client, family, and service providers in order to agree on goals and to plan, mobilize, coordinate, and monitor services.

There have traditionally been many different career paths leading to the role of case manager, and professionals from many disciplines can contribute within this role. As the complexities of the role become better understood, it is clear that much of the foundational knowledge required for care management practice is provided within the existing educational programs that prepare health and human service professionals. Standards developed within the disciplines of social work and nursing and the opinions of other experts support the position that a baccalaureate degree in a health or human service profession supplemented by significant experience in working with particular client groups is the most desirable minimum preparation for case management practice (Bower, 1992; Case Management Society of America, 1994; Geron & Chassler, 1994; National Association of Social Workers, 1992). Some studies have demonstrated the effectiveness of case managers with master's level preparation (Cronin & Makelbust, 1989), and master's degrees focusing on this area of practice have been developed (Haw, 1995). Many experts believe that in-service education for case management should be supplemented, or replaced by, interdisciplinary credit programs or continuing education focused on the specialized knowledge, skills, and values required for effective practice in the case management role.

The field of case management is relatively new, but research to identify or confirm client needs, case managers' skill requirements, the effectiveness of interventions, and the outcomes of case management is beginning to influence and improve case management practice (Austin, 1983; Chamberlain & Rapp, 1991; Fleishman, 1990; Franklin et al., 1994; Holloway et al., 1995; Lamb, 1992; Lemire & Austin, 1996; Rothman, 1992; Smith, 1998). Professionals entering this field have the opportunity to benefit from and participate in ongoing research.

Summary

Traditionally, services have been provided and organized to accommodate the organizational boundaries of professions, agencies, and funding organizations. The result for clients and their families has often been frustration, inconvenience, and discontinuity of care. The use of case management to coordinate care within professional disciplines, departments, programs, agencies, and regions can help to improve continuity of care. But the achievement of integrated service may require more fundamental redesign of service delivery strategies and structures with the needs and experiences of the client as the focus.

In this chapter, the origins, development, and terminology of case management have been introduced. Models and issues in service delivery have been discussed and illustrated through case studies. The need for improving the integration of services has been highlighted. A reduction in expenditures can be expected if targeting and assessment enable high-risk client groups to be identified and appropriate services to be provided. Eliminating duplications in service and developing services to meet unmet needs also results in reduced costs, because many of the services now missing from delivery systems are "low-tech" services that provide information, support, and community-based services to clients or their informal caregivers. The process of case manager and the practice of expert case management from many professional disciplines offer a demonstrated means of improving continuity of care and service integration in which client and family advocacy remains a goal and cost reductions occur as a by-product (Austin & McClelland, 1996).

Current professional standards offer expert guidance in the design of the case manager role and in the requirements for practice. Interdisciplinary education, collaboration, and research will continue to develop in the field of case management and will provide ongoing guidance in the development of evidence-based standards and strategies. Professionals entering the work force or wishing to redirect their careers will find challenging opportunities in case management positions in numerous program settings and in new boundary-spanning roles that will inevitably develop in response to consumer demand.

References

A brief look at rehab outcome measures for case managers. (1994). Case Management Advisor, 49–51.

Applebaum, R., & Austin, C. (1990). Long-term care case management: Design and evaluation. New York: Springer.

Austin, C. D. (1983). Case management in long-term care: Options and opportunities. Health and Social Work, 8(1), 16–30.

Austin, C. D. (1992). Have we oversold case management as a "quick fix" for our long-term care system? Journal of Case Management, 1(2), 61–65.

Austin, C. D., & McClelland, R. W. (1996). Introduction: Case management: Everybody's doing it. In C. D. Austin & R. W. McClelland (Eds.), Perspectives on case management (pp. 1–16). Milwaukee, WI: Families International.

Beatrice, D. F. (1981). Case management: A policy option for long-term care. In J. J. Callahan & S. S. Wallack (Eds.), Reforming the long-term-care system (pp. 121–161). Toronto: Lexington Books.

Bower, K. A. (1992). Case management by nurses. Washington, DC: American Nurses Association.

Brooks, D. N., Campsie, L., Symington, C., Beattie, A., & McKinley, W. (1986). The five-year outcome of severe head injury: A relative's view. Journal of Neurology, Neuroscience, and Psychiatry, 46, 870–875.

Carswell-Opzoomer, A. (1990). Occupational therapy: Our time has come. <u>Canadian Journal of Occupational Therapy, 57</u>(4), 197–204.

Case Management Society of America. (1994). CMSA proposes standards of practice. <u>Case Manager, 5</u>(1), 59–71.

Chamberlain, R., & Rapp, C. A. (1991). A decade of case management: A methodological review of outcome research. <u>Community Mental Health Journal, 27</u>(3), 171–188.

Church, J., & Lawrence, S. (1999). Community health centres: Innovation in health management and delivery. In J. M. Hibberd & D. L. Smith (Eds.), <u>Nursing management in Canada</u> (2nd ed.) (pp. 219–236). Toronto: W. B. Saunders.

Cioschi, H. M., & Goodman, C. L. (1994). A lifetime case management model for persons with spinal cord injury. <u>Journal of Case Management, 3</u>(3), 117–123.

Cohen, E. L., & Cesta, T. G. (1997). <u>Nursing case management</u> (2nd ed.). Toronto: Mosby.

Cook, J. V. (1995). Innovation and leadership in a mental health facility. <u>American Journal of Occupational Therapy, 49</u>(7), 595–606.

Cronin, C. J., & Makelbust, J. (1989). Case-managed care: Capitalizing on the CNS. <u>Nursing Management, 20</u>(3), 38–47.

Dring, R. (1989). The informal caregiver responsible for home care of the individual and cognitive dysfunction following brain injury. <u>Journal of Neuroscience Nursing, 2</u>(1), 42–45.

Dyck, D. (1996). Managed rehabilitative care. <u>American Association of Occupational Health Nursing, 44</u>(1), 18–27.

Erlen, J. A., & Mellors, M. P. (1998). Managed care and the nurse's ethical obligations to patients. In E. C. Hein (Ed.), <u>Contemporary leadership behaviour: Selected readings</u> (5th ed.) (pp. 118–123). Philadelphia: Lippincott.

Everett, B., & Nelson, A. (1992). We're not cases and you're not managers: An account of a client-centered professional partnership developed in response to "borderline" diagnosis. <u>Psychosocial Rehabilitation Journal, 15</u>(4), 49–60.

Fleishman, J. A. (1990). Research issues in service integration and coordination. Community-based care of persons with AIDS: Developing a research agenda. <u>Conference Proceedings, U.S. Department of Health and Human Services, Agency for Health Care Policy and Research. Washington, D.C., Public Health Service,</u> 157–167.

Franklin, J. L., Solovitz, B., Mason, M., Clemons, J. R., & Miller, G. E. (1994). An evaluation of case management. <u>American Journal of Public Health, 11</u>(3/4), 269–282.

Geron, S. M., & Chassler, D. (1994). The quest for uniform guidelines for long term care case management practice. <u>Journal of Case Management, 3</u>(3), 91–97.

Gilbert, M., & Counsell, C. M. (1995). Coordinated care for the SCI patient. <u>Spinal Cord Injury Nursing, 12</u>(3), 87–89.

Gordon, S., & McCall, T. (1998). Helping your patients manage managed care. In E. C. Hein (Ed.), <u>Contemporary leadership behaviour: Selected readings</u> (5th ed.) (pp. 326–333). Philadelphia: Lippincott.

Haw, M. A. (1995). State of the art education for case management in long term care. <u>Journal of Case Management, 4</u>(3), 85–94.

Heater, B. C. (1998). The current health care environment: Who is the customer? In E. C. Hein (Ed.), Contemporary leadership behaviour: Selected readings (5th ed.) (pp. 307–313). Philadelphia: Lippincott.

Holloway, F., Oliver, N., Collins, E., & Carson, J. (1995). Case management: A critical review of the outcome literature. European Psychiatry, 10(3) 113–118.

Kane, R. A. (1992). Case management in health settings. In S. Rose (Ed.), Case management and social work (pp. 170–203). New York: Longman.

Komplin, J. (1995). Care delivery systems. In Y. Wise (Ed.), Leading and managing in nursing (pp. 410–435). Toronto: Mosby.

Koska, M. T. (1990). Case management: Doing the right thing for the wrong reasons. Hospitals, 64, 28–30.

Krupa, T., & Clark, C. C. (1995). Occupational therapists as case managers: Responding to current approaches to community mental health service delivery. Canadian Journal of Occupational Therapy, 62(1), 16–22.

Lamb, G. S. (1992). Conceptual and methodological issues in nurse case management research. Advances in Nursing Science, 15(2), 16–24.

Lamb, G. S., & Stempel, J. E. (1994). Nurse case management from the client's view: Growing as insider-expert. Nursing Outlook, 42(17), 7–13.

Lemire, A., & Austin, C. D. (1996). Care planning in home care: An exploratory study. Journal of Case Management, 5(1), 32–40.

McClelland, R. W. (1996). Managed care. In C. Austin & R. W. McClelland (Eds.), Perspectives on case management practice (pp. 203–218). Milwaukee, WI: Families International.

McClelland, R., Austin, C., & Schneck, D. (1996). Practice dilemmas and policy implications. In C. Austin & R. McClelland (Eds.), Perspectives on case management practice (pp. 257–278). Milwaukee, WI: Families International.

Mohr, W. K., & Mahon, M. M. (1998). Dirty hands: The underside of marketplace health care. In E. C. Hein (Ed.), Contemporary leadership behaviour: Selected readings (5th ed.) (pp. 124–131). Philadelphia: Lippincott.

More, P. K., & Mandell, S. (1997). Nursing case management (p. 92). New York: McGraw-Hill.

National Association of Social Workers. (1992). Case management in health, education and human service settings. In S. M. Rose (Ed.), Case management and social work practice (pp. 21–28). New York: Longman.

Nelson, M. (1993). The race for victory in rehabilitation case management. Rehabilitation Nursing, 18(4), 253–254.

Nikolaj, S., & Boon, B. (1998). Health care management in workers' compensation. Occupational Medicine: State of the Art Reviews, 13(2), 357–379.

Perrow, C. (1970). Organizational analysis: A sociological view (p. 76). London: Tavistock.

Raiwet, C., Halliwell, G., Andruski, L., & Wilson, D. (1997). Care maps across the continuum. Canadian Nurse, 93(1), 26–30.

Roberts-DeGenarro, M. (1987). Developing case management as a practice model. Social Casework: The Journal of Contemporary Social Work, 68, 466–470.

Roberts-DeGenarro, M. (1993). Generalist model of case management practice. Journal of Case Management, 2(3), 106–111.

Rothman, J. (1992). Guidelines for case management: Putting research to professional use. Itasca: F. E. Peacock.

Shapiro, E. (1995). Case management in long-term care: Exploring its status, trends, and issues. Journal of Case Management, 4(2), 43–47.

Smith, J. (1998). Experiences of caregivers in arranging services for survivors of traumatic brain injury. Unpublished master's thesis, University of Alberta, Edmonton, AB.

Smith, J., & Smith, D. L. (1999). Service integration and case management. In J. M. Hibberd & D. L. Smith (Eds.), Nursing management in Canada (pp. 174–194). Toronto: W. B. Saunders.

CHAPTER 6

Attitudes Toward Disability

Roseanna Tufano

Health professionals have a profound impact on a person's physical and psychological recovery. Attitudes, beliefs, and perceptions regarding disability are an inherent part of the rehabilitation process. In the therapeutic relationship, staff and clients continuously influence each other with their attitudes, affecting treatment in positive and negative ways.

Many factors contribute to the development of attitudes and beliefs toward disability. This chapter addresses a variety of topics from both the health professional and client perspectives. The reader will learn about the different sources from society that influence each of us, shaping our thoughts, feelings, and behaviors toward persons with disabilities. Ethnic beliefs will also be discussed as sources of influence, highlighting how our family of origin significantly affects our views about health. Popular theories and models in health care are summarized, assisting the reader to recognize the significant formulations they make about wellness, "normalcy," and illness. Common reactions and anxieties associated with disability are discussed, including how the use of language contributes to both positive and negative perceptions within health care and society. After the description of these varied sources that influence our personal and professional beliefs, the reader will find a practice exercise to encourage reflection about the different topics and theories described while encouraging the application of the various strategies needed to incorporate positive attitudes toward disability. It is my sincerest hope that you will find these suggestions readily applicable in the rehabilitation treatment process.

What Is an Attitude?

An attitude is a state of mind, a thought, or a feeling about something. People can verbally describe and express their attitude regarding a particular matter, or they can demonstrate it nonverbally through body language. In everyday encounters with other people, we are accustomed to listening to verbal statements and words while paying minimal attention to nonverbal language. Through the process of socialization, people have learned to use spoken language to gain attention and acceptance from the listener. Simply stated, we all have the ability to tell someone what they want to hear.

Health professionals know that body language should never be ignored in therapeutic communication because it provides significant information about the client's feelings and thoughts. An astute professional pays attention to both the spoken words and body language of a client, noticing if the verbal and nonverbal messages are congruent. For example, a client's attitude toward the rehabilitation process may be interpreted as genuine when he verbally tells you, "Yes, I want to get better," and also shows you his level of commitment by being punctual for all treatment sessions. In this example, the client's spoken and unspoken messages are consistent and match each other. Similarly, a health professional is perceived as genuine and trustworthy by the client when what is *said* verbally during treatment sessions and what is *shown* in the treatment process are consistent.

A person's internal mood state is often unconsciously shown in his or her attitude. We all project our feelings and thoughts about ourselves into the environment and onto others. A person who is happy and satisfied with him- or herself tends to project an optimistic and accepting attitude toward others. On the other hand, someone who bears self-hatred and personal intolerance tends to project hate, prejudice, and pessimism toward others.

Health professionals must learn to identify both their clients' attitudes toward disability as well as their own. Effective professionals are open and conscious about their own feelings and beliefs that involve regarding the client as a person, not just a diagnosis. Once professional staff are comfortable with accepting their own positive and negative attitudes, they can accept the clients' range of feelings and beliefs as well. The therapeutic relationship is an interactive process. Attitudes that originate from both the health professional and client have the potential to equally and significantly influence treatment outcome.

Attitudes Toward Disability

Research on the impact of attitudes toward disability continues to be conducted by sociologists, psychologists, and health professionals of varied disciplines. It is a significant topic for all rehabilitation staff to understand because societal attitudes continue to shape the self-image and self-concept of persons with disabilities.

Rousch, a physical therapist, has studied the impact of attitudes on health care. She believes that health professionals are in a unique position to change the way our society views people with disabilities. In her 1986 article, "Health Professionals as Contributors to Attitudes Towards Persons with Disabilities," Rousch proposes that health professionals need to pay more attention to their use of language and stereotypes. She writes that attitudinal barriers continue to limit and challenge the rehabilitative relationship in negative ways. She proposes that health professionals should become facilitators of positive regard and nonjudgmental acceptance within the therapeutic process. Rousch is describing an attitude for health professionals that is based on a philosophy known as "humanism."

It is clear from both research and narrative personal accounts that assumptions and stereotypes about clients are barriers that limit and negatively influence treatment outcomes. However, health professionals can have a significant and positive impact by using respectful and nonjudgmental attitudes, both spoken and unspoken, when directly communicating with clients or about them to others in society.

Ethnic Influences from Our Family of Origin

A significant source to the development of our belief systems is ethnicity. Studies have shown that ethnic values and group identification remain with families for several generations after immigration. Ethnicity is defined as a sense of belonging with a group who regard themselves as sharing a common ancestry, real or fictitious. Ethnic patterns influence many aspects of our lives, including what we eat, how we work, what we celebrate, and how we feel about sickness, health, and death.

In 1969, Zborowski published a significant study identifying how different ethnic groups respond to physical illness. For example, he found that patients who were of Italian and Jewish descent tended to report their "pain," while the Irish and white Anglo-Saxon Protestant groups did not. Persons of Irish descent tended to view pain as punishment for sins and took full responsibility for its origin. Zborowski also realized that many medical personnel viewed the expressiveness to pain shown overtly by Jewish and Italian patients as "exaggerated."

We all have developed certain beliefs and attitudes about illness and disability from our families of origin. As health care providers, we must first identify our own internalized beliefs about health care to appreciate the attitudes of our clients. Professionals must consider the sources of these beliefs and check out their validity and truthfulness with our clients, because they significantly influence our professional roles and behaviors. An effective way to develop some personal insight is to identify why you have chosen to become a health care provider and what you gain by fulfilling this role. For example, if your reason for becoming a health professional is to "help" others in need, what will be your reaction and attitude when a client refuses your "help"?

Treatment Models That Influence a Health Professional's Attitudes

Humanism is a philosophy that emerged in the early 1900s. Two well-known humanists are Abraham Maslow and Carl Rogers. The philosophy of humanism proposes that all persons are innately good and contain the ability to self-direct and to make choices that satisfy their own personal needs. Humanism also postulates that individuals have the innate desire to grow and to seek the meaning of their existence. Persons strive to reach their potential, to self-actualize, and to attain a sense of personal completeness.

Rogers focused much of his research on the therapeutic relationship. His approach is known as *person-centered* or *client-centered* therapy. Rogers believed that all human beings have the basic need to be positively regarded by others, which contributes to a feeling of acceptance and belonging. When a therapist offers positive regard to a client, he or she offers an unconditional attitude of acceptance, which includes the client's strengths and shortcomings. Clients feel appreciated for *who* they are, and their efforts are recognized and positively reinforced even when recovery is not possible, such as with terminal illnesses.

Rogers stressed that unconditional positive regard is significant to a young child's development because it fosters self-actualization or a sense of personal completeness. Health professionals and clients who may not have received this level of acceptance from their families and significant others appear intolerant, judgmental, and critical of others. In actuality, such persons are really unable to accept aspects of their own selves. We cannot tolerate in others what we cannot tolerate about ourselves. On the other hand, children who are raised with positive affirmations and unconditional regard develop strong, healthy egos. They are naturally sensitive to others, conveying an openness to differences because they appreciate the unique aspects, or humanness, of every person.

Health professionals who value their clients as people first, rather than cases to be solved, incorporate the humanistic philosophy into their work. From this perspective, clients are invited to assist in the everyday problem solving and decision making of their treatment care. They are encouraged to make choices about their treatment whenever possible, including the identification of personal needs, wants, and goals that they want to achieve in rehabilitation. They feel empowered and accepted within the rehabilitative process. The establishment of rapport and trust within the therapeutic relationship is a priority to the health care provider who seeks to gather information about the client's values and treatment goals as part of the assessment process. Health professionals who practice the humanistic philosophy are concerned about the impact of disability on the person's life and future adjustment, not just the immediate needs of the day.

Another significant approach that influences health care professionals is the biomedical model. This scientific approach focuses on the disease processes and pathology associated with disorders or illness. The focus of the medical model is to alleviate symptoms and find cures based on scientific evidence from research. Treatment is given in a medically prescriptive manner and designed to improve the malfunctioning physical components of disease and disorders. The biomedical model provides an objective and structured way to deliver health care, a necessary and effective mission. Therefore, within the context of its very definition and core, the biomedical model focuses on the physical entities of disability rather that the psychosocial impact of a disability.

Some rehabilitation staff who work from this biomedical perspective may become inclined to refer to their patients as a "diagnosis" or a "case" that requires treatment implementation. These health care providers may consider their role as performing treatment *to the patient* instead of facilitating the promotion of health *with the person*. When health professionals refer to someone as "the paraplegic," "the stroke victim," or "the schizophrenic," they strip away any semblance of personhood and dignity. While this may not be the health care worker's intent, calling a person by their diagnosis is a form of disregard to that client and encourages the prevalence of negative attitudes within the medical community.

It is truly one of our greatest challenges as health professionals to balance both the humanistic philosophy and biomedical model within the course of rehabilitation. An example of a type of formulation that serves to include both the biological and psychosocial aspects of a client is the biopsychosocial model. Within the biopsychosocial model, a client is understood from a variety of influential components that include the biological origins of disease as well as the social implications from one's environment and interpersonal experiences. From this approach, a vital concern for all health professionals is to recognize and clarify how family and societal attitudes contribute to one's disability, and how these perceptions affect both the physical and emotional course of recovery for clients within the rehabilitation process.

Stigma

A stigma, otherwise defined as a mark or label, has a negative connotation. When a person is stigmatized, he or she is branded in disgrace or shame.

Social scientists have conducted many studies regarding how attitudes of able-bodied persons, who make up the majority of our population, view persons with a disability, who are the minority. Many of these attitudes are formed from assumptions made about disability without experiencing one. Some of the typical emotional reactions toward someone with a disability include pity, guilt, and anxiety.

Some people assume that it is a sign of weakness to need medical attention. They fear that they may become helpless and dependent on the medical community or seem different and abnormal from the rest of society. Often, persons with a disability are not viewed as having a separate identity from their diagnosis. Disability and self-identity are mistakenly merged and associated together as synonyms for one's self-concept. For example, labeling someone as "the manic depressive" suggests that this mental disorder is one's personality and source of personal identity rather than a separate condition. This particular negative stigma serves to invalidate a person with associations of "craziness" and "mental incurability." Labeling encourages us to generalize our thinking rather than to individualize. Generalized associations are formed and get attributed to all persons with the same diagnosis from one single experience. These labels serve to further segregate and negatively discriminate a minority group of people from the general population.

Another distressing assumption within our society is that someone's disability is the sole reason that prevents integration into the community. This narrow-minded belief suggests that the "impairment" is to blame for the various types of obstacles experienced by persons with physical or emotional challenges. From this assumption, obstacles such as architectural barriers, the economy, legal issues, and cultural beliefs are ignored and not even considered even though they are all created by humankind. This reasoning process is linear, or one sided, and an example of cause-and-effect thinking. In other words, disability causes problems in society. This assumption fails to view the relationship between the person and his or her environment as a constant interactive and systemic interchange that is highly influenced by feedback from one to the other.

How do these attitudes perpetuate within our society? Jones et al. (1984) reported from their studies that when someone sees a person with a "disability," this leads to feelings of vulnerability and thoughts of death from the observer. Anxiety and the realization of lack of control enter one's consciousness or awareness. When members of society, including health professionals, do not have adequate coping mechanisms, they may disown their anxious thoughts and feelings by projecting them onto others. Common examples of projections include stigmatizing, stereotyping, and labeling in efforts to minimize the impact of a person with a disability. The action of putting down another, whether it is through verbal expression or outward behavior, allows one to feel "normal" and subsequently "in control" of him- or herself. This power burst to one's ego is short lived, however. Soon, this person must find another source to put down and control in order to cope with the increasing anxiety that once again begins to emerge into one's awareness.

Aesthetic and Existential Anxiety

Livneh (1982) defined the concepts of "aesthetic" and "existential" anxiety as significant components in the formulation of attitudes. Both of these concepts reinforce negative perceptions of others and reinforce stigmatizing of persons with disabilities.

Our society places high value on physical beauty and attractiveness. Those persons who are preoccupied and stressed about their own appearance are also sensitive to the physical differences of others. "Aesthetic" anxiety occurs when someone becomes fearful and worried about his or her own physical vulnerabilities when noticing someone else whose traits are perceived as unappealing. Studies show that people ineffectively cope with their anxiety in several ways. One attempt to deal with this anxiety is to shun or avoid the person with these noted physical differences. Deliberately ignoring or neglecting to regard others can be just as hurtful as calling them derogatory names. Another faulty coping strategy is to disempower persons with a disability by labeling them as insignificant and not meeting up to the standards of "normal" people in society. Another example of a destructive coping mechanism used by some is to increase one's own self-esteem by demeaning the value of those around him or her. Lastly, some people pursue supernormal physical characteristics as a way to decrease "aesthetic" anxiety. Such examples include addictive exercising to maintain a certain body weight and physique, consumption of steroids, and cosmetic and plastic surgery solely to enhance one's physical appearance with little consideration for the possible risks associated with this decision.

"Existential" anxiety is defined by Livneh (1982) as fear of potential or functional loss that would interfere with having a satisfactory life. This type of anxiety occurs when an able-bodied person "identifies with" or is in "agreement with" the assumed feelings of a person with a disability. A statement that reflects "existential" anxiety is "I would rather be dead than be confined to a wheelchair like Louis for the rest of my days!" This attitude is reflective of the belief that only persons with high physical performance can be happy and feel satisfied in this life.

The effect of "existential" anxiety is to associate persons with disabilities as helpless and dependent, incapable of controlling their own destiny. It is common for sympathy to be expressed toward persons with disabilities as a form of "existential" anxiety. When health professionals sympathize with a client, they are in agreement with the feelings and experiences of this person. Consider the following example of sympathy:

John is a 22-year-old rehabilitation professional who is working with his client, Louis, who has a C6 spinal cord lesion from a diving accident. Louis is feeling depressed and pessimistic about his future. Louis is also 22 years of age. After the session, John states to his fellow colleague, "I feel sorry for Louis. He is only 22 years old and will never be able to walk again, swim, or play sports, or have a normal relationship. His whole life is ruined!"

This expression of pity serves to demean and disempower the client. The health professional is projecting his own fears and anxieties onto the client as he imagines what it would feel like to have a disability. This statement further stigmatizes that Louis is an invalid who has little possibility for a happy social life because he has a spinal cord injury.

As a first step, therapists and rehabilitation staff must identify their own personal attitudes and biases toward clients. Unless health professionals are consciously aware of their own feelings, it is common to project them onto a client. The most effective, therapeutic way to communicate feelings within a professional relationship is through empathic statements, not sympathetic ones. Empathy is a counseling skill that connotes understanding of the client's feelings and behaviors rather than the health professional's sympathies or projections. It is a statement that conveys respect for the client as defined by the humanistic philosophy. Empathic statements have two components. One part identifies the *feeling* expressed by the client, and the other part describes the *content* that contributes to this feeling.

Health professionals do not need to agree with the behaviors and feelings expressed by clients, but they should always be capable of understanding and validating them. An example of an empathic statement that could be made to the same client in the earlier example is the following:

I understand that you are feeling depressed about your future. There are many changes in your daily routines that you will have to make. You believe that you will not be able to participate in the activities that once gave you pleasure. I am here to help you adjust both physically and emotionally to your injury. I believe that we can work on your rehabilitation goals together and find new ways to assist you in doing the things that you like to do.

These empathic statements validate the client's feelings, attitudes, and behaviors without judging whether they are accurate or "right" for Louis to express in treatment. Effective health professionals know how to empower and support the person, even when giving constructive, negative feedback about related treatment issues. They are aware of their personal attitudes toward disability when working with clients, being careful not to project biases, prejudices, stigmas, stereotypes, and anxieties onto the clients and their significant others, nor among society.

Defining a Disability

Health professionals within the medical environment have great influence on how disability is defined. Written documentation is a critical and necessary aspect of our jobs, and it takes many forms, such as chart writing, messages to colleagues, insurance claims, case study reports, incident reports, research analysis, and published articles. Along with the daily expectations of written documentation, health professionals talk with many different people in numerous formal and informal conversations. These people may include colleagues, clients, and their significant others, insurance companies, students, and paraprofessional staff. The actual words used in this correspondence create an image of the described person. Health professionals should consistently use respectful language in all daily communication to promote a positive impression of their clients.

The following is a review of the terms most often found in written and verbal health care correspondence.

Impairment. "Any loss or abnormality of the psychological, physiological, or anatomic structure or function" (World Health Organization, 1980). Impairments include the residual effects of a disease or injury that may or may not be permanent. Examples include a speech impediment, a hearing loss, a weak knee, or paralysis.

Disability. "Any restriction or lack of ability to perform an activity in the manner or within the range considered to be normal for a human being" (World Health Organization, 1980). Disabilities result from impairments and are long-term conditions that can be reversible, stable, or progressive (Livneh, 1982; World Health Organization, 1980). Examples include inability to speak, limited range of motion, and psychomotor retardation.

Handicap. "A disadvantage for a person, resulting from an impairment or disability which limits or prevents fulfillment of a role that is normal for that individual (consider age, gender, social, and cultural factors). A person's social and occupational roles are interrupted; conditions are usually irreversible and socially stigmatized" (World Health Organization, 1980). The word *handicap* originated from "cap in hand," a beggar's term. Examples of handicaps include mental retardation and chronic mental illness.

"Person First" Language

"Person first" language evolves from the humanistic philosophy. Individuals are identified as a person first, distinctly regarded and respected apart from the disability that he or she may possess. Emphasis is placed on a person's potentials and abilities rather than what someone is unable to do.

The Association for Persons with Severe Handicaps, TASK, initially adopted this "person first" philosophy (Bailey, 1992). A true benefit from

TABLE 6.1
Stigmatic Language Versus "Person First" Language

Stigmas	*"Person First"*
An AIDS victim	A person with AIDS
The CP child	A child who has cerebral palsy
The paraplegic	A man with paralysis of his lower body
The TBI	Person who has incurred a brain injury
The lunatic	Person with a mental illness

AIDS = acquired immunodeficiency syndrome; CP = cerebral palsy; TBI = traumatic brain injury.

this adoption is that many other groups and advocacy organizations have continued to promote similar concepts. In an effort to influence society's perceptions in a positive way, organizations such as United Cerebral Palsy and the National Easter Seal Society continue to educate others about "person first" language. Table 6.1 gives examples of the language of stigmas versus "persons first" language.

The concept of personhood affects more than the words we use in language. This philosophy promotes respect and concern for all persons within our society and models a humane and positive view for others to emulate. An effective health professional always addresses the client in a respectful manner within direct treatment sessions and during all correspondence to significant others and colleagues.

Summary

The formulation of a person's attitudes and beliefs regarding disability is contingent on various influential sources. Some of these factors are external sources that we learn from our environment, such as society's use of language, the media's stereotyped images of persons with disabilities, or the theoretical bases that constitute medical treatment and rehabilitation. Other sources are internal and assimilated into our belief system, such as our values about humankind and health, and our tolerance to differences.

Rehabilitation is an interactive process in which both the client and health care professional constantly influence each other in the therapeutic relationship. Each of us has unique perceptions about wellness and illness, normal and abnormal behaviors, and what constitutes a positive and negative body image. Our emotional reactions and anxieties about our own well-being can easily be projected onto others if we do not recognize and identify their existence within ourselves. Common expressions of sympathy and pity are efforts to alleviate our own discomfort when viewing a person with a disability. Often, our perceptions about this person are inaccurate and our attitudes are based on previously learned images or prior experiences. Concerned health professionals always directly check out their perceptions with those of their clients rather than forming assumptions based on external or internal influences. Health care workers know that faulty beliefs and stereotypes reinforce the development of negative attitudes toward persons with disabilities, and they make direct efforts to change these attitudes into positive ones.

An effective health professional is concerned about the person first and how rehabilitation and treatment could be collaboratively arranged for the client. With the knowledge of various treatment models, the health professional provides unconditional positive regard and individualized care, always conscious to present a positive attitude within this process. The client's feelings are acknowledged in the form of empathy, not sympathy, with the intent to empower and assist the client to accept and adjust to one's disability.

Finally, health professionals recognize that they are role models for others within the medical community, as well as society in general. They are aware of the power of their language when describing persons with disabilities and subscribe to defining disability in a positive, humane manner. Effective health professionals are dedicated to personal reflection and change regarding their own attitudes, beliefs, and perceptions, which significantly affect the rehabilitation process. In essence, they demonstrate a commitment to clients that offers a nonjudgmental and unconditional regard for the *person*, regardless of the disability.

Exercises

The following questions will assist you in reflecting about the various topics discussed in this chapter. You are invited to answer them individually or as part of a group exercise.

1. What present attitudes do you have about people with physical and emotional disabilities? Now consider how these attitudes have originated. Who suggested them to you? What personal and familial experiences have shaped the development of your attitudes and beliefs? How has your ethnic identification contributed to your beliefs?

2. Why do you want to become a health professional? What personal or professional experiences have influenced this career decision? What do you hope to accomplish in this role?

3. What model of health care practice seems to suit your personality and professional style? Explain why.

4. Give an example of a situation in your life when you experienced either "aesthetic" or "existential" anxiety. Specifically, what were you anxious about? How did you cope with this anxiety?

5. Practice giving constructive feedback and empathizing with a client who is refusing to participate in your suggested treatment plan.

6. What term do you think is more respectful: *disability* or *handicap*? State your reasons for your answer. What do you think about a sign labeled "handicap parking"? Identify other common labels and stereo-typed messages in our society.

7. When is it respectful to use the word *normal*? How can the term *normal* infer a negative stigma? Give examples to support your answers.

8. Generalizations and labels such as the "chronic mentally ill" strip away a person's individuality, connoting negative associations. How can you refer to groups without categorizing the people negatively? Give examples of negative group connotations and how you can change these phrases into neutral or positive ones.

9. Certain verbs and nouns negatively focus on one's limitations and depict a passive and demeaning image of the person. Examples are "suffering with . . ." and "a victim of. . . ." What other words and phrasing can you think of that convey passive and demeaning images? Change the words in these phrases to sound more neutral and non-judgmental.

10. A common way of describing an impairment or condition is to use a form of the verb "to be" in the phrasing. An example is: "Mary *is* floppy." This wording suggests that Mary's personal identity is syn-onymous with the condition of floppy tone. List common phrases that you recall in which persons and their conditions are not differen-tiated. Next, substitute forms of the verb "to have" in the phrasing to distinguish the person's identity from the disability. Example: "Mary *has* the floppy tone that is a condition of cerebral palsy."

References

Bailey, D. (1991). Guidelines for authors. Journal of Early Intervention, 15(1), 118–119.

Jones, E. E., Farina, A., Hastorf, A.H., Markus, H., Miller, D. T., Scott, R. A., and French R. de S. (1984). Social stigma: The psychology of marked relationships. New York: Freemen.

Livneh, H. (1982). On the origins of negative attitudes toward people with disabilities. Rehabilitation Literature, 43, 338–347.

Roush, S. E. (1986). Health professionals as contributors to attitudes toward persons with disabilities. Physical Therapy, 66(10), 1551–1554.

World Health Organization. (1980). International classification of impairments, disabilities and handicaps (ICIDH). Geneva, Switzerland: Author.

Zborowski, M. (1969). People in pain. San Francisco: Jossey-Bass.

CHAPTER 7

Cultural Diversity and Health Behavior

Renè Padilla

The population seeking health care in today's society is of unprecedented diversity. The last two decades have been characterized by a dramatic shift in the demographic makeup of many nations. For example, because of rising immigration from non-European countries, it is expected that by 2056 the average U.S. resident, as defined by census statistics, will be of non-European descent (Henry, 1990). In addition, the general population is growing older, and the older population is larger in proportion to the rest of the population. Between 1980 and 1996, the percentage of the youth population, ages 15 through 25, fell from 18.8% to 13%, with the highest proportional increase in the population aged 65 and older (Commission on Work, Family, and Citizenship, 1997). This diversity has been an important factor fueling the transformation of many North American institutions, including government, education, and health care.

The economy, for example, is firmly global in scale, reducing once-giant corporations to simply one of many players in the world market. The acquisition of raw materials, manufacturing processes, and distribution of goods is done worldwide, so that it is difficult to define what products are national or foreign, or even to find importance in that definition. We increasingly interact with people from other nations in matters of trade, and political events occurring in other countries have a much more profound effect on our own political agenda than they used to (Reich, 1992).

In the family, too, profound changes in organization and structure are seen. For instance, in 1942, 60% of families could be described as "nuclear" families, consisting of two parents and their children. The social value was that the father's role was to leave the home every day to support the family and earn money, and the mother's role was to stay home and raise the children. Today, less than 10% of American families match that ideal (Rosen, 1999). It is estimated that divorce or separation disrupts two-thirds of all marriages in the United States, and the single-parent household is becoming the norm (Hetherington et al., 1999). Often, this single parent is a mother living in poverty with more than one child. Increasingly, this mother is a teenager, although poverty is not limited to this type of family (Kennedy et al., 1996). Another growing family configuration is one in which two adults of the same sex, committed to one another over time, are raising children who may be biologically related to one or the other adult, or who may have been adopted by them (Johnson & Keren, 1998). Clearly, the family pattern that was once considered normal and that guided the policies of our institutions is now a minority pattern.

Transition can also be observed in the institutionalized churches of all faiths. Once largely steeped in Judeo-Christian heritage, North American society is now home to a growing number of faiths that are unfamiliar to many people. Buddhism, Islam, and other religions of the East and Middle East are growing as new immigrants bring their religions with them. Similarly, so-called New Age religious sects seem to have proliferated, while, at the same time, conservative or fundamentalist branches of mainline Catholic, Protestant, and Muslim religions have become the fastest-growing religious organizations. The tension between so-called liberal and conservative elements of the organized church is becoming one of the most profound social conflicts of contemporary life.

North American schools have been part of this social transformation as well. In 1976, for example, 24% of the total U.S. school enrollment was nonwhite. By 1984, this percentage had grown to 29%, and by 1996, children of color made up almost one-third of all students enrolled in public schools. It is projected that by 2020, children of color will make up 46% of children in school (Hodkinson, 1997). In California, Arizona, New Mexico, Texas, and Colorado, students from so-called minority groups already make up more than 50% of the school population. These children often find themselves in the uncomfortable position of being the majority in a world whose rules are set by a more powerful minority (Cushner et al., 1996).

All the changes discussed so far are inevitably reflected in health care. About two decades ago, futurist Alvin Toffler predicted that by the end of the century, we would witness profound changes in our basic institutions, and that these changes would constitute a fundamental shift in the nature of our civilization. He stated that we would move away from what he called "second wave" institutions, characterized by reliance on standardization, synchronization, specialization, centralization, and a value on "bigness," toward "third wave" institutions, characterized by individualization, choice, diversity, and a value on "smallness" (Toffler, 1980). Many elements of Toffler's predictions now seem quite evident in the health care delivery system, where an enormous array of consumers with widely different needs are demanding individualized options of care at the same time that third party payers are insisting on trimmed-down treatment programs that discourage duplication and overlap of services.

Rehabilitation professionals face a particular challenge in this environment. At the same time that they are responsible to provide cost-effective and efficient treatment, they are also being asked to provide ethical and relevant treatment. Treatment must make a difference in the client's ability to function in everyday life. In other words, the social relevance of rehabilitation professions to a great extent is measured by the degree to which they provide for meaningful changes in client's lives. Within this context, it is essential for rehabilitation professionals to become culturally literate. This chapter will address the idea that culture encompasses people's values and beliefs and, in many respects, the ways in which they find meaning in their lives. Cultural literacy means, among other things, that the professional be sensitive to the client's particular cultural background and consider it in treatment. It also means, however, that the professional must be aware of his or her own culture and recognize the ways in which it supports or interferes with the therapeutic process. "Meaningful" treatment is one in which the client's perspective determines what is significant or functional. The rehabilitation professional is charged with adapting his or her approach to meet the client's perspective.

It is important to note that although culture has a significant influence over many aspects of people's lives that have important implications for their health, culture is by no means the only such influence. Culture is only one of many factors—including individual (age, gender, size, appearance, personality, intelligence, and experience), educational (formal and informal), and socioeconomic (social class, economic status, and occupation)—that have an effect on a person's health status (Helman, 1997). Furthermore, culture must always be seen in its particular historical, social, economic, political, and geographic contexts. In other words, any person's culture, at any point in time, is always influenced by many other factors, and it is impossible to isolate "pure" cultural determinants of health. Thus, culture should never be considered in a vacuum, but as only one component in the complex mix of influences over a person's life.

In the next sections of this chapter, I examine more in depth the concept of culture and the various dimensions that may have influence over a person's health status. I conclude with some specific strategies that rehabilitation professionals may wish to consider when planning therapeutic interventions. The objectives of this chapter are:

1. To understand culture and the culture-learning process.
2. To recognize dimensions of culture that have an impact on health behaviors.
3. To discuss strategies rehabilitation professionals may use to understand the cultural perspective of clients.
4. To infuse the practice of rehabilitation with cultural sensitivity and relevance.

Culture

One of the greatest difficulties found when beginning to explore concepts related to culture is the lack of agreement that exists about the term. Many different disciplines study culture, including anthropology, sociology, education, psychology, business, and the military. Consequently, there are literally hundreds of definitions of culture. What all these definitions seem to have in common, however, is the notion that culture determines, to a large extent, our thoughts, ideas, ways of interacting, and material adaptations to the world around us. One of the most famous definitions of culture is anthropologist E. B. Taylor's, who in 1871 wrote that culture is "that complex whole which includes knowledge, beliefs, art, morals, law, custom and any other capabilities and habits acquired by man as a member of society" (Leach, 1982). Other definitions emphasize the ideational nature of culture, describing it as made up of "systems of shared ideas, systems of concepts and rules and meanings that underlie and are expressed in the ways that human beings live" (Keesing, 1981).

Webb and Sherman (1989) described culture in a functional way that this chapter uses to understand the assumptions of culture. They wrote:

> Cultures solve the common problems of human beings, but they solve them in different ways. . . . Each provides its people with a means of communication (language). Each determines who wields power and under what circumstances power can be used (status). Each provides for the regulation of reproduction (family) and provides a system of rules (government). These rules may be written (laws) or unwritten (customs), but they are always present. Cultures supply human beings with an explanation of their relationship to nature (magic, myth, religion, and science). They provide their people with some conception of time (temporality). They supply a system by which significant lessons of the culture (history) can be given a physical representation and stored and passed on to future generations. This representation usually comes in the form of dance, song, poetry, architecture, handicrafts, story, design, or painting (art). What makes cultures similar is the problems they solve, not the methods they devise to solve them.

From this definition we can deduce that culture is a type of "lens" through which individuals perceive and understand the world they inhabit and learn how to live within it. A person is not born with this lens; it is not contained within his or her genetic makeup. Rather, a person is born *into* culture. The lens is learned over time through the process of *enculturation*. Four important assumptions inherent in this understanding are that culture is constructed, shared, both objective and subjective, and both conscious and unconscious.

Unlike most animals, humans are not born with the genetic programming that automatically prepares them to use the environment to find food and shelter. In short, humans do not know how to survive without other people to care for them and teach them. Consequently, humans must discover effective ways of interacting, both with their environment and with each other. They must learn to *construct* the knowledge, including the rules for living, that will enable them to survive. Culture encompasses this knowledge, as well as the ways in which it is presented (e.g., litera- ture, art, rituals) and the meaning it has for us. Thus, the concept of cul- ture refers to things, both physical and mental, that are constructed by human beings. For example, when we look out to a snowy mountainside, both the snow and the mountain occur naturally in nature, and neither is considered culture. How we think about and what we do in the natural environment, on the other hand, depend greatly on our culture. Thus, a snowy mountain may be seen as a good place to build a ski lodge, to take photographs, or to hunt. These three activities are expressions of the underlying knowledge, attitude, values, and behavior patterns we have about the natural environment.

Culture is not only constructed, it is socially constructed. As human beings interact with each other, they come to *share* cultural ideas and understandings as a group. In this way, people recognize the knowledge, attitudes, and values of one another, and, to a great extent, come to agree on which cultural elements are more important than others. In other words, individuals acquire the cultural lens of the society they inhabit to learn how to live in it. Without such a shared perception of the world, the cohesion and continuity of any human group would be impossible.

The shared cultural identification is transmitted from one generation to the next through formal and informal means. Formal means include schooling, religious training, and education into a profession. Informal means are those in which values and beliefs are transmitted indirectly or without formal instruction. Gender identification, for example, in North American culture is most often learned by imitating people around us rather than by formal education. Television and film are also very powerful informal socializing agents in many cultures of the world.

A third assumption we can make about culture is that it has both *objective* and *subjective* elements (Triandis, 1972). Objective elements include the numerous visible or physical artifacts people create, including clothing, food, and furniture. Subjective elements, on the other hand, are the invisible, intangible aspects of peoples' lives, such as attitudes, values, beliefs, behavior norms, learning styles, and hierarchy of roles. These dimensions of culture have been likened to an iceberg: What can be seen above the surface of the ocean (objective culture) is only about 10% of the whole, whereas 90% of the iceberg lies beneath the surface (subjective cul- ture) (Cushner et al., 1996).

Finally, objective and subjective culture are related to what authors describe as *conscious* and *subconscious* culture (Hall, 1984; Harris, 1989; Peacock, 1986). Conscious culture is that part of culture that we are aware of, can describe, and about which we can talk. Unconscious culture, on the other hand, affects our behavior and thoughts without our awareness. Using the same metaphor of the iceberg, we can say that conscious culture is the 10% that is visible above the surface, and unconscious culture is the hidden 90%. It is the subjective and unconscious part of culture that, concealed below the surface like the iceberg, is the most meaningful to the individual. This part of culture continually operates at the subconscious level, shaping the person's perceptions and responses to those perceptions. At the same time, unconscious culture can be potentially the most dangerous dimension, leading to numerous intercultural misunderstandings without us even knowing the source of the problem.

Culture-Learning Process

Because it is socially constructed, objective and subjective, and conscious and unconscious, culture is very dynamic. Although a group may share some general cultural features in common, each individual in that group contributes uniquely to that shared meaning. Each individual in a society is in the course of "learning" culture, and consequently is at a different point in this process. Both shared and individual events in people's lives shape what the person learns and how he or she learns it. For example, two children might be born a year apart into the same family. These children might be cared for at home until the older reaches schooling age. This child is sent to her first year of schooling, while the second child remains at home. The context of life, at least temporarily, is changed for the first child. At school she must begin learning to deal with a larger group of children, to behave appropriately in a classroom, and to deal with educational materials. She also has the opportunity to observe how other children interact with adults in authority, such as teachers and parents. When the first child returns home, she has experienced events that the second has not. This experience has moved her further along in the culture-learning process. However, she is not a passive recipient of culture-learning. When she returns home she might re-enact her school experiences while playing with her sibling. In this way, the second child has a completely unique experience about schooling. The first child did not have an older sibling that did the same for her. Consequently, although during play both children are relating to each other around the topic of school, their contexts of experience are quite different. Each has his or her unique image of school. Each learns and shares culture from a unique perspective.

This example also illustrates why the boundaries of culture are often vague. Although superficially individuals in a society might seem to behave in the same way, to some degree each is acting on the basis of their own perception of what they have learned as culture. Consequently, cultures are never really homogeneous, and one should always avoid using generalizations in explaining people's beliefs and behaviors. Generalizations have, in many cases, led to the development of stereotypes, and then usually to cultural misunderstandings, prejudices, and discrimination. Individuals within a culture, and cultures as a whole, are never static.

Rather, they are constantly being influenced by other groups around them and, in most parts of the world, are in a constant process of adaptation and change. In addition, individuals and groups may creatively generate culture without external influence.

To better understand the complexity of culture and the culture-learning process, it is helpful to consider the various contexts within which people socially construct culture. Krefting and Krefting (1991) suggest viewing culture as a series of mutually influencing social levels. Within each level there might be a number of subgroups, each with their own concepts, rules, and social organization. Although each of these subcultures is developed from the larger culture and shares many of its concepts and values, each also has unique and distinctive features of its own. These levels include the individual, the family, the community, and the geographic region.

At the individual level are the relational, one-to-one interactions through which people learn and express their unique perception of culture. These include personal attributes, such as sense of humor, coping style, sense of personal space, and role choices. At the family level are the beliefs and values shared within a primary social group. It is in this group that most of a person's early socialization takes place, which includes such dimensions as gender roles and family structure. At the community level are the various secondary groups in which the person participates, such as school, neighborhood, profession, and church. Finally, at the regional level are the cultural elements that a person shares with people in a broader geographic area, such as language, mass communication media, holidays, and ethnicity.

In most cultures, the family and community levels have the greatest influence on the individual. Through socialization, people learn the patterns of behavior that are expected at each level. They also learn which options of behavior are unacceptable. Furthermore, there may be differences and even contradictions within subcultures at each level. For example, a person may learn in his or her family that competition with siblings is unacceptable, yet attend a school that encourages competition among its students. How people deal with these apparent contradictions depends on how their culture has taught them to handle discrepancies. In some cultures discrepancies are tolerated, whereas in others they are not. In the cultures in which contradictions between subcultures are discouraged, people may have to choose one subculture over the other. For example, in some cultures allegiance to a religious sect takes primacy over allegiance to family.

The four levels of culture serve as primary lenses through which people learn about the surrounding cultural world and through which they form their cultural identity. One aspect of the "cultural lens" is that in all societies, it contributes to the division of people into different categories, each with their own name. These categories become sources of cultural identity. All cultures have elaborate ways of moving people from one category to another, and also of confining people to the categories into which they have been placed (Helman, 1997). For example, in many instances, rehabilitation constitutes the process of moving people from the category

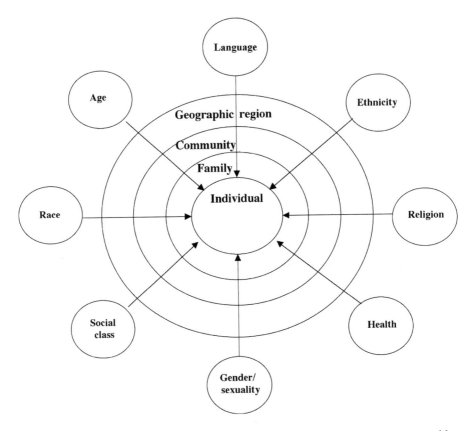

FIGURE 7.1. Sources of cultural identity. The four levels of culture act as a filter of cultural identity.

of disabled to able. Although this chapter focuses mainly on issues related to culture and health, it is important to again note the interrelationship between the various sources of cultural identity. These sources include race, ethnicity, gender/sexuality, age, religion, language, health, and social class (Lynch, 1998). Figure 7.1 illustrates the dynamics of cultural identity.

Although the word *race* refers to "a clustering of inherited physical characteristics that favor adaptation to a particular ecological area" (Yetman, 1991), in many ways it is also a cultural category. Different societies define different sets of physical characteristics when referring to the same race. Furthermore, groups of people may possess physically identifiable characteristics that in one society are selected to make racial distinctions, whereas in another they are ignored or overlooked as irrelevant. In addition, the term has been used to refer to many characteristics that are not physical, as in the case of language (the "English-speaking race"), religion (the "Jewish race"), or nationality (the "German race"). Consequently, it has been argued that race as a biological concept is of little value because there are no "pure" races (Yetman, 1991). Instead, race is understood as a categorization of characteristics based on the particular values of a society. This categorization is important not because of biology but because of the cultural meaning it has. In other words, the concept of race is relevant solely within the particular culture in which it is defined. For example, in the United States, skin color and the shape of the lips are important differing criteria. However, in much of Latin America, stature and eye color are more important than skin color, so that someone defined as black in Georgia or Michigan might be considered white in Ecuador or Bolivia.

Ethnicity is similarly defined culturally. This term refers to the knowledge, beliefs, and behavior patterns shared by a group of people with the same history and the same language. Ethnicity is associated with a sense of "peoplehood" or loyalty to a "community of memory" (Bellah et al., 1985). It is also associated with a particular geographic region, although an ethnic group need no longer exist in that region to feel a sense of belonging to it. For example, at the beginning of the twentieth century, Jewish people were dispersed throughout the world. Their common identity was traced back to the land of Palestine, even though the great majority of Jews had never been there. This common identity associated with the geographic region was the basis for the founding of the nation of Israel after World War II. Jews from around the world converged in the region after being persecuted out of the nations where they had been born and raised.

Ethnicity should not be confused with nationality, however. Nationality is a categorization based on citizenship of a country and may or may not include a shared ethnicity. Israel, for example, was formed by Jews of many different nationalities (e.g., Polish, Russian, and German), but Arabs and Palestinians are other ethnic groups that also are part of that nation. Like Israel, most nations include members who vary in ethnicity. Although in the United States we are accustomed to the idea of multiple ethnicities and racial makeups, we sometimes are unaware that the same reality exists for most other countries. Thus, we tend to identify all people from Mexico as Mexican, from Germany as German, or from Japan as Japanese. We are surprised when we come across Brazilian citizens of German ethnicity, Peruvian citizens of Japanese ethnicity, or British citizens of Moroccan ethnicity. Tragically, the misconception that a nation is made up of only one ethnicity, or that one's own ethnicity is superior to all others, has given rise to many wars within and between nations.

Gender is defined based on the cultural meanings associated with male and female reproduction. These meanings are expressed through socially valued behaviors, or roles, that are assigned according to gender. These culturally assigned behaviors become so accepted that eventually they are thought of as natural to that sex. Consequently, gender is what it means to be male or female in a society. Gender roles, then, are those behaviors thought to be normal in that society when carried out by the assigned gender. As in the case of cultural definitions of race and ethnicity, the particular behaviors considered male or female vary greatly from society to society. They vary further within a society based on ethnicity, social status, religion, and so on. Ultimately, any social or psychosocial trait can be "genderized" in favor of one sex or another (Benedict, 1989). What in one society may be considered a naturally female trait, such as submissiveness, in another may be considered male (Brislin, 1993). In a related way, sexuality is also culturally defined on the basis of accepted behavior within a society. In spite of growing evidence that one's sexual orientation is, in part, a function of innate biological characteristics (LeVay & Hamer, 1994), persons who deviate from socially approved norms are often ostracized and even physically abused. The prevailing view in many cultures is that sexuality is bimodal: Only male and female are identified as possibilities. In other societies, such as the Lakota Sioux, other options are available. In that society, for example, males who have predominantly female characteristics are accorded high honor as possessing multiple talents (Brislin, 1993).

Age is culturally defined both by length of life and the state of physical and mental development a person has attained. Different societies measure chronologic age in different ways, such as by calendar years; by major natural or social events; or by natural cycles, such as phases of the moon. Likewise, mental and physical development is measured differently in different societies. Although most societies seem to view development in stages, what is considered normal in each stage varies widely. For example, in most Western cultures, adolescence is an identified cohort group between childhood and adulthood. In many non-Western societies, however, the adolescent cohort may not exist at all (Schweder, 1991).

Shared ideas about the relationship between humans and a deity form the basis of the cultural definition of religion and spirituality. The deity figure is perceived, in essence, to be greater than oneself. These beliefs usually include a shared set of rules for living (moral values) that enhance the relationship between the person and deity or deities. In many cultures, the deity is anthropomorphic (humanlike), whereas in others the deity takes on the characteristic of various life-energies or the earth itself (Bauman, 1999). Religious identity may include membership in an organized religion (e.g., Islam, Christianity, Judaism, and Buddhism) or loose affiliation with spiritualistic groups. At any rate, religious affiliation can engender intense loyalty, community, and pride in a shared history. The cultural meaning of religion is often expressed through a rigid sense of righteousness and virtue, and consequently can be a powerful determinant of behavior.

Language is "a shared system of vocal sounds and/or nonverbal behaviors by which members of a group communicate with one another" (Gollnick & Chinn, 1990). Most cultural knowledge is acquired through language, making it one of the most important sources of cultural learning. Brain research has shown that humans are born with a predisposition to learn whatever spoken language or sign system used around them (Chomsky & Peck, 1987). This learning in early childhood almost seems automatic and effortless. Language has meaning in its verbal properties (the words we use to name objects, people, and ideas) and its nonverbal properties (norms regarding interpersonal space, gestures, and so on). Language is the literal representation of the experience of a society or social group in its surroundings. In other words, through its verbal and nonverbal meanings, language gives us an insight into another person's life (Chomsky, 1995).

As with the other sources of cultural identity discussed so far, health is also defined by a particular group's view of what physical and mental states constitute being "healthy." For many years, the medical profession has guided the dominating cultural definition of health in the Western world. In the traditional medical model, health has been defined as the absence of disease or illness (Purnell & Paulanka, 1998). In many cases, this definition of health has been equated with "normalcy." Consequently, disabilities (such as mental retardation, deafness, blindness, and even cerebral palsy) are deemed as states of ill health, when in fact it is quite possible to be a healthy person with blindness or mental retardation. The management of states of ill health in the United States and in most of the industrialized world is highly biomedical, although increasingly "alternative" systems—such as acupuncture, naturopathy, and faith healing—are becoming available and gaining acceptance. Ironically, models of health deemed "alternative" in Western societies are the dominant models in other societies (e.g., China), and biomedicine may be considered to be the less-accepted "alternative" (Purnell & Paulanka, 1998).

A related issue to the cultural construct of health is the notion of ability or disability. Ability is defined according to a society's view of what it means to be physically, mentally, and emotionally "able." Depending on the society, the category of disability can include a wide variety of physical or mental characteristics, such as intelligence, impaired movement, or sensory or neural disturbances (Holcomb, 1997). The cultural meaning of disability is often related to the public's perception of the needs of the disability itself. For example, the desire of deaf people to have a shared system of communication has resulted in the development of sign language as well as some degree of shared values and traditions among its members—in other words, the development of a "deaf culture." Some studies have indicated that the public's perception of deaf people can be less than positive because they require an interpreter or, in other words, "special" services (Brown & Gustafson, 1995). It is clear that the reaction to disability greatly depends on the society's norms of what is acceptable special care.

Finally, almost every society has its own set of criteria for ranking its members in a stratified hierarchy. There is an enormous diversity in the criteria that societies use to determine social class. However, a prevalent value is associated with wealth. Other criteria, such as power, influence, and level of education are related to economic resources. Consequently, many experts consider social class as the most significant culture-learning factor (Wright, 1997). Class structure varies from society to society, and even within a society. In some societies the class structure is fairly rigid. In India, for example, one is born into a particular social class, and one tends to remain in that class for life. In other societies, class structure is not as rigid, and it is possible to move from one social class to another. In the United States, for example, it is almost a social expectation that individuals "move up" in class as their education and careers progress. This expectation has even engendered the perception that something is "wrong" with the person if he or she does not advance. On the other hand, in societies that do not place value on leaving one's social class, attempts to do so are considered wrong and consequently are discouraged. In most societies, however, social class to a large extent determines the opportunities one has in life. Thus, health status is very much related to socioeconomic level because illness and poor nutrition may result from poverty, unemployment, psychological stress, alcohol abuse, poor sanitation, inadequate housing, and lack of money to pay for medical care (Helman, 1997; Vanneman & Cannon, 1988).

In many cultures, socioeconomic factors are closely associated with professional level. Professions are based on, or organized around, a body of specialized knowledge (the content) not easily acquired and that, in the hands of qualified practitioners, meets the needs of or serves clients (Sargent & Johnson, 1996). Members of a profession often organize themselves to sanction entry into the profession and to limit competition. In many ways, professions can be considered subcultures, as they often contain explicit and implicit rules of behavior based on shared values and ideologies among members. For example, the North American health care system seems to be based on certain assumptions and premises (Kleinman, 1980). These premises conclude that health care is *physician-centered* (the doctor, not the client, defines the nature of the client's problem via diagnosis) and is *specialist-oriented* (specialists rather than generalists get higher rewards). In addition, it can be said that this system is *single-case-centered* and is *quantitative* (based on quantifiable biological processes) (Sargent & Johnson, 1996). The assumptions often subconsciously guide the approach health professionals take toward their clients, frequently requiring the client and his or her problem to adapt to the framework of the professional. In addition, clients often comply, because to some degree they accept these basic assumptions, or because they associate professionalism with socioeconomic status and power (Lynch, 1998).

Culture-Learning Associated with Health

In the next section I discuss in more detail several dimensions of health that are particularly related to cultural interpretation. Rehabilitation professionals should make a special effort to understand these dimensions from the perspective of their clients and adapt evaluation and treatment methods accordingly. The professional must keep in mind that culture is only one of many complex influences on what people believe and on how they live their lives. It is possible to overemphasize the importance of culture when interpreting how clients present their symptoms. Underlying physical and mental disorders may go untreated when the professional ascribes behaviors and symptoms to the client's culture and fails to thoroughly analyze the situation (Kleinman, 1980).

The two most important strategies rehabilitation professionals can use are asking questions and observing behavior carefully. The values and beliefs that encompass "culture" direct clients in their particular way of showing their symptoms, both verbally and nonverbally. In addition, these values and beliefs direct how the client perceives and interprets the behaviors of health professionals (Sargent & Johnson, 1996). Therefore, rehabilitation professionals must be oriented to the client's culture to provide relevant and meaningful treatment. This cultural orientation should include an understanding of the client's beliefs about the body, health, and healing. In addition, it is important to understand the client's thinking and communication styles, as well as some of the value systems that might influence the outcome of their care. All these dimensions are intimately related to each other, and often it is futile to attempt to determine where one dimension ends and another begins.

Beliefs about the Body

In all societies, the body is the focus of many beliefs regarding its structure, function, and social and psychological significance. The individual acquires this notion of *body image* as part of growing up in a particular family, social group, and culture. The body image of each person can be considered an individual variation of body image within each of these groups. Some important dimensions of body image to consider include beliefs about the body's structure and function, beliefs about the body's optimal size and shape, and beliefs regarding boundaries of the body (Brislin, 1993; Hall, 1990).

The inner structure of the body is a matter of speculation for most people, particularly for those who have not had the benefit of an anatomic education. Personal theorizing and experience, as well as inherited folklore, usually form the basis for beliefs about how the body is constructed. These beliefs can be called the *inside-the-body image* and are particularly important to understand because they strongly influence people's perception and presentation of bodily symptoms, as well as their response to medical treatment. People's knowledge of the structure and function of the body varies greatly, and many only vaguely are aware of the location of most internal organs (Pearson & Dudley, 1982). For example, many people believe the heart occupies most of the thoracic area or that the stomach occupies the whole abdomen. Others believe humans have two livers on opposite sides of the body, or that the gallbladder is concerned with urination. These discrepant beliefs may lead a person with a vague discomfort anywhere in the abdominal area to report "stomach trouble" or someone with thoracic discomfort to report "heart problems." Interestingly, people's internal body image is not static, and age, experience, education, and illness contribute to its transformation throughout life. Often during illness people may refer to a particular body organ as an "it," something alien to their body. For example, people blame symptoms, such as diarrhea or vomiting, on a weak or unreliable organ, such as an "irritable bowel" or "weak stomach," thus separating their identity from the illness or symptom. Psychogenic symptoms also often are attributed to a poorly working brain (Purnell & Paulanka, 1998). What is important to understand in these depersonalized reports of symptoms is the person's sense of lack of control over them, which may lead to hopelessness or excessive dependence on health personnel.

Related to people's beliefs about the structure of the body are their assumptions about how the body works or functions. These beliefs are probably more significant in their effect on the person's behavior. There are many cultural beliefs regarding the body's physiology. For example, the belief that the normal working of the body depends on the harmonious balance between two or more elements or forces has many cultural variations throughout the world. These forces may be both internal or external to the body, or both, and may be related to elements in nature or supernatural forces. In Latin America, for example, the "hot-cold theory of disease" supposes that health is strengthened or weakened by the effect of heat and cold on the body (Foster, 1994). Thus, many people shy away from ice cubes in their drinks or from being outside in the cool evening breeze without a heavy coat. In Ecuador, for example, many people have the belief that breathing cold air may cause one to get the flu (*resfrio*) and do not feel comfortable in air-conditioned environments. The hot-cold theory does not only refer to temperature. Certain foods or states of health may be associated with a symbolic hot or cold power. If one has a "hot illness," it can be balanced by consuming a "cold food" or "cold medicine." In certain regions of Central America and Mexico, for example, pregnancy is considered a "hot" state, and consuming hot foods is thought to produce an ill-tempered baby. The classification of which condition or food is hot and which is cold varies throughout the regions, and what is considered hot in one subgroup may be considered cold in another. In addition, how these elements work to balance each other may be thought of differently. Among the people of northern Guatemala, menstruation is thought to be hot and is treated by consuming hot foods rather than cold. Cold foods (such as fruits and vegetables) are avoided for fear that they will thicken or clot menstrual blood. Yet in other groups, people may consume hot or cold foods or medicines to prevent illness, such as some people in Puerto Rico who consume garlic, chocolate, and cinnamon to avoid getting colds. These beliefs ultimately may lead people to consume a less nutritional diet, depleting their bodies from needed vitamins and becoming malnourished. In addition, these beliefs may lead people to avoid taking needed medications if they do not associate them with the corresponding hot or cold condition. Variations of the "hot-cold theory" exist throughout the world and include traditional Chinese medicine, the ancient Indian Ayurvedic system, and the Moroccan humeral model, to name a few.

Culture-based beliefs about how the body works are too numerous to discuss in detail here. Other examples include the notion of the body as "plumbing" (in which people literally imagine the internal body as composed of a series of interconnected tubes from the mouth to the anus), and the notion of the body as a machine (in which people imagine the body as a series of independent parts that somehow work together). The essential reductionism of modern Western medicine, with its advances in diagnostic technology, has reinforced in many people the belief that the body is composed of many progressively smaller pieces. Consequently, this "medical body" is also a culturally based explanation of how the body works. What is important to emphasize, however, is that these various conjectures lead people to accept the types of treatment that conform to their cultural beliefs and reject those that do not. Although some of these beliefs may actually prove harmful (such as avoiding foods with high nutritional value), they should be seen as metaphors that help the person make sense of his or her body. It is often helpful for the rehabilitation professional to begin explaining the goals of treatment from within the client's cultural beliefs and gradually provide education toward a more realistic perception of one's physical self. Naturally, what is "more realistic" is, in itself, also a cultural metaphor. Consequently, rehabilitation professionals must balance the need to protect the client from harm and the client's right to maintain his or her cultural integrity.

Another important dimension of culture has to do with beliefs about what the body should look like and how it should be used. In almost every society, the human body has a social dimension in addition to the physical (Hall, 1984). Social dimensions of the body have to do with ideal size, shape, adornment, and interpersonal boundaries. Culturally defined notions of beauty direct people to value certain features and to modify their bodies through means such as diet, tattooing, piercing, and clothing. In the Western world, there tends to be high value placed on slimness in women; consequently, much of their time, energy, and resources are spent to reduce their weight to "attractive" dimensions (Althen, 1988). In contrast, in parts of West Africa, daughters in wealthy families often are sent to "fatting-houses" to become plump and pale, which is the body shape associated with fertility and beauty in that culture. To conform to culturally defined standards of "beauty," people use orthodontics to straighten their teeth, undergo plastic surgery, use wigs, paint their fingernails, and undergo various forms of ornamental mutilation, such as piercing their ears, nose, eyebrows, and other body parts. The most widespread form of bodily mutilation is male circumcision (Helman, 1997). All these modifications to the body ultimately are based on the symbolism groups of people share within a culture regarding the social dimensions of the body.

The social body not only communicates culturally defined aesthetic values, it also communicates status and power. Clothing is of particular importance in this regard. In the Western world, designer-brand clothing and jewels are worn as a display of wealth. The white laboratory coat and starched uniforms health workers wear not only serve the practical purpose of cleanliness, but indicate these peoples' membership in a prestigious, powerful professional group as well. Likewise, the graduation gown, wedding dress, and mourning shawl are indicators that the person is in a process of transition in status (e.g., from student to professional, from single to married, from married to widowed). In Western health care settings, the cultural significance of clothing for the client is often subordinated to convenience for the health professional. Thus, in most hospitals, clients are required to wear gowns that identify their status as patients and in which they feel exposed and self-conscious, rather than being permitted to wear the clothes they would normally wear if they were at home.

To some degree or another, every human being's sense of identity extends beyond the border of the skin. We are surrounded by a series of "symbolic skins" that represent boundaries of relationships. For example, Hall (1984) identified four invisible layers or concentric circles of space that surround bodies of middle-class Americans. These include intimate distance (0–18 in.), personal distance (18 in. to 4 ft), social distance (4–12 ft), and public distance (12–25 ft or more). Only those people who have a very close relationship with the individual may enter the intimate circle, while friends may enter the personal space. Impersonal business transactions occur within social distance, whereas no social or personal interaction is expected to occur within public distance. Although the exact distance of each of the layers identified by Hall may vary from individual to individual and from culture to culture, it is an important consideration for the rehabilitation professional to include in his or her approach toward clients. Depending on their particular sense of boundaries, clients may feel invaded when the rehabilitation professional crosses these invisible skins without first obtaining permission to do so. A person's sense of boundaries includes the language used in social interactions. For example, in some cultures the expectation is that when meeting someone for the first time you refer to them by the equivalent of "Mr." or "Ms." in addition to their last name. Calling someone by their first name without having first built an intimate relationship would be considered overstepping of boundaries. This often is particularly true when speaking to older members of that culture.

In addition to language, a sense of boundaries includes which body parts may be touched under various circumstances. In some cultures, even strangers might greet with a kiss on the cheek, whereas in others, that would constitute a terrible offense. In American culture, it is acceptable for someone to enter a room of people and simply state a general greeting to the whole room. In contrast, in many Latin American cultures, the expectation is that the person shakes hands and greets everyone individually. Because the rehabilitation process often involves a large amount of tactile contact between professional and client, professionals become sensitized to touch and often do not consider the impact it has on the client. Professionals should not assume that the client feels as comfortable or unconcerned with physical touch as they do. For example, some people in groups from India may feel embarrassed when being touched on the feet, as that is considered a very dirty part of the body. Similarly, people from the Arabic Peninsula may feel offended if someone touches them with their left hand, as that is the hand reserved for assisting oneself with bodily functions. Uncomfortable feelings may be so intense that the client is completely unable to attend to the rehabilitation process.

Beliefs about Health and Healing

Beliefs about the body's structure and function are closely related to beliefs about how the body maintains health or overcomes states of ill health. Food in particular has long been recognized as a central feature of each culture because of the broad range of symbolic meanings it occupies in each society (Levi-Strauss, 1970). In the hot-cold theory discussed earlier, certain functions of the body are classified as fitting either of those categories. These categories are related to a parallel classification of foods. Therefore, depending on the condition, the person might consume or avoid foods of the opposite category to restore the balance between hot and cold.

In addition to the "hot-cold" or parallel type of classification, other types of classification systems have been identified, including food versus nonfood, sacred versus profane food, food used as medicine, and social foods (Helman, 1997). These classification systems are evidence that diet is often based on cultural criteria rather than nutritional value. It is quite possible that several of these classification systems coexist in a single culture. These categorizations are important for the rehabilitation professional to consider, because they may severely restrict the types of foodstuffs the patient is willing and able to eat.

The classification of food versus nonfood refers to the substances each culture considers edible and which ones not. For example, frogs' legs are considered edible in France, but not usually in Latin America, whereas guinea pigs are considered a delicacy in many Andean countries, but not usually in the United States. Definitions of food versus nonfood are often based on historical associations but to some degree are flexible, because under conditions of famine or while traveling in a different country, for instance, many people would consider eating something they do not typically associate with food.

Religious beliefs further limit the types of foodstuffs one may ingest or even come in contact. Examples of these restrictions include the Catholic temporary abstinence from eating meat during Lent or the Jewish permanent prohibition of pork. As with the classification of food and non-food, the categories of sacred and profane are flexible, so that there may be times when a particular food is considered sacred and others when it is considered profane. Some foods may even be associated with particular rituals, including rituals perceived as necessary for healing from illness. There are more secular versions of the sacred versus profane food classification, such as what is considered "whole food" and "junk food" in the United States, and the modern vegetarian movement in the West.

Food classification systems often overlap, as in the case of foods considered to be medicines and medicines considered to be food. The hot-cold classification system has already served as an example of food being used to restore health. In these and other societies, special diets may be seen as a form of "medication" to deal with various physical and emotional illnesses. The American folk illness of "high blood" (referring to high volume of blood rather than high blood pressure), for example, is treated with a diet of lemon juice, vinegar, pickles, and sour oranges, among other foods. The counterpart illness of "low blood" is treated with a diet high in red meat, red wine, and beets. If the client confuses the diagnosis of high blood pressure with "high blood," he or she may increase the ingestion of foods high in salt, thus aggravating his or her hypertension. As with all food classification systems, what is considered medicinal in one culture may be seen as ordinary food or not food at all in another.

Definitions of what constitutes health and illness vary between individuals, families, and cultural groups. For most, however, health is seen as more than the absence of unpleasant symptoms. Usually there is some way of explaining health as a balance in the relationship between humans, between humans and nature, or between humans and the supernatural world. The term *explanatory model* (EM) was first used by Kleinman (1980) to refer to the ways in which both patients and health practitioners "offer explanation of sickness and treatment to guide choices among available therapies and therapists and to cast personal and social meaning on the experience of sickness." To understand a person's EM, it is very important to consider the context of that explanation. *Context* refers to the social and economic organization as well as the dominant ideology (or religion) of the particular society in which the person developed the EM. Exploring the EM provides important information regarding how the person perceives what is happening to him or her, why it has happened, and why it is occurring at this moment in time. In addition, this exploration provides information about what the person believes would happen if nothing were done, what effects the illness or symptom has on other people, and what should be done about it. In Western health care, too often the health practitioner is the only one permitted to offer an EM in the form of a medical diagnosis. Understanding the client's EM, however, may ultimately be the key in designing a meaningful therapeutic program that will be followed through to the end.

Examples of EMs include *mal de ojo* and *susto* in much of Latin America. In the first case, the belief is that the symptom or illness was caused by an enemy's curse. In the second case, the belief is that wandering spirits snatch the person's strength at vulnerable times. In both these cases, there are elaborate ways to counteract the effects of the illness, which may include hiring a folk healer to perform a particular ritual, wearing amulets, or eating specific foods. Variations of these themes exist throughout the world, as in *tabanka* in Trinidad, *koro* in China, and *amok* in Malaysia. EMs exist in every culture, including industrialized ones. In the United States, moralistic EMs for illnesses such as acquired immunodeficiency syndrome (AIDS) have come about, ascribing the disease as punishment from God for nonmainstream lifestyles.

As stated earlier, EMs often include an indication of what should be done to manage or counteract the illness. This may include ways in which the person should help him- or herself, or ways through which to obtain help from other people. Examples of caring for oneself include taking the day off from work and staying home, or taking a home remedy. Other solutions may involve other people, such as asking for advice from a friend or neighbor who has had a similar experience, or consulting a priest or local folk healer. In addition, a physician may be consulted if one is available. Three overlapping sectors of health care have been identified, including the popular sector, the folk sector, and the professional sector (Kleinman, 1980). Each sector usually has its own way of explaining and treating illness, although often these sectors overlap. It is important to note that people associate certain illnesses with certain sectors and may not feel fully healed or cared for until they receive the culturally sanctioned treatment.

The popular sector is lay and nonprofessional. Usually, this is where ill health is first recognized. In this sector, treatment is not paid for and may be initiated by patients themselves or by relatives, friends, or neighbors who have had a similar experience. Home remedies have their origin in this sector. Secular or sacred healers who are not part of the "official" medical system comprise the folk sector. These healers receive some type of payment for their service, although not always in monetary form. There is a wide variety of these healers in any society, and generally they share similar cultural beliefs, values, and world views as the population in the communities they serve. An important feature of folk healing is that it usually involves the patient's family, and even community, in some way. In contrast, the professional sector, recognized as the "official" health system, is typically focused on the individual patient. The professional sector is usually protected and regulated by laws, and although its members may come from the communities they serve, they often have a dramatically different set of values, beliefs, and world views by virtue of their indoctrination into their profession. In the Western Hemisphere, this legally sanctioned professional healing sector is based on a biomedical EM.

It has been estimated that only approximately 10–25% of health care in the world occurs in this sector because of the long-standing low availability of physicians in many parts of the world (World Bank, 1993; World Health Organization, 1987). Even in industrialized nations, poverty often severely limits the contact that many people may have with the professional health sector. It is clearly evident, therefore, that rehabilitation professionals must become very familiar with folk and popular healing beliefs and practices to gain crucial insight into the client's world of meaning.

Thinking Styles

As indicated in the previous discussion, few individuals are perfect representatives of their culture. This is particularly evident when referring to cultural *cognitive styles*. This term refers to thought patterns that are very general and indicate the way people approach ideas and process information, rather than the specific content of thoughts. Although evidence suggests that cultural groups fall into open-minded and closed-minded categories (Hecht et al., 1989), it is important to remember that communication takes place between individuals, not cultures. Therefore, understanding these generalizations is useful only when the knowledge serves to improve communication between the rehabilitation professional and client rather than to predict it.

People with an open-minded cognitive style tend to seek out more information before making a decision and are likely to admit that they do not have enough information or need to learn more before forming their final opinion on a matter. They tend to ask many questions and want to hear about alternatives before reaching conclusions. People with a close-minded cognitive style tend to look only at a narrow range of data and ignore the rest. These people tend to take this approach because they function under strict rules of behavior or because their cultural assumptions are very strong. Studies have shown that most cultures tend to produce closed-minded citizens (Morrison et al., 1994; Peacock, 1986). This probably happens because one of the very functions of culture itself is to set boundaries and pattern people's lives. Because cognitive style is the result of habit, it tends to be automatic and subconscious.

Working with both open-minded and closed-minded people poses interesting challenges to rehabilitation professionals. Open-minded people may require an extended amount of time and information to make a choice. A young man with recent paraplegia who wants to see all possible options of wheelchairs before making his choice, or a middle-aged woman who wants to hear about all options of exercise to strengthen her right shoulder after a cycling accident are both examples of open-minded cognitive styles. These people may become offended if they perceive the professional as cutting the interaction short or limiting the choices available to the client. Closed-minded people, on the other hand, may be impatient when given prolonged explanations of treatment options and distrust a rehabilitation professional who appears indecisive in his or her desire to explore all available options. In this way, both open- and closed-minded styles may lead to ineffective treatment. When well understood, cognitive style can enhance treatment by reframing the open-minded client's approach as growth-producing exploration, and the closed-minded client's approach as focused determination.

It is important to note that the professional also approaches the therapeutic relationship from the perspective of an open- or closed-minded cognitive style. Consider, for example, the case of a dietitian working with a devout Hindu patient. This patient is appalled when offered ground beef as a dietary option to increase protein intake. Her religious beliefs have narrowed her view, so she does not even consider the goal of increasing protein intake but rather focuses on the inappropriate request. The dietitian as well has focused solely on the need to increase protein intake, without taking into account other information about the client. A closed-minded approach on both sides has created a possibly unnecessary conflict. Ultimately it is the professional's responsibility to be flexible and offer appropriate alternatives so that the client can maintain cultural integrity. The dietitian, for example, could have met with the client and first explained the goal of increasing protein intake, and then offered two or three alternative foods, including beef.

A related aspect of cognitive style is the way in which people process information, which can be divided into *associative* and *abstractive* processing styles (Hall, 1990). Personal experience serves as a filter of new data for those people who think associatively. In other words, new information can only be understood in terms of similar past experience. These people require concrete and often visible examples before feeling secure in their understanding of a unit of information. In contrast, people who think abstractly consider hypothetical situations or use their imagination to gain understanding. All cultures produce both associative and abstractive thinkers, but typically associative thinkers are more common (Morrison et al., 1994).

As with the open- and closed-minded characteristics, associative and abstractive thinkers each have both strengths and weaknesses. Associative thinkers are often skeptical of unfamiliar or untried approaches in therapy and need several demonstrations and practice sessions to learn a particular skill. Once these people see concrete results, however, they become invested in the process. Their skepticism or reluctance may try the rehabilitation professional's patience, but when satisfied, these clients become the best advocates for the professional's service. Abstractive thinkers, on the other hand, may appear confused and uninvolved when they do not understand the long-term objectives of therapy or the ultimate purpose of a particular therapeutic approach. They may become overwhelmed when presented with too many details to remember. These clients appreciate it when rehabilitation professionals explain the basic rules or principles of therapy and then permit them to apply those principles for themselves in various situations. In their own ways, both associative and abstractive thinkers attempt to gain understanding of the situation to exert control or mastery over it. They simply use different approaches to achieve this end.

Communication Styles

Cultures vary in the ways that members derive meaning from social inter-action and communication. Communication is one of the most complex human endeavors because of the intricate intermingling of language, emotion, values, personality, and experience. The primary function of language is to transmit information. This transmission occurs through both verbal and nonverbal means. The resulting meaning of the communication appears to depend on the relationship between the amount of information relayed and the shared experience, or context, between the people involved in the transaction (Lynch, 1998). Accordingly, the more context people share, the less information they need to communicate verbally and explic-itly. Experiences shared in the past have taught them what each other's gestures, tone of voice, and words mean. For example, a couple that has been married for 50 years probably does not have to explicitly communi-cate their emotional state to each other in verbal form. After 50 years of living together, they are able to surmise each other's mood from their tone of voice, eye contact, rate of speech and respiration, walking pattern, and so on. They may have become so accustomed to each other that this inter-pretation of meaning may come subconsciously or automatically, and they may even describe it as "intuitive." Most likely, however, when first mar-ried it was necessary for them to communicate more with each other ver-bally to resolve or avoid miscommunications. Only after building context with each other for a prolonged period of time has their awareness of each other's communication style become second nature.

Cultures differ in the way they rely on information or context for com-munication. Hall (1984) noted that high-context cultures rely more on shared experience and history than on verbal communication. This means that in these cultures, during communication, more emphasis is placed on nonverbal cues and messages than on the words that are spoken. High-context cultures tend to rely on hierarchy and be more formal and rooted in the past. Thus, these cultures tend to provide more stability for their members because they change slowly (Hecht et al., 1989). When words are used in high-context cul-tures, communication is more indirect, and meaning is conveyed more through stories that imply the teller's opinion than through unambiguous speech (Benedict, 1989).

In contrast, members of low-context cultures tend to rely more on the spoken word, and their communication is more direct, precise, and logi-cally linear. These people often do not take into account gestures and non-verbal cues. To people of low-context cultures, the unarticulated moods and meanings that are so important for people from high-context cultures may go completely unnoticed. However, people from low-context cultures seem to be more comfortable with change, although they may lack a sense of continuity and connection with the past (Hecht et al., 1989).

Cultural miscommunication is commonplace because of the difference in value placed on context. Individuals from high-context and low-context cultures are likely to respond quite differently to similar situations. For example, a rehabilitation professional may routinely begin his or her treatment sessions by asking clients how they are feeling and what activities they have done in the last week. Once clients have answered these questions, the professional introduces the tasks to be accomplished during the present session. A client from a high-context culture may find this introductory interaction insufficient, whereas a client from a low-context culture may find it superfluous.

Value Systems

Every culture has a complex set of explicit and implicit value systems that help its members differentiate between right and wrong or good and evil. Thinking and communication styles—as well as beliefs about the body, health, and healing—have their basis in these underlying value systems. These values systems are assumptions that characterize each culture. For example, American culture has been characterized by a valuing of individualism and privacy, belief in the equality of all persons, and informality in the interaction between people. Other salient values of American culture include an emphasis on the future, change, progress, materialism, punctuality, and achievement (Althen, 1988). Although there are many value systems operating in any culture, this section addresses what is accepted as truth, locus of decision making, sources of anxiety reduction, issues of equality/inequality, and the use of time. The root assumption in all these value systems is, however, that they are right and should be the standard against which all human behavior is measured.

What Is Accepted as Truth

People from different cultures arrive at a sense of truth in different ways. These ways can be narrowed down to fact, faith, or feeling. People who act on the basis of fact want to examine objective evidence that supports a particular course of action before accepting it. These people may also stop participating in an activity if they do not see clear evidence of its benefit. On the other hand, people who act on the basis of faith use a belief system derived from a religious or political ideology to determine what is good and bad. Options for action are evaluated in comparison to the tenets of the ideology. An example of this is the person who refuses a needed blood transfusion because his or her religion specifically forbids it. Another example of action based on faith is when someone who has a chronically debilitating disease refuses to use a wheelchair to avoid fatigue because they value self-sufficiency above all else. Finally, people who act on the basis of feeling are those who "go with their gut instincts" and choose a course of action because they have an intuition that it is the right one rather than because they have analyzed it objectively or measured it against an ideological standard. When these people are confronted with a choice over something that makes logical sense over something that feels right, they choose the latter. Logic is then used to confirm the choice after it has been made. Interestingly, this cultural approach is the most common (Morrison et al., 1994). It is easy to see how easily conflicts may arise between people who use different approaches to arrive at "truth."

Locus of Decision Making

This value system represents the degree to which a particular culture prizes individualism as opposed to collectivism. Individualism is related to the degree to which a person takes only him- or herself into consideration when making decisions. Collectivism, on the other hand, is related to the degree to which a person must abide with the consensus of a group when making a decision. Pure individualism or collectivism are actually rare. In most cultures, people take into account the opinions of others when making decisions, but are not strictly bound to the desires of the group. Many cultures, however, expect the individual to consider what is best for the family when making a decision. In other societies, the person may be expected to consider larger social groups than one's family. An example of individualism might be the client who is tired of being in the hospital and wants to be discharged regardless of the added strain it may produce on his family. An example of collectivism in a similar situation is the client who postpones discharge as long as possible to avoid burdening her family. Another place in which individualism and collectivism may be evidenced is in various clients' need for privacy. Individualism tends to engender a high need for privacy and personal space, whereas collectivism reduces this need.

Sources of Anxiety Reduction

An important belief system that rehabilitation professionals should consider is what clients believe they should do to relieve stress. Most people turn to one or more of four basic sources of stability and security: interpersonal relationships, religion, technology, and the law (Hall, 1990; Harris, 1989; Morrison et al., 1994). Clearly people undergoing rehabilitation are under stress as they must make important health-related decisions or must adapt to a traumatic event or limitation in function. Consequently, it is important for rehabilitation professionals to know where their clients usually go for advice and help. If a client usually seeks assistance from a family member or a priest, for example, professionals should make every effort to make sure that these people are included in team discussions as early as possible in order for them to be able to give the client informed advice. Similarly, if the client finds comfort in religious observances or rituals, it is important that rehabilitation professionals facilitate this process. It is not as crucial that the professional understand all the nuances of the client's religion so much as that they acknowledge and appreciate the importance it has for the client. Finally, people who rely on technology as a source of anxiety reduction may seek additional diagnostic tests to confirm or refute a diagnosis, or may want additional medications or adaptive devices to relieve their stress. Rehabilitation professionals must carefully consider if any equipment prescribed is truly essential for functioning, or if it has been ordered solely to relieve anxiety. Other methods of anxiety reduction may ultimately be more beneficial for the client.

Issues of Equality/Inequality

All cultures make some form of division of power, whether on the basis of financial resources, gender, race, or professional status. Disadvantaged groups exist in all cultures. Members of advantaged classes may appear arrogant to rehabilitation professionals because they have a sense of entitlement to care and treat the professionals as servants. Members of disadvantaged groups, on the other hand, may view the professional with suspicion or may accept any instruction out of fear of retaliation through withdrawal of services. An understanding of how the client views the distribution of power between women and men may be particularly helpful for rehabilitation professionals. In most cultures, men are more likely to be obeyed and trusted when they occupy positions of authority (Bateson, 1989). This value may make a tremendous difference in how the client responds to the professional or other caregivers. Because roles of men and women are culturally determined, they tend to operate subconsciously in both clients and professionals.

Use of Time

In each culture, the use of time is constructed uniquely. Through conscious and subconscious means, time is used as a language, as a way of handling priorities, and as a way of revealing how people feel about one another. Cultures can be divided into two large categories according to how time is patterned: monochronic and polychronic (Hall, 1984). As with any value system, the potential for conflict is high between people who approach life from a monochronic perspective and people who approach life from a polychronic perspective. People from monochronic cultures tend to organize their lives with a "one-thing-at-a-time" mentality. In these cultures, time is viewed as a commodity that can be squandered if not handled carefully. Adages such as "time is money" and "waste of time" are characteristic of monochronic cultures. In addition, adherence to schedules is very important in these cultures, and people may become offended if made to wait for an appointment. People from monochronic cultures tend to prefer to have the rehabilitation professional's undivided attention, and it is important to them that time be used efficiently.

In contrast, people from polychronic cultures organize their lives around social relationships rather than schedules. For them, the amount of time spent with someone is directly related to the value they place on that relationship. People from these cultures may feel rushed by schedules and often are late for appointments because they come across acquaintances whom they did not want to offend by rushing off. Whereas people from monochronic cultures tend to prefer to keep social "chit-chat" at a minimum when concentrating on a work or therapy task, people from polychronic cultures enjoy doing many things at a time, including maintaining a conversation while engaged in a therapeutic activity. People from polychronic cultures may feel offended when required to make therapy appointments on time or when they are not squeezed into the schedule when they arrive without an appointment.

Integrating Cultural Sensitivity into the Rehabilitation Process

From the discussion in this chapter, I conclude that culture is not a separate realm of human experience, but rather that it is a filter through which most of life is interpreted. Although I have highlighted issues of culture that have particular importance for health and the work of rehabilitation professionals, these by no means are the only issues that may have an impact on the therapeutic process. Because each individual has his or her unique cultural perspective, and because the boundaries of each culture are hazy at best, the integration of cultural sensitivity in rehabilitation is an ongoing, never-ending process. Two basic principles direct this process.

Principle 1: Professionals are under the influence of their own culture. Being culturally sensitive means first that rehabilitation professionals themselves acknowledge that they organize their own lives through the filter of their own culture. Their choices of work schedule, clothing, food, treatment strategy, and even words are greatly colored by the cultural perspectives they have learned as individuals, as members in a family or other social group, and as professionals in a particular discipline. Rehabilitation professionals must be committed to examining the ways in which their own cultural perspectives influence their therapeutic encounters with clients and be willing to adapt or change to the benefit of the client. Table 7.1 lists some suggested questions rehabilitation professionals should reflect on to recognize how their own cultural values and beliefs may affect their work. If rehabilitation professionals do not examine their

TABLE 7.1
Reflection Questions for Rehabilitation Practitioners

1. What do I believe my own "culture" is? When someone asks me what culture I am from, how do I answer?
2. What is my "ethnicity"? In what ways does this heritage make me different from others around me?
3. How do I believe men and women should behave? What behaviors do I consider masculine and which feminine? How did I arrive at these conclusions?
4. What are my religious beliefs? What do I think about the notion of a "deity"? How does my belief (or lack thereof) in a deity affect how I relate to others? What behaviors does my belief require?
5. What is my primary language? What are my values regarding people who do not speak my language?
6. What does it mean to be "healthy"? What do I consider "normal" health? What are my standards of physical and mental health? What are my beliefs about how someone should go about becoming healthy when they are sick?
7. What are my values about how goal oriented people should be? What types of life goals do I have? Do I tend to plan in the long term or short term?
8. What values or beliefs about being a professional do I have? Where did I learn these values? Who else holds these values? What are the attitudes I believe professionals should demonstrate toward their clients?
9. How do I explain to others how the body works? What kinds of words or metaphors do I use to describe how the body works? What do I believe the "ideal" male and female bodies looks like? What do I believe appropriate uses of the body are? What do I consider to be "personal body space"? Whom do I permit to enter that space? Under what circumstances?
10. What are my favorite foods? What animals and plants do I not consider to be food? How do I react when I hear about someone eating one of these? Is there anything I eat that others would consider "unusual"?
11. When confronted with the need to make a decision, do I usually like to get more information about the issue, or do I prefer to make the decision based on the available information and then change it as information becomes available?
12. Is it easier for me to learn something new if I can associate with a similar past experience or when I mentally analyze the information? Do I learn best by doing or thinking?
13. How comfortable am I telling the intimate details of my life to someone I do not know? What parts of my life am I comfortable disclosing and which not? Are there people I would and people I would not talk to about personal matters? What makes the difference?
14. How do I know something is "true"? Do I accept the voice of recognized authorities or do I prefer to verify truth for myself? What do I believe is the role of emotion in the acceptance of truth?
15. What do I do when I am feeling stressed or anxious? Do I tend to rely on activities or on other people to relieve my stress? How does this change with different kinds of stress?
16. What is my typical use of time? Would others describe me as "organized and efficient" or as "relaxed and laid back"? How do I usually respond to interruptions? Do I prefer to handle several tasks at one time, or do I prefer to deal with only one?

values, it is likely that they will unconsciously devalue people who do not hold the same beliefs (Krefting & Krefting, 1991).

Principle 2: Cultural sensitivity should neither be predictive or prescriptive. When discussing culture, there is the inherent danger that professionals come to believe that they know enough to predict the attitudes, values, and behaviors of clients, and consequently do not wait for the clients to disclose their cultural perspectives. The professional may also make choices of therapeutic interventions based on what he or she thinks the client will appreciate, without first confirming the cultural interpretation with the client. These attitudes on the part of the professional are essentially prejudiced because they are based on the assumption that the professional can categorize the client and can read the client's mind from the status of "expert." Rehabilitation professionals must understand that ownership of culture resides with the client, and that it is the professional's responsibility to draw it out and integrate it as much as possible in the treatment process. Rehabilitation professionals could ask their clients to respond to most of the same questions presented in Table 7.1 by modifying them and making them applicable to their clients. In this way, treatment is more likely to take into account the client's preferences and help the professional be aware of potential interpersonal problems with the client. Kleinman (1984) suggested health professionals ask clients eight questions to gain a sense of the client's EM. These questions appear in Table 7.2.

In addition to these basic principles, rehabilitation professionals should consider the following suggestions while evaluating and treating their clients. Naturally, the list of suggestions presented here is not exhaustive. The professional is encouraged to continue adding to this list as he or she finds success.

Pay attention to the client's communication and cognitive styles. If the client asks many questions, routinely offer more information—do not wait for the client to ask. Make sure you frequently ask the client if he or she has any questions. If the client seems impatient with conversation, make a question-and-answer period a formal part of the treatment session. For example, you can explain to the client that the first and last 5 minutes of the session will be used to discuss any questions.

Include the client's sources of anxiety reduction early in the treatment process. The more comfortable the client feels, the more likely he or she will invest in therapy. Including sources of anxiety reduction may mean scheduling treatment sessions when a family member or priest can be present. If the source of anxiety reduction is an activity, this activity can be made a goal of treatment. For example, if a client feels relieved when he or she walks in the garden, treatment can be focused on the incremental steps required to walk in the garden. In this way, the rehabilitation professional is more likely to address what is meaningful to the client.

TABLE 7.2
Eliciting the Client's "Explanatory Model"

---

1. What do you call the problem?
2. What do you think caused the problem?
3. Why do you think the problem started when it did?
4. What do you think the sickness does? How does it work?
5. How severe is the sickness? Will it have a short or long course?
6. What kind of treatment do you think you should receive? What are the most important results you hope to receive from this treatment?
7. What are the chief problems the sickness has caused?
8. What do you fear most about the sickness?

Adapted from Kleinman, A. (1980). Patients and healers in the context of culture. Berkeley, CA: University of California Press.

Adapt the evaluation or treatment strategy before you attempt to adapt the client's context or ask the client to adapt his or her behavior. Because the client's context is likely to be a source of stability and reduction of stress, it is important to maintain it unchanged as much as possible. For example, although it may seem more practical and efficient to remove furniture from a room to help a client with cognitive deficits find his or her way to the bathroom, the lack of familiar landmarks may create further problems.

Conclusions

This chapter provides the reader with a general framework to guide the shared exploration of culture between rehabilitation professionals and clients. Like any culture, the therapeutic relationship is socially constructed. By considering cultural values, rehabilitation professionals are likely to make intervention more meaningful and thus more useful to the client. In addition, by analyzing their own cultural values and preconceptions, rehabilitation professionals are more likely to avoid misunderstandings that can interfere with the client's progress of the effectiveness of intervention. The ultimate benefit of being sensitive to cultural perspectives is the appreciation of human diversity, vitality, and creativity.

References

Althen, O. American ways (pp. 23–48). Yarmouth, ME: Intercultural Press.
Bateson, M. C. (1989). Foreword. In R. Benedict (Ed.), Patterns of culture (pp. vii–x). Boston: Houghton-Mifflin.

Bauman, G. (1999). The Multicultural riddle: Rethinking national, ethnic, and religious identities. New York: Routledge.

Bellah, R. N. Madsen, R., Sullivan, W. M., Swindler, A., & Tipton, S. M. (1985). Habits of the heart: Individualism and commitment in American life (pp. 152–155). New York: Harper & Row.

Benedict, R. (1989). Patterns of culture (pp. 223–250). Boston: Houghton-Mifflin.

Brislin, R. (1993). Understanding culture's influence on behavior (pp. 130–172). Ft. Worth, TX: Harcourt Brace Javonovich.

Brown, P. M., & Gustafson, M. S. (1995). Showing sensitivity to deaf culture. ASHA, 37(5), 46–48.

Chomsky, N. (1995). Language and thought. Wakefield, RI: Moyer-Bell Ltd.

Chomsky, N., & Peck, J. (1987). The Chomsky reader. New York: Pantheon Books.

Commission on Work, Family, and Citizenship (1997). American youth: A statistical snapshot. Cited in F. J. Macchiarola & A. Gartner, Caring for America's children (2nd ed.) (p. 21). New York: Academy of Political Science.

Cushner, K., McClelland, A., and Safford, P. (1996). Human diversity in education: An integrative approach (2nd ed.) (pp. 3–22, 49–80). New York: McGraw-Hill.

Foster, G. (1994). Hippocrates' Latin American legacy: Humoral medicine in the new world (pp. 35–59). Langhorne, PA: Gordon & Breach.

Gollnick, D., & Chinn, P. (1990). Multicultural education in a pluralistic society (3rd ed.) (p. 211). New York: Macmillan.

Hall, E. T. (1984). The dance of life: The other dimensions of time (pp. 3–10, 153–193). New York: Anchor Books.

Harris, M. (1989). Cows, pigs, wars and witches: The riddles of culture (pp. 3–10). New York: Vintage Books.

Hecht, M., Andersen, P., & Ribeau, S. (1989). The cultural dimensions of nonverbal communication. In M. Assante & Gudykunst A. (Eds.), Handbook for international and intercultural communication (pp. 35–77). Newbury Park, CA: Sage.

Helman, C. G. (1997). Culture, health and illness (3rd ed.) (pp. 1–11). Oxford: Butterworth–Heinemann.

Henry, W. (1990, April 9). Beyond the melting pot. Time, p. 28.

Hetherington, E. M., Law, T. C., & O'Connor, T. G. (1999). Divorce: Challenges, changes, and new chances. In A. S. Skolnick & J. H. Skolnick (Eds.), Family in transition (10th ed.) (pp. 163–172). New York: Addison Wesley Longman.

Hodkinson, H. (1997). All one system: Demographics of education—Kindergarten through graduate school (2nd ed.) (pp. 30–33). Washington, DC: Institute of Educational Leadership.

Holcomb, T. (1997). Development of deaf bicultural identity. American Annals of the Deaf, 2, 89–93.

Johnson, T. W., & Keren, M. S. (1998). The families of lesbian women and gay men. In M. McGoldrick (Ed.), Re-visioning family therapy: Race, culture, and gender in clinical practice (pp. 320–329). New York: Guilford Press.

Keesing, R. (1981). Cultural anthropology: A contemporary perspective (p. 518). New York: Holt, Reinhart & Winston.

Kennedy, M., Jung, K., and Orland, M. (1996). Poverty, achievement, and the distribution of compensatory education services (pp. 98–104). Washington, DC: U.S. Government Printing Office.

Kleinman, A. (1980). Patients and healers in the context of culture (p. 106). Berkeley, CA: University of California Press.

Krefting, L., & Krefting, D. (1991). Cultural influences on performance. In C. Christiansen & C. Baum (Eds.), Occupational therapy: Overcoming human performance deficits (pp. 101–124). Thorofare, NJ: Slack, Inc.

Leach, E. (1982). Social anthropology (pp. 38–39). Glasgow: Fontana.

LeVay, S., & Hamer, D. (1994) Evidence for biological influence in male homosexuality. Scientific American, 270, 44–49.

Levi-Strauss, C. (1970). The raw and the cooked (pp. 65–90). London: Jonathan Cape.

Lynch, E. W. (1998). Conceptual framework: From culture shock to cultural learning. In E. W. Lynch & M. J. Hanson (Eds.), Developing cross-cultural competence (2nd ed.) (pp. 23–45). Baltimore: Paul H. Brooks Publishing Co.

Morrison, T., Conaway, W., & Borden, G. (1994). Kiss, bow, or shake hands (pp. x–xiii). Holbrook, MA: Bob Adams, Inc.

Peacock, J. (1986). The anthropological lens: Harsh light, soft focus (pp. 44–81). London: Cambridge University Press.

Pearson, J., & Dudley, H. (1982). Bodily perceptions in surgical patients. British Medical Journal, 284, 1545–1546.

Purnell, L. D., & Paulanka, B. J. (1998). Transcultural health care: A culturally competent approach. Philadelphia: F. A. Davis Company.

Reich, R. (1992). The work of nations (pp. 10–32). New York: Vintage Books.

Rosen, D. (1999). What is a family? Nature, culture and the law. In A. S. Skolnick & J. H. Skolnick (Eds.), Family in transition (10th ed.) (pp. 53–63). New York: Addison Wesley Longman.

Sargent, M., & Johnson, T. M. (1996). Handbook of medical anthropology. Westport, CT: Greenwood Press.

Shweder, R. A. (1991). Thinking through cultures: Expeditions in cultural psychology (pp. 113–155). Cambridge, MA: Harvard University Press.

Toffler, A. (1980). The third wave. New York: William Morrow and Company.

Triandis, H. (1972). The analysis of subjective culture (pp. 10–37). New York: Wiley-Interscience.

Vanneman, R., & Cannon, L. (1988). The American perception of class: Labor and social change. Philadelphia: Temple University Press.

Webb, R., & Sherman, R. (1989). Schooling and society (2nd ed.) (pp. 49–50). New York: Macmillan.

World Bank (1993). World development report: 1993. New York: Oxford University Press.

World Health Organization (1987). Hospital personnel and hospital establishments. Geneva, Switzerland: Author.

Wright, E. O. (1997). Class counts: Comparative studies in class analysis theory (pp. 20–53). New York: Cambridge University Press.

Yetman, N. R. (1991). Majority and minority: The dynamics of race and ethnicity in American life (pp. 3–41). Boston: Allyn & Bacon.

CHAPTER 8

Team Approaches
to Geriatric Rehabilitation

Janet E. McElhaney and Marion C. E. Briggs

Challenges and Opportunities in Geriatrics

A major challenge facing not only health care, but world economy in general, is the aging of the population. Currently, 12.7% of the U.S. population is older than 65 years of age, and this is projected to increase to 16% by 2020 (U.S. Bureau of the Census, 1993). Projections from these statistics indicate that the population older than 85 years will double during that time period. Currently, more than one-third of persons in the United States aged 85 years and older require long-term institutional care. At this rate of growth, the health care system will be overwhelmed by the needs of this age group. Effort must be focused not only on understanding the secrets of successful aging, but also on developing strategies to educate health care professionals about how to prevent the progression of frailty in older adults.

Our challenge is to understand how to maintain health throughout the aging process. We understand that the components of good health are fundamentally related to socioeconomics, nutrition, exercise, education, and psychosocial support and have little to do with the health care system per se. In an era in which health reform remains highly controversial, this at least is good news. Disease prevention through vaccination and other means is both more cost-effective and more likely to maintain health status than is disease treatment or rehabilitation. Table 8.1 identifies the determinants of health for the general population, and Table 8.2 identifies the most reliable determinants of health in the older adult population.

Older adults do, of course, experience problems requiring hospital care. A certain proportion of adults would require hospital care even if effective health promotion and disease prevention strategies were com-

TABLE 8.1
Population Determinants of Health

Income and social status
Social support
Education
Employment and working conditions
Physical environments
Biology and genetic endowment
Personal health practices and coping
Healthy child development
Health services

Data from Federal, Provincial, and Territorial Advisory Committee on Population Health (1994). Strategies for population health: investing in the health of Canadians. Ottawa, Ontario: Author.

TABLE 8.2
Determinants of Health for Seniors

Lifestyle
    Maintaining social ties
    Maintaining physical activity
    Good nutrition
    Self-esteem and sense of control
Socioeconomic environment
    Conditions, opportunities, and amenities available to those with financial means
    Longest life expectancy not found in wealthiest countries, but in those with the
        smallest spread of income and smallest proportion of the population in rela-
        tive poverty
    Lack of education and lifelong learning opportunities may be a significant
        predictor of dementia
    Social support and safe living conditions are critical
Absence of or minimal chronic disease
Opportunity for health promotion

Data from Minister of Public Works and Government Services, Canada (1996). What determines health: National forum on health (pp. 54–55). Ottawa, Ontario: Neena L. Chappell.

mon. Even though the population older than 65 years represents 12.7% of the total population, increased hospitalization rates, medication use, and frequency of medical visits mean that this same population consumes more than one-third of the total health resources (Levit et al., 1996). Efforts to make health services efficient and effective remain important, as do discussions about rationing of care, but promotion of health and prevention of

TABLE 8.3
The (New) Goals of Medicine

The prevention of disease and injury and promotion and maintenance of health
The relief of pain and suffering caused by maladies
The care and cure of those with maladies, and the care of those who cannot
  be cured
The avoidance of premature death and the pursuit of a peaceful death

---

Data from The Hastings Center (1996, November/December). The new goals of medicine: An international project of the Hastings Center. The Hastings Center Report (special supplement).

disease hold the real promise for both controlling costs and improving quality of life years. Concerted effort is needed by clinicians and educators as well as researchers and policy makers to focus resources and effort toward prevention. Failure to do that will result in a predictable dilemma in which the benefit of health services for older adults will have to be balanced against the direct and "opportunity" costs of those services. *Direct costs* are those attributed to providing care to older adults. *Opportunity costs* consider services or interventions that would have been provided to others if funds had not been allocated to older persons. Older adults will be at increasing risk of marginalization as ever more scarce health resources are focused toward those whom society values more highly and who hold greater political and economic influence than do most of the elders.

While these challenges are great and sometimes even overwhelming, it is within geriatrics that the greatest opportunities exist to reform the goals of medicine to include significant focus on health promotion and disease prevention. Table 8.3 shows the new goals of medicine recently defined in an international collaborative involving intense discussion among top medical leaders in 14 countries. These "new" goals reflect the truth in which geriatrics has always been grounded: that effective health maintenance and disease prevention is the cornerstone of the ability to meet emerging challenges. Medicine's greatest challenge and its focal point to date has been to understand the causes and cures of disease, and many challenges remain in that arena. Yet that relatively narrow focus has distracted both attention and funding from discovering ways to prevent chronic illness. If we fail to make a conscious shift toward health promotion and disease prevention in the older adult population, the needs of the elderly will completely overwhelm health service resources as the proportion of persons aged 65 years and older increases.

Key to that effort is the concept of "compression of morbidity" (Hebert, 1997). That concept acknowledges that there are few effective means of prolonging total years of life, and consciously focuses effort toward increasing the number of *healthy* years of life. These efforts have become an urgent priority and are creating an opportunity that must be seized to influence policy makers, funding agencies, researchers, clinicians, and educators to begin to focus on programs and services that prevent disease and disability. It must be understood that the health of the population older than 65 years is heterogeneous. Only 10–20% of older adults have no chronic diseases; this subset is classified as "successfully aging." We understand that the determinants of health are both genetic and environmental, but we do not understand how to unravel the secrets to successful aging. The remaining 80–90% of older adults have one or more underlying chronic diseases; only 10–20% of this group is readily identified as frail. The balance of this "usual aging" population remains at risk for developing functional dependence. Prevention of disability will promote maintenance of a satisfying quality of life and compress morbidity.

To underscore this critical notion, we need to understand what interventions will be effective in delaying frailty to the last years of life, thus compressing morbidity into a shorter time frame. It is important to emphasize that whatever interventions are used, very small, if any, gains are made in longevity—extending life is not our chief aim. The real possibility for significant impact is in improving quality of life. Geriatric specialists speak of this concept as adding "life to years, rather than years to life." Clearly, if we can maintain health, especially during the later years, we will also achieve a significant reduction in overall costs of providing health care over the span of one's life. To patients, this would be an incidental gain, secondary to achieving lasting good health. To policy makers and funders, reduced cost of care may be a more compelling reason to support interventions that will achieve effective health maintenance.

Team Approach

Geriatrics has traditionally taken a multidisciplinary approach to understanding and managing the problems of older adults, especially those who have become frail. Frailty can be defined as functional dependence from a variety of causes (e.g., dementia, arthritis, stroke, heart disease, sensory changes) and presents a risk for further functional decline during acute illness. It is particularly important to identify and aggressively treat the reversible components of that functional decline and support independence in the context of the client's social network. This requires each discipline on the team to bring to the task their unique clinical philosophy and skills and the ability to collaborate effectively. In this way, we can prevent duplication and gaps in service and spend health resources wisely. The development of a flexible, skilled, and seamless geriatric service delivery team ensures that appropriate and comprehensive approaches to meeting the needs of frail older adults are identified.

In its desire to provide good care, the team must be careful not to impose their own goals and values and inadvertently disenfranchise the patient's autonomy and independence. It is possible to do "too much" and create in our patients a sense of helplessness and dependence that derives from meeting our own need to be needed as health care professionals, rather than appropriately supporting the patient's ability to fully exercise his or her own capacities. Part of what often distinguishes beginning from experienced professionals is the appropriateness of decisions made when choosing from everything that *can* be done, those interventions that will actually help a patient. This comment is not to be critical of beginning professionals. It simply indicates another strength of the team approach. Professionals from different disciplines and different levels of experience can mentor and guide one another. More seasoned professionals can mentor appropriate choice of interventions, and new professionals can help those who are more experienced to continue to learn and think when repetitive clinical patterns may put continuous learning and creativity at risk.

Barriers to Health Maintenance

Traditional holistic health models have recognized the interdependent nature of physical, mental (or cognitive), and social spheres in influencing health behavior and experience of health. Older adults themselves have asked that a fourth sphere be given equal priority: that of spiritual issues (personal observations). Consequently, our model for considering health includes the four spheres depicted in Figure 8.1. Health in each sphere and integrated interaction between all spheres reflect a healthy overall state of being, even in the presence of disease. Consider as an example how this model might apply to a patient experiencing pain. Figure 8.2 shows the elements of pain from the perspective of each of the spheres, and it is easy to see how different assessment and management approaches might emerge from each. Determining the total approach that makes most sense can be complex—but then, people (including older people) are complex, so this should not surprise us.

The team approach should identify in each sphere both the needs and capacities of patients and their families. Members of the health care team need not address identified needs if the patient and family have the skills, resources, and will to manage specific areas. Well-intentioned health care teams may provide more services than are helpful or welcome unless they carefully identify capacities along with needs.

Geriatric Assessment

We have already indicated two cornerstones of geriatric practice: use of the multidisciplinary approach to assessment and management and an orientation to health promotion and disease prevention aimed at compressing morbidity. The application of this approach has been variably

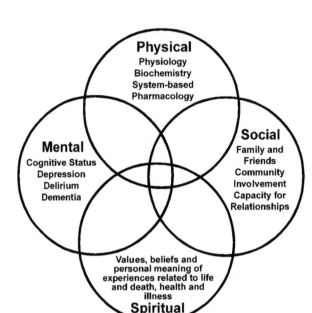

FIGURE 8.1. The model for considering health includes these four spheres.

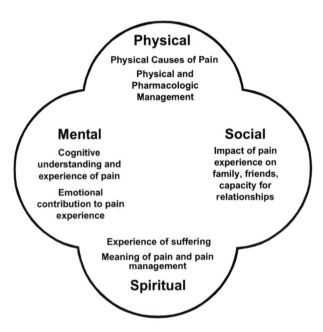

FIGURE 8.2. The elements of pain from the perspective of each of the spheres in Figure 8.1.

successful from a perspective of cost-effectiveness, depending on the setting and the targeted population (Stuck et al., 1993). Another cornerstone of geriatric practice is an orientation to making the important distinction between dynamic and stable frailty (Buchner and Wagner, 1992). Inevitably, some older adults become frail, and it is in assessing and managing this subset of older adults that the medical subspecialty of geriatrics is particularly helpful. All segments of the population older than 65 years benefit from the general approaches described in this chapter, but identifying and managing dynamic frailty is of crucial importance to preventing functional decline in at-risk older adults. In addition to preventing frailty in at-risk older adults, this issue is also pertinent to rehabilitation approaches when frailty is present.

Dynamic frailty is defined as an acute change in function that is often due to intercurrent illness or iatrogenic disorder. Dynamic frailty is often reversible if its causes and effects are managed aggressively and quickly. Delayed and inadequate treatment of any acute change in function is a serious problem and can lead to increased nonreversible frailty that could have been prevented. Chronic disease is by definition not reversible, even though it may increase the risk of acute illness and dynamic frailty. Hence, functional impairment or frailty caused by chronic disease is not reversible and is called *stable frailty*. When dynamic frailty is superimposed on chronic disease and frailty, the impact is much greater than either alone. Distinguishing between dynamic and stable frailty is a key component in geriatric assessment because it identifies those problems that should be aggressively managed and defines the goals of rehabilitation and other interventions needed to reverse the dynamic frailty. To describe the geriatric assessment process, one must first determine the target population.

Geriatric patients cannot be defined completely by age. Any older adult can become frail and develop complex needs. Rather than using age criteria, the combination of functional dependence and multiple medical, psychological, and social issues is a better indicator of the need for a geriatric approach to management. Most often, geriatric patients (that is, frail older adults) have multiple chronic medical conditions and diminished physiologic reserve. Poor health outcomes are often seen after acute illness as a result of the combined risk of losing functional status and being undertreated by health care providers with limited geriatric training and experience. Advanced age, inadequate or absent social support, and recurrent hospital admissions are very-high-risk factors for catastrophic events that may ultimately result in the need for nursing home placement.

Functional status is defined by evaluating the degree of independence in measures of instrumental activities of daily living (IADLs) and activities of daily living (ADLs). These tests measure the physical, cognitive, and social aspects of health and have been shown to be reliable and accurate measures of functional status. Subtle changes in any of these measures or

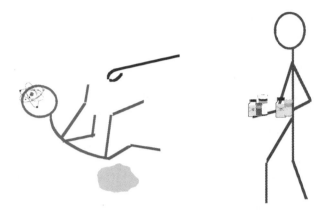

FIGURE 8.3. These geriatric giants represent common threats to functional indepen-dence in older adults: confusion, falls, incontinence, polypharmacy, and some level of dependence in activities of daily living and instrumental activities of daily living.

in behavior and independence reported by a client or caregiver are warning signs of an acute problem. Less experienced care providers, or those not trained to be alert to these signs, may misinterpret changes as part of the normal aging process and thus miss opportunities for early intervention. Thus, the expertise of multiple professions must be coordinated to deliver effective geriatric care. Multidisciplinary assessment continues to be a cor-nerstone of geriatric medicine. Our focus is on identifying acute challenges to independence in individual patients and developing strategies that effec-tively manage reversible components. In this way, the team supports the highest possible level of independence for the longest possible time, even in the presence of one or more chronic illnesses.

There are numerous standardized scales used to assess function in the various spheres that we have outlined. The mix and detail of assessment scales clearly depend on the nature of the problem and the setting in which care is being provided. Although it is beyond the scope of this chapter to list all the scales and indications for their use, the undergraduate student is encouraged to gain experience using many different scales and to become aware of the subtle differences in their use.

Disease Presentation in Older Adults: Geriatric Giants

Common disease presentations in frail older adults include confusion, incontinence, falls and immobility, polypharmacy, and functional decline. Collectively, these conditions are known as the *geriatric giants* (Figure 8.3). It is important to remember that even though these conditions are common, they are not normal in older adults. They demand a response, just as fever from an infection or chest pain from a heart attack would demand a response. Failure to take appropriate measures quickly may affect the older adult's ability to return to previous levels of independence in IADLs and ADLs; hence, response to these acute conditions in older adults is of critical importance to success in rehabilitation. The appropriate management of these geriatric giants in the acute care setting is best accomplished through a team approach that includes the at-home caregivers and focuses on early mobilization and return to functional independence. This alternative to traditional medical models of care has been shown to improve clinical outcomes for frail older adults with acute illness (Naughton et al., 1994; Palmer et al., 1998).

Factors Influencing Rehabilitation

The presence of comorbidity and the complexity of problems in older adults does affect "rehab-ability." Underlying chronic conditions are not only disabling but increase the risk of iatrogenic complications of treatment. This is a major challenge to the recovery of the patient and can present a barrier to effective treatment. In an attempt to avoid adverse effects, providers may err on the side of undertreating frail older adults. Sometimes this undertreatment is also based on assumptions that the patient is only experiencing a "normal" decline in function. Undertreatment of painful conditions is particularly common and disturbing. Approaches that appropriately medicate as well as offer nonpharmacologic management options must be developed and promoted. The involvement of a skilled geriatric team can greatly expand options for management in a way that saves money and improves the quality of life.

Table 8.4 shows the conditions for which the potential impact on function is great and for which it then makes sense to take aggressive rehabilitation measures without limiting the legitimate role for rehabilitation for any disabling condition (Hoenig, 1993). Successful management of disabling conditions includes aggressive management of prevalent chronic conditions before the onset of disability. This would include the conditions for which dramatically effective interventions are known (Cassel & Sigell, 1998). In addition, the application of rehabilitation care maps, clinical practice guidelines, and other standardized protocols prevent or improve common disabling conditions such as incontinence, confusion, immobility and falls, and polypharmacy. The most effective protocols have been developed using a team approach, and the necessary course of care can be delivered by anyone. These protocols do not replace the added "magic" of the team but are an alternative strategy for managing populations of older adults when skilled geriatric resources are limited.

TABLE 8.4
Prevalence and Efficacious Treatment of Leading Causes of Disability in Older Adults

Leading Causes of Disability in Older Adults (Ranked in Descending Order of Impact)	Medical Treatments Demonstrated to Be Effective in Older Adults	Prevalence (% in 55+ Population)
Cardiovascular disease	Treatment of hypertension	4.7
Hip fracture	Fall prevention program	2.4
Visual impairment	Cataract surgery	11.0
Osteoporosis	Hormone replacement therapy	2.7
Atherosclerosis	Treatment of hypertension	7.5
Diabetes	Management of type 2 diabetes	8.9
Ischemic heart disease	Bypass surgery/angioplasty	12.1
Arthritis	Hip/knee replacement	43.7
Cancer	Breast cancer surgery	6.2
Other circulatory conditions	—	10.2
Hearing impairment	—	28.1
High blood pressure	Treatment of hypertension	40.3
Vision disease	—	15.0

Adapted from Hoenig, H. (1993). Educating primary care physicians in geriatric rehabilitation. Clinics in Geriatric Medicine, 9, 883–893; and Verbrugge, L. M. (1991). Physical and social disability in adults in primary care research: Theory and methods. In H. Hibbard, P. A. Nutting, & M. C. Grady (Eds.), Primary care research (pp. 31–58). Washington, DC: U.S. Department of Health and Human Services.

Team Approach: Types of Teams

For the purposes of this chapter, we identify and distinguish four types of teams: functional, multidisciplinary, interdisciplinary, and transdisciplinary. Although team language is widely used in literature describing collections of health providers serving common patient cohorts, definitions of these teams are inconsistent. Without trying to claim the "right" definition, we describe what we mean by these various types of teams and then discuss the settings in which we believe the various team constellations are most appropriate.

Functional Teams

The functional approach to team operation is arguably not a team at all but describes a situation in which each professional is consulted independently, usually through a physician's order, to provide service directly to a patient. The organizing principle is the discipline. Members of the discipline are hired by and follow the policies of a "home" department of their peers (e.g., the physical therapy department). The department supplies service to patients located in in- or outpatient units, or in the home department of the discipline involved. There may be little or no consultation between disciplines, except as required for scheduling and coordination or information sharing. Team or family conferences are rare—an exceptional event, rather than a routine one—and conflicts arising between members of different disciplines are likely to be directed to an administrative level for resolution. Professional boundaries are strong and are often rigid and fiercely protected.

Multidisciplinary Teams

"Patient-focused" models of care have challenged the traditional functional approach. But many clinical areas (e.g., geriatrics, rehabilitation, intensive care units, and rheumatology) began to use multidisciplinary approaches even before patient-focused care became a common health reform strategy. In multidisciplinary teams, the organizing principle (i.e., how staff are organized and human resources allocated) remains functional: physical therapy department hires, trains, pays, and supervises physical therapists; nurses hire nurses; occupational therapy hires occupational therapists; and so on. But these functional departments generally assign one or more staff to a particular patient program or population. Members of many disciplines work together (at least clinically) and consult one another regarding the management of individual patients, even though they remain administratively aligned with a home department.

Multidisciplinary models are often called *matrix structures*, because there are really two organizational structures: an administrative one that remains functional (or unidisciplinary), and a clinical one that is organized around a particular patient population and that establishes the organizational possibility of collaboration among disciplines—mostly around the needs of individual patients. Professional boundaries often remain strongly intact in multidisciplinary teams and can become a source of conflict, because various disciplines work more closely with each other and become more aware of areas of professional overlap. Protection of professional turf can become a distracting focus and may consume energy and resources that could be more usefully applied to ensuring seamless, cost-effective, and rational care to patients.

Interdisciplinary Teams

Interdisciplinary team models begin to reflect a move along the continuum toward organizing staff and other resources around the needs of a particular patient population, rather than along disciplinary lines. Here, the clinical program head is at least involved in—and may be independently responsible for—recruiting staff from all disciplines to work with a defined patient population. Members of individual disciplines may have some organizational links with their own discipline, but these are generally weaker than the alliance with the clinical program. Professionals function on a day-to-day basis as members of a team that includes many disciplines. The team is responsible for not only managing individual patient care plans, but also for establishing general policies and priorities for a patient population. Team meetings to establish policy and address issues of interdisciplinary collaboration and patient/family conferences are standard operating procedures for these teams. Collaboration occurs on a broader spectrum, and team members feel more aligned both clinically and administratively with their team than with the home department. The home or functional department link is generally for the purpose of professional standards and education and not for the purpose of hiring, orienting, scheduling, clinical service, program planning, and development. Still, disciplines within interdisciplinary teams remain professionally distinct, and although there is some role blending that creates flexibility in meeting clinical demands, the real strength in interdisciplinary teams lies in close collaboration between unique professionals serving unique functions. Professional boundaries are not held as strongly, and some intentional cross-training may allow members of one discipline to provide limited services traditionally reserved for another.

Transdisciplinary Teams

Transdisciplinary teams move farthest along the continuum of role blending and overlap. The focus here is more on providing a consistent approach to care and less on who provides the care. Nursing, physical therapy, occupational therapy, recreational therapy, and social work (and many others) may all be represented as disciplines within the transdisciplinary team. However, roles are not as strictly defined along professional discipline lines, and staff increasingly blend roles to reduce the distinctions between them in favor of approaching clinical care with consistency. Cross-training and "multiskilling" as educational techniques for developing these teams are emphasized over discipline-specific training that occurs distinct from the team. Although the focus is on blending roles and reducing distinctions between disciplines, each discipline is still recognized for its unique contributions and still contributes unique approaches and techniques. Table 8.5 summarizes these team characteristics.

What Is "Best"?

Recent health care reform strategies have emphasized patient-focused care and cross-training, holding out the transdisciplinary model as cost-effective, efficient, and generally better than other models of team-oriented care. Critics of these reform strategies have expressed fear that these models diminish professionalism and reduce overall quality of care by focusing exclusively on cost and failing to recognize the value of highly trained, specialized health care professionals. It is our belief that each of the team mod-

TABLE 8.5
Team Configurations

Type of Team	Organizing Principle	Policies Are Developed For/By	Interdisciplinary Collaboration	Role-Blending
Functional	Discipline	For and by the discipline	Limited	Limited
Multidisciplinary	Discipline; team leader functions as head of clinical service; does not hire, train, or supervise staff in other than own discipline	For the discipline by the discipline; for a defined patient population, by the team	Moderate	Limited; roles remain distinct
	Patient group; team leader involved in hiring members of all disciplines; relationship with home department focused on professional standards and education	For the discipline and the patient group by the team; some link to home department may be retained	Significant; it's the way business is done	Moderate; distinct roles are maintained, but overlap becomes more intentional
Transdisciplinary	Patient group; weak relationship with home department; home department may not exist	Collaborative policy development for and by team with focus on serving patient needs	Significant	Significant; distinct roles are recognized, but there is intentional overlap in roles and functions

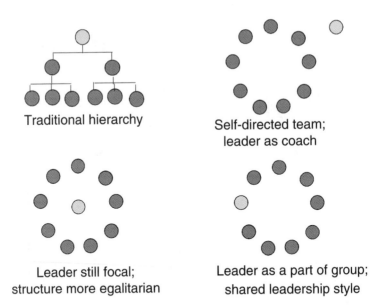

FIGURE 8.4. Common team leadership styles.

els described has advantages and disadvantages and that no single model of team operation is best in all circumstances. In the following section, we describe common geriatric settings and propose the team model that may be best suited to each. Nevertheless, we caution the reader to understand that issues well beyond patient type and setting for care influence the team structure that works best.

Decisions about organizing and managing care and distributing resources to most effectively meet the needs of defined populations of patients within geriatrics need to be context sensitive and resist the one-size-fits-all approach. Institutional administrative styles and the experience that each individual professional brings to a specific clinical situation all influence what the best team fit will be, along with the patient type and care setting. In selecting the approach to be used, consideration of how the total environment will support and facilitate—or resist—the selected approach is critical to success. The type of team does not necessarily define requirements for leadership. Regardless of the type of team (multidisciplinary, interdisciplinary, or transdisciplinary), leadership can be structured hierarchically (not inherently a bad thing, despite consistently bad press) or along various forms of shared leadership and decision making, as depicted in Figure 8.4. Again, like team configuration, there is no single leadership style that is "best"—rather, there are options to consider in light of the specific context in which leadership is required.

Orthostatic hypotension

Dehydration

Malnutrition

Delirium

Depression

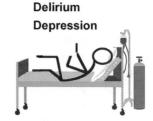

Decreased endurance

Pneumonia

Deconditioning

Contractures

Pressure sores

Constipation/urinary retention

Urinary/fecal incontinence

FIGURE 8.5. Effects of bedrest.

Geriatric Care Settings

Acute Care of the Elderly Units

Acute care of the elderly units (Palmer et al., 1998) have been designed to deliver a more comprehensive and holistic model of care for older adults in a hospital setting. These units are structured to aggressively manage medical problems, while encouraging early functional recovery and prevention of the typical iatrogenic complications of hospitalization. This would include the complications of bedrest (Figure 8.5) and hazards associated with invasive medical lines (e.g., intravenous lines, catheters, and oxygen), which restrict mobility and limit participation in activities of daily living. Interdisciplinary team approaches that bring to bear the specialized knowledge of each discipline are key to the aggressive medical and rehabilitation management of these very high-risk patients (Kresevic & Holder, 1998). The interdisciplinary team is able to collectively move away from a purely medical model of care that is typical of the hospital environment but which is actually hostile to the recovery from dynamic frailty for at-risk older adults.

Geriatric Rehabilitation Programs

Specialized geriatric rehabilitation programs target the complex older patient who experiences acute functional decline due to an acute illness being superimposed on disability associated with multiple chronic medical conditions. Identifying and managing dynamic frailty is the key issue requiring rehabilitation in this patient population. These patients are often also challenged by social isolation and cognitive disturbances and have limited physical, cognitive, and social resources to manage their declining independence. It has been demonstrated that appropriate targeting and timing of interventions for this heterogeneous patient population does affect the outcomes that may be achieved. For example, patients with mild cognitive dysfunction or extreme fatigue after an acute illness may not have the capacity to engage in aggressive rehabilitation programs, although over the long run, significant gains can be made. In other words, these patients are at risk of experiencing what may seem to be a "failed" trial of rehabilitation, which in fact may have more to do with the timing of interventions than whether the goals can be achieved at all.

Older patients with a stroke or hip fracture could be admitted to specialized units or to a more general geriatric rehabilitation unit. Decisions regarding the appropriate placement need to include an assessment of capacities in all spheres of function (physical, mental, social, and spiritual). One would expect, for example, that otherwise well persons or persons with a single syndrome (e.g., stroke) or problem (e.g., hip fracture repair) would do well in a problem-specific unit with heterogeneous age groupings. An older adult whose overall condition is more complex—and who either has or is at risk of developing chronic functional impairment—would likely do better in a unit specialized in the care of the older adult with these complex challenges.

The multidisciplinary or interdisciplinary approach is likely to be the most appropriate to the rehabilitation setting, where specialized, experienced professionals work together with the patient and family to achieve the best possible medical and functional outcome. On a geriatric rehabilitation unit, individual team members need advanced skills and experience in geriatric care to deal with the management of these frail older adults. The decision to structure a team in an interdisciplinary or a multidisciplinary model is more related to organizational culture than on any inherent advantage of one over the other in terms of meeting patients' needs.

Patients appropriate to a geriatric rehabilitation setting are challenging to manage and have complex problems because of multiple underlying chronic diseases that need to be managed in the context of the acute problem for which a rehabilitation program has been implemented. Team members need to be highly skilled in managing the geriatric giants, as well as determining the goals of rehabilitation and how they affect discharge planning. The individual goals of rehabilitation and the discharge plan should be determined in collaboration with the patient as an integral part of the team. Distinguishing between the treatable components that will improve during rehabilitation and the chronic irreversible problems determines the level of support needed to achieve the highest level of independence, particularly once the patient has been settled in his or her discharge destination. The rehabilitation approach is used to make the important distinctions between what can be fixed and what support is needed for those problems that cannot be fixed. The ultimate goals should reflect the best possible outcome in terms that are meaningful to the patient and that consider the necessary balance between independence and safety, quality of life, and appropriate management of potentially life-threatening circumstances.

At the point of transition back to the community, the appropriate team approach needs to evolve to a more transdisciplinary model to reflect the changes in patient needs once acute problems have been managed and the health status is again more stable. At discharge, highly specialized skills may remain important to continued aggressive management of acute and chronic conditions but increasingly may be focused through a transdisciplinary approach. Planning for the needs of the patient must be a dynamic process that includes ongoing assessment and reevaluation of the care needs and appropriate intervention architecture as the anticipated improvement in functional independence is realized.

Geriatric Home Care

Not surprisingly, the assessment of need is key to identifying the type and configuration of services that may be required in a home setting. Required care may be *restorative* (aimed at improvement), *assistive* (aimed toward providing assistance to overcome some chronic problem), or *supportive* (aimed at identifying and supporting the patient's own capacity to manage some chronic problem). Because the care setting is the patient's home, it is helpful to limit the number of team members who interact with the patient and his or her family on an ongoing basis. Transdisciplinary teams are important to this setting, even while we preserve and make good use of the unique contributions that each team member has to offer. Case management would be an example of how the necessary providers and skills can be coordinated in a cost-effective manner that avoids duplication of services and also avoids overwhelming the patient and his or her family. Home care teams also need to understand and include the capacities of the informal caregiver and be conscious of ways to incorporate these caregivers into the team.

It is important to develop specific goals for home care management and to consider those goals in determining the team members to be involved with ongoing service provision for a given person. If we identify restorative goals to reverse a problem, involving the team member with the right specialized training (a nutritionist or physical therapist, for example) is important. As goals move closer to being assistive or supportive, it may be that a personal care attendant is the best choice for ongoing management, coupled with periodic visits from a nurse or social worker for more detailed assessment of current status. Home care teams should be flexible and creative and seek to provide the necessary care with as few people as possible. There is great risk that well-intended home care services will "medicalize" the life experience of clients—particularly those with high needs. We should resist this and remain conscious at all times that we are entering a person's home and life in a way that can be very invasive—even violating. Particularly when supportive roles are indicated, caution should be exercised to avoid "taking over" or disenfranchising patients in areas where the intention is to support capacity rather than assist incapacity. When possible, we suggest a transdisciplinary approach that makes liberal use of cross-trained workers and carefully monitors improvements. As new capacity is achieved, interventions can be reduced, and increased independence can be facilitated. Promoting self-efficacy in these frail older adults and enhancing informal caregiver relationships heightens self-esteem and strengthens the role of that person as a member of their own care team.

Geriatric Care in the Nursing Home Setting

The goal of geriatric care in the nursing home is to create a home, not to "medicalize" the life of a frail older adult. While members of the team should assist patients in spheres of incapacity, it is important to recognize that the goal is largely maintenance of function rather than improved function. It is perhaps in the nursing home population that we find it most difficult to avoid either over- or undertreating these very frail people. It is often the case, for example, that reports of pain are overlooked and not treated appropriately. Even patients with severe cognitive dysfunction can experience and express pain—the expression of pain may not be verbal.

Our ability as health professionals to recognize and promote individual capacity in the context of often profound disability is very important to our ability to continue seeing these frail older people as valuable in their own right. Assisting these patients to continue making decisions and participating in their own life is both challenging and rewarding. Matters of valuing life and promoting dignity take on special importance in this population. Older adults do not necessarily see themselves and their bodies as an observer might. Instead, they may see themselves from the perspective of who they have been in their lives.

The job of the professional in this setting is not so much about aggressive treatment as it is about ensuring that we can see and value older persons for whom they believe they are. It is our view that one of the most important interventions is the "hello." The "hello" intervention means stopping for a moment to actually look at someone and listening to what they have to say. It means understanding that the nursing home is not actually a home for nurses, but a home for older people who are unable to manage without the support offered in such an environment, and who, if they had a choice, would rather not need such extensive care. Older adults often experience significant functional decline and die when their "homes" are institutions and their closest "family" (at least the people they see most) are strangers to them. Health care workers are warned about the dangers of becoming "involved" and about the need to remain "objective" (usually meaning distant), yet few people would choose to live their lives with people who acted that way. Compassion is part of what the "hello" intervention is about and should liberally inform interactions and care.

Transdisciplinary teams are an effective way of delivering care in this setting, where the professional skills required are directed to the more social aspects of caring rather than to highly specialized skills aimed toward improving health. Expected outcomes do not generally anticipate discharge to a more independent setting, which is not to say that discharge never happens or that it is not a laudable goal. Surely, discharges can and do happen from nursing home settings and are always a cause for celebration. Realistically, though, care is more often custodial in nature, and the creation of a warm, nurturing, and respectful atmosphere is what makes the biggest difference to the residents' quality of life.

Outpatient Setting

In the outpatient setting, the team approach needs to be much more flexible. There are many examples of care delivery models for older adults who are ambulatory. The methods for evaluating effectiveness in these programs are highly variable; analyses of cost-effectiveness must particularly be viewed with some skepticism. In fact, some studies have shown that comprehensive geriatric assessment in the day hospital setting may introduce additional systemwide costs and offer uncertain effectiveness clinically (Siu et al., 1994). On the other hand, a randomized trial of outpatient geriatric evaluation and management has demonstrated improved quality indicators but may not reduce health care use or overall costs (Toseland et al., 1997). In part, the pitfall of these studies is that they are not targeted to early intervention for acute problems. Functional gains in restorative outpatient programs for the management of chronic conditions may be minimal, simply because of when they were studied. Thus, it may be difficult to demonstrate the benefit of a geriatric intervention unless it is timed to the moment of risk rather than to the time when functional losses or recovery have already occurred.

The transdisciplinary approach potentially offers a more cost-effective approach to the initial assessment of needs and even to ongoing interventions for reversible components. We have incorporated this concept into a geriatric outpatient model of care that links the team approach to the primary care physician to manage risk of functional decline during an acute illness. We have demonstrated that early intervention reduces the complexity of the acute problem and simplifies the care plan required to prevent or curtail the functional losses that may ultimately result from that episode of illness (McElhaney et al., 1998). Combined team approaches may also be useful in this setting where a "core" transdisciplinary team (e.g., nurse, Licensed Practical Nurse, Physical Therapist) initially assess patients and as necessary call on the specialized services of a multidisciplinary team (e.g., occupational therapist, social services, speech pathology, respiratory therapy).

Summary

The aging of the population is most dramatically realized in the older-than-85-years age group. Effective interventions to prevent the increased health care demands raised by the disability experienced in this population are key to avoiding an economic crisis in health care. The cornerstones in geriatrics include the multidimensional, multidisciplinary, holistic assessment of the individual; the multidisciplinary team approach to management of acute change; and the support to maintain independence. The recognition of dynamic frailty and effective interventions that include timely and accessible services for older adults are critical for compression of morbidity in this population. Improvements in quality of life indicators generally translate into more cost-effective care. However, we continue to strive for the optimal team in the right setting at the right time to serve the needs of the individual patient.

References

Buchner, D. M., & Wagner, E. H. (1992). Preventing frail health. Clinics in Geriatric Medicine, 8, 1–17.

Cassel, C. K., & Sigell, L. C. (1998, May). Medicare for the 21st century: The goals of health coverage for our aging society. Paper presented at the annual meeting of the American Geriatric Society, Seattle.

Hebert, R. (1997). Functional decline in old age. Canadian Medical Association Journal, 157, 1037–1045.

Hoenig, H. (1993). Educating primary care physicians in geriatric rehabilitation. Clinics in Geriatric Medicine, 9, 883–893.

Kresevic, D., & Holder, C. (1998). Interdisciplinary care. Clinics in Geriatric Medicine, 14, 787–798.

Levit, K. R., Lazenby, H. C., Braden, B. R., Cowan, C. A., McDonnell, P. A., Sivarajan, L., Stiller, J. M., Won, P. K., Donham, C. S., Long, A. M., & Stewart, M. W. (1996). National health expenditures, 1994. Health Care Financing Review, 17, 220.

McElhaney, J. E., Genge, T., & McKim, R. (1998). Acute risk management clinic for seniors. Journal of the American Geriatric Society, 9, S94.

Naughton, B. J., Moran, M. B., Feinglass, J., Falconer, J., & Williams, M. E. (1994). Reducing hospital costs for the geriatric patient admitted from the emergency department: A randomized trial. Journal of the American Geriatrics Society, 42, 1045–1049.

Palmer, R. M., Counsell, S., & Landefeld, C. S. (1998). Clinical intervention trials: The ACE unit. Clinics in Geriatric Medicine, 14, 831–849.

Siu, A. L., Morishita, L., & Blaustein, J. (1994). Comprehensive geriatric assessment in a day hospital. Journal of the American Geriatrics Society, 42, 1094–1099.

Stuck, A. E., Siu, A. L., Wieland, G. D., Adams, J., & Rubenstein, L. Z. (1993). Comprehensive geriatric assessment: A meta-analysis of controlled trials. Lancet, 342, 1032–1036.

Toseland, R. W., O'Donnell, J. C., Engelhardt, J. B., Hendler, S. A., Richie, J. T., & Jue, D. (1997). Outpatient geriatric evaluation and management. Medical Care, 34, 624–640.

U.S. Bureau of the Census (1993). Population projections of the United States by age, sex, race and Hispanic origin: 1993–2050. In Current population reports (pp. 25–1104). Washington, DC: U.S. Government Printing Office.

CHAPTER 9

Sexuality in Rehabilitation: Options and Alternatives

Benita Fifield and *Shaniff H. Esmail*

> Sexual health is the integration of the somatic, emotional, intellectual, and social aspects of sexual being in ways that are positively enriching and that enhance personality, communication, and love (World Health Organization, 1975).

Since 1975, there has been a considerable increase in sexual health care curricula for health professionals of all disciplines, resulting in more effective sexual rehabilitation services for clients. Despite these improvements, surveys still show that most health professionals do not consider themselves competent to provide sexual health care, and many are unsure of their role in such services (Anderson, 1992; Conine, 1984). Clients report varying degrees of satisfaction with the sexual health services they receive. Many state that they were not asked about their sexual concerns during rehabilitation (Rodocker & Bullard, 1981). The aim of this chapter is to assist rehabilitation professionals to improve the quantity and quality of these services.

This chapter includes selected definitions of human sexuality and sexual health, a rationale for the provision of sexual information and counseling at all levels of health care, information on basic sexual physiology and common dysfunctions, and some examples of specific counseling interventions and strategies suitable for use by rehabilitation professionals in various disciplines. These strategies are intended to complement and expand—not replace—the primary traditional roles of the various health disciplines. Our goal is to provide such professionals with the knowledge, skills, and attitudes that will enable them to incorporate sexual aspects of health into their regular duties. When clients' needs go beyond this level, referral should be made to a sex therapist or a counselor, services normally found outside the hospital setting. Such personnel have the expertise required to assist clients with more complex sexual and relationship concerns. In our experience, only a minority of patients in rehabilitation require this specialized level of intervention.

Defining Sexuality

Sexual behaviors and lifestyles vary greatly from culture to culture and on an individual basis; what is acceptable for some is unthinkable for others. Attitudes toward these matters are influenced by factors such as education, laws, ethnicity, family, peer groups, personal experience, and religion. Personal values are most affected by whichever of these factors are most important to the individual. Despite the diversity of behaviors and lifestyles found in all communities, most members of Western society give strongest support to the long-standing value of sex for procreation, or at least sex in a committed, long-term, heterosexual relationship. Sexologists call this the *reproductive bias* in attitudes. There are laws in many countries against sexual behaviors that are nonprocreative, such as oral-genital sex, anal sex, and same-sex relationships. In general, according to the law in Canada, two consenting adults in private may participate in any consensual activity. However, simply making a behavior legal does not necessarily prevent those who practice it from being stigmatized by community members who may hold different views.

It is important to establish that in this chapter, sexuality is addressed as a broad concept that includes, but is not limited to, reproductive issues. Sexuality is a major component of who we are as individuals, not simply what we do sexually. We are all sexual beings from birth to death. Our needs and manner of expressing sexuality are unique to each of us based on factors such as gender, age, personality, socialization, and ethnicity.

Sexuality can be described from three aspects:

1. Behaviors—what we do sexually
2. Emotions—how we feel about ourselves and our intimate relationships
3. Knowledge and beliefs—how much information we have about human sexuality and how our own and others' beliefs affect our use of that information

Integration of these aspects of sexuality contribute to the overall health of individuals (World Health Organization, 1975).

Dailey (1984) described sexuality as having five components: sensuality, intimacy, sexual identity, reproduction, and sexualization.

Sensuality relates to our need to be aware of and accept our own body through all of our five senses. Knowledge of sexual anatomy and physiology is important in embracing and owning our body and developing a positive body image. Part of being sensual is our attraction to others. Dailey suggested that we each have an "attraction template," a cluster of certain attributes that get our immediate attention and attract us to others. This template starts early in life and "kick starts" our sexuality, often through fantasy. It could be stated that the brain is perhaps our most important sexual organ as it governs how we feel about ourselves and others and guides our behaviors. Our thoughts or opinions about our sexuality and our relationships with others can lead to feelings of guilt, shame, pride, and joy. It is suggested that most sexual counseling involves treatment of the mind rather than the body. Another important factor in sensuality is what Dailey describes as "skin hunger," that is, our need for touch. Although many consider North America to be a rather touch-phobic society, we all need physical contact with others. It has been shown that both psychological and physical well-being are enhanced by positive touch. Conversely, those deprived of positive touch may be more likely to have low self-esteem and general health concerns (Montagu, 1978).

Intimacy is described as our need and ability to experience emotional closeness to another human and to have that emotional closeness predictably returned in kind. This usually involves physical intimacy as well, but not necessarily. True intimacy involves being vulnerable through genuine caring, open communication, and appropriate emotional risk taking. Intimacy in sexual relationships requires an ability to communicate openly by giving feedback and instructions to each other, knowing and trusting that you will be heard.

Identity is another part of being a sexual person and is a continual process of discovering who we are in terms of our sexuality. We become aware of our gender at approximately 3 years of age; however, it is through our socialization, education, and life experiences that we develop our full sexual identity. Part of our sexual identity is our orientation—that is, which gender(s) we are attracted to sexually. In addition, the roles that we play as men and women are affected by our perceptions of masculinity and femininity.

Reproductive aspects of sexuality are often the most readily discussed issues as they conform to the reproductive bias referred to earlier. However, as lifestyles in our society change and more alternatives regarding conception and child rearing are sought—such as single parenthood, adoptions by gay persons, and in vitro fertilization—differences in beliefs and values produce conflict among us. Society sets moral standards of behavior through religious, legal, and cultural systems. However, individuals have the right to make their own choices based on their particular values. For individuals to make informed choices, there is a need for greater public education regarding medical reproductive technology and the effects of sexually transmitted diseases on both general and reproductive health.

Sexualization is the term used by Dailey to describe our use of sexuality to influence, control, and manipulate others. It is important to stress that although much of this component of sexuality may be viewed as negative, there are also positive aspects. Our style of dress, general appearance, and body language can be used to show respect for others and to enhance our personal and business relationships. However, those same elements can be used to coerce and harass others. Sexual messages, both positive and negative, are prominent in advertising, movies, talk shows, and print media and often lead to misconceptions about healthy sexuality. It is important that sexual health education includes a balance of positive aspects of sexuality as well as negative ones, such as assault and abuse.

These five components—sensuality, intimacy, identity, reproduction, and sexualization—are affected by an environment in which sociocultural influences such as family, ethnicity, and religion influence the quality of their development. It is important to look at the five components as an integrated whole. Each component influences and is influenced by all other components. The greater the integration of the five aspects in an individual, the more positive his or her "sexual beingness" (Dailey, 1984).

> Readers are encouraged to review their own sexuality using the five-component framework, with special attention to how the components overlap. If significant changes were to occur to one or more of the components because of disability or illness, how would they affect your sexuality? Increasing your awareness of all components of your own sexuality will enable you to better understand your clients' situations.

Need for Sexual Health Care in Rehabilitation

If we accept the premise that sexuality is an integral part of our total personality, not limited simply to our reproductive behaviors, it follows that all rehabilitation clients have the potential to have sexual concerns. The type and intensity of their concerns vary depending on their personality, age, previous experience, and the type of disability they have. However, it can be assumed that concerns fall into certain aspects, such as physical ability, emotional reactions and self-esteem, amount of sexual information, and stability and type of existing relationships.

As health professionals, you will meet clients and colleagues whose sexual values are unlike your own. While it is not necessary for you to change your values, it is important that you learn to respect other peoples' choices. In situations in which the differences of values are extreme and you choose not to discuss the issues with clients, it is your responsibility to acknowledge their concerns and refer them to another professional. Although instances of reportable behaviors, such as child abuse, are relatively rare in your practice, you should know where to find assistance for your client and yourself. Knowledge of the *Diagnostic and Statistical Manual of Mental Disorders*, fourth edition and the criminal code will help you differentiate between behaviors that are different but acceptable and those that are unacceptable (American Psychiatric Association, 1994; Dailey, 1988; Rodrigues, 1989; Rozovsky & Rozovsky, 1982).

Health professionals should have a positive attitude toward sexuality and objectivity in counseling. In addition, they must have knowledge of biological and psychological aspects of human reproduction, sexual behaviors, sexual dysfunction, and sexual diseases (World Health Organization, 1975). Because sexuality is a value-laden topic, it has been shown that acquisition of knowledge alone is insufficient in the preparation of professionals to provide sexual health services. Discussion and review of values and attitudes and opportunity to develop skills in communication and nonjudgmental sexual counseling are imperative. Basic sexuality curricula for all health disciplines should include the following:

1. Sexual values, past and present; influence of religion and culture
2. Communication skills and sexual language; taking a sexual history
3. Reproductive anatomy and physiology; sexual response; sexual dysfunction
4. Psychosexual development through the life cycle; male and female roles
5. Sexual lifestyles; role of sex in relationships and families; orientation
6. Possible effects of illness and injury on sexuality; sexually transmitted diseases; sexual assault and abuse
7. The role of the health professional as a sexual advocate, educator, and counselor
8. Sources of specialized sexual health services for referral

An overview of some of these topics is presented in this chapter. The reader is encouraged to explore other resources for further information.

Love and Relationships

The ability of couples to adjust to changes in their lives that affect their intimate relationship—such as having children, different careers, or illness and disability—depends in part on the quality and the developmental stage of their relationship. It is necessary for rehabilitation professionals to understand the developmental nature of intimate relationships to assess fully the effects of such changes on the lives of their clients, as well as in their own lives.

There are many ways of describing the development of long-term relationships. We have chosen four stages for elaboration here. Although they are described as a progressive sequence, the timing and stability of each stage depends on many factors. Couples may experience difficulties that result in a return, at least temporarily, to an earlier stage of development. Some couples may in fact never reach the later stages as described here.

The initial stage of attraction is that of *romance*. The two individuals sense the possibilities of creating a shared future together. It is characterized by intense emotions, especially passionate love. The relationship is the primary focus of their lives and is unstable in that there is a fear of rejection or of losing the love of the partner. Because of this fear, there is a reluctance to criticize or acknowledge any shortcomings in the partner (Sternberg, 1988).

As the relationship continues, a period of *power struggles* is inevitable (Hendrix, 1988). No two persons conduct their lives in exactly the same manner. When two people begin to share their lives with each other, there is a period when they must adapt to recognize and validate the priorities and needs of the other person as well as their own. Learning to say who they are and what they want as individuals is an important skill in this stage.

As the relationship reaches a stage of *stability*, the individuals learn to take more responsibility and expand their own sense of identity through interaction with each other. This stage should highlight their ability to recognize that there are three components to a couple: you, me, and us (Satir, 1972).

Mature or compassionate love is characteristic of the *commitment* stage. There is a conscious decision to work at the relationship for life. Trust is at a higher level, and the relationship feels strong and secure. There is more opportunity for each person to find their place in their community outside of the relationship. They experience themselves as interdependent and learn to live with paradoxes and insoluble dilemmas.

Most difficulties in relationships are about individual resistance to getting emotionally closer to our partner or being more independent of him or her (Schnarch, 1997). When significant changes occur, such as illness or disability, these may upset the fragile balance of interdependence of a couple. One person may have to care for his or her partner as well as take on more jobs or household-related duties. The health professional's understanding of the developmental stage and quality of the client's relationship, together with provision of appropriate support services, is important in assisting the couple to find a balance that meets the needs of both partners.

The reproductive bias leads many professionals to assume that all their clients are heterosexual. This may prevent bisexual individuals, homosexual men, and lesbian women from receiving the health services they need. For example, if a disabled male patient is not married and says he is not involved with a woman at present, do not assume that there is no need to provide advice on his sexual abilities—he may be in a relationship with a man. Orientation is about who we are attracted to sexually and romantically—same and/or other gender—and involves feelings, values, and behaviors. Bisexual, gay, and lesbian individuals and couples struggle with similar relationship issues as those who are heterosexual and need an equal variety of services and support (Hawkins, 1998). When they are ill or injured, they require health care congruent with their orientation and lifestyle. Appropriate ways of asking about this aspect of sexuality are discussed later in the chapter.

Although most people experience intimate sexual relationships at some time in their lives, there are those who choose, either temporarily or for all of their life, not to be involved in a sexual relationship. There are several terms, such as *celibate* and *abstinent*, which are associated with people who refrain from sexual activity because of religious or personal beliefs. It is important that rehabilitation professionals respect and validate individuals who make such choices. For some, celibacy excludes all forms of sexual stimulation, either with others or alone; but for many, sexual relations with other individuals are excluded, but self-pleasure and masturbation are acceptable.

Sexual Pleasure and Function

A good knowledge of sexual anatomy and the physiology of normal sexual response is needed as a basis for understanding client concerns about their sexual function and pleasure.

Sensual or sexual pleasure involves all our senses: touch, sight, hearing, smell, and taste. Individuals should be encouraged to explore ways of increasing involving all of their senses to enhance their sexual pleasure through the use of massage, candlelight, music, perfumes, and favorite foods. Pleasuring of one's body in a sensual way—for example, taking a warm bath or shower, or relaxation through meditation, movement, or dance—is a helpful way to learn about and accept one's own body and enhance relationships. Self-pleasure is often associated with sexual thoughts and fantasies. Such fantasies may occur when alone or with a partner and may be shared or kept to oneself. Some may involve rehearsal for situations likely to occur and others may allow for exploration of events unlikely to be achieved, or even not wanted in actuality.

Masturbation is usually defined as touching and stimulating one's own genitals. Although medically it is now considered to be a normal behavior that is appropriate throughout an individual's life, there is a wide range of attitudes toward masturbation. Some believe it to be a part of normal sexual release and eroticism and a way to learn about one's body. Others believe it to be dirty, selfish, unnecessary eroticism, nonprocreative, unhealthy, and therefore an unacceptable behavior. Even if accepted, masturbation is often considered to be a substitute for "the real thing" (intercourse) and acceptable mostly in given situations—such as when single or during the absence or illness of a partner. It is a difficult subject for many to discuss, but it should be included in sexual counseling, together with other sexual behaviors and topics (Rathus et al., 1997).

Many of these sensual activities discussed may be done with a partner. These activities are sometimes categorized as foreplay; however, they are an important part of sexual pleasure and fulfillment regardless of whether they are followed by sexual intercourse.

Sexual response is highly individual, however, certain common patterns exist. The most widely recognized terminology is that of Masters and Johnson (1966) who described four stages in both women and men: *excitement, plateau, orgasm*, and *resolution*. Kaplan (1974) suggested three phases—*desire, excitement*, and *orgasm*—to be a more accurate and useful description.

Sexual *desire* is the drive and interest level for sexual activity. Testosterone is the hormone that influences desire level in both men and women. Desire arises in the brain and is strengthened by fantasy and by appropriate stimulation of all the senses. When sexual desire is high, excitement occurs easily. When it is low, more physical stimulation is needed to attain the same level of arousal. Low or high desire is not necessarily a dysfunction in itself, but it may cause difficulties in a relationship if the partner has a different sexual appetite.

During sexual *excitement*, both genders experience increases in muscle tension, heart rate, and blood pressure. Sex flush and nipple erection often occur and are especially noticeable in women. In women, there is engorgement of the clitoris, labia, and vagina, together with vaginal lubrication, elevation and enlargement of the uterus, and breast enlargement. Men experience penile erection, enlargement and elevation of the testes, and sometimes Cowper's glands secretions.

The *plateau* stage is marked by continued increase in muscle tension, hyperventilation, and elevated heart rate and blood pressure. In women, the clitoris withdraws under its hood, the labia minora deepen in color, the orgasmic platform forms in the vagina, the uterus is fully elevated, and the areolas become swollen. In men, the corona becomes fully engorged, the testicles continue both elevation and enlargement, and the Cowper's glands are active.

During *orgasm*, involuntary muscle spasms occur throughout the body, most significantly in the vagina and the penis. Blood pressure, heart rate, and respiration rate peak. Orgasm is slightly longer in duration in women. Male orgasm typically occurs in two stages: emission and expulsion.

In *resolution*, the body returns to its nonexcited state, a process that may take several hours, depending on a number of factors. Kaplan suggests this is simply a state of nonresponse, not a phase of the cycle.

Although there are more similarities than differences in the sexual responses of men and women, certain important primary differences remain. As a group, women demonstrate a wider variability in their sexual response patterns. Multiple orgasms occur with greater frequency in women, more often while masturbating than during coitus. The presence of a refractory period in only the male cycle is one of the most profound differences between the sexes. This period, in which the man is unable to be aroused, varies greatly in time but usually lengthens as the man ages.

Sexual Dysfunction

A sexual dysfunction is defined as any disorder that makes normal arousal and sexual response difficult or impossible. Several dysfunctions are reviewed briefly here in regard to causes, course of the problem, and brief treatment interventions. Dysfunctions should be differentiated from paraphilias—in which arousal and response are dependent on unusual objects or behaviors, but physiologic response is intact. An example of a dysfunction would be difficulty obtaining or maintaining an erection, whereas an example of a paraphilia would be a voyeur (one who attains sexual arousal by secretly watching other people). It should be noted that conditions that are categorized as dysfunctions in the literature or by clinicians may not be of concern to an individual or couple.

Sexual dysfunction may result from organic, psychogenic, or cultural and interpersonal factors. *Organic* causes include physical trauma, illness, developmental differences, drug use, and hormone changes. Any possible organic cause should be investigated before other causes are explored. *Psychogenic* factors are associated with low self-esteem, lack of confidence, conflict of personal values, history of abuse, anxiety, and lack of sexual information. *Cultural* and *interpersonal* sources may be a result of problems arising from the conflict between predominantly repressive societal sexual values and the sexual feelings and desires of the individual or couple. Other sources may be a general lack of sexual experience, insufficient sexual information, or lack of communication skills (Rathus et al., 1997).

When evaluating clients' sexual concerns, it is important to examine the course of the problem and to determine if the problem has always existed, if it is a recent and consistent change, or if it is situational. Situational dysfunctions occur in given circumstances only—for example, with a specific partner or in a specific place. Dysfunctions may be primary (present all of life) or secondary (occurring now or sometimes).

Early treatment methods focused on Freud's psychoanalytic model. In the 1960s, Masters and Johnson introduced the behavioral approach, and later Kaplan used a combination model, which she called psychosexual therapy (Kaplan 1974, Masters et al., 1982). Today, most practitioners use an eclectic approach, which allows them to individualize their therapy and counseling to meet the needs of their clients. Common sexual dysfunctions and their causes and treatment are outlined in Tables 9.1, 9.2, and 9.3.

Sexuality and Persons with Illness or Disability

There are more similarities than differences between the sexual concerns of able-bodied people and those with illness or disability; however, for the latter, the causes of their concerns may relate to their disability. Because sexuality is usually associated with youth, beauty, and ability, it is not unusual for people with disabilities to be viewed as asexual by society. These attitudes, together with the attitudes of the disabled individual, greatly affect sexual potential. Any illness or disability has the potential to affect a person's sexuality in many ways. It is useful to group the aspects of a person's sexuality that may be affected by illness or disability into three categories:

- *General*: Self-esteem, body image, attitudes toward self and others, past/current sexual relationships
- *Function*: Arousal, potency, orgasm and ejaculation, fertility, pregnancy and delivery
- *Behaviors*: Self-pleasure and masturbation, choices of sexual activities, positioning for sexual activities, use of assistive devices

These areas of sexual concern or difficulty may be experienced by people with physical disabilities, psychiatric illness, psychological dysfunctions, intellectual impairment, or a combination of one or more of these. It is beyond the scope of this chapter to discuss all of these specifically. However, provision of sexual information and opportunity for discussion of concerns is relevant to any client population. Readers are encouraged to modify the ideas presented here to meet the needs of their own particular client population.

Factors that affect sexual adjustment include whether the condition is congenital or acquired, mild and localized or severe and systemic, stable or progressive, and visible or invisible. Additional factors are the degree and constancy of pain, the degree of bladder and bowel control, the status of the person's current relationship or if they are looking for a relationship, and the attitudes of significant others in their social network. These factors are no different from those that affect every other aspect of adjustment to illness or disability, but they are often overlooked when assessing sexual adjustment (Sandowski, 1989).

From the social and interpersonal point of view, there is an important characteristic of any disability that is often not addressed—that is, whether the disability or illness is visible to others in a public situation. Consider the differences in a social encounter with someone with a spinal cord injury using a

TABLE 9.1
Sexual Dysfunctions for Both Men and Women

Sexual Dysfunctions	Possible Causes	Possible Treatment Strategies
Sexual desire disorders		
Low or inhibited sexual desire. Lack of interest, does not initiate, does not respond, but normal physiologic function. Most common report. Difficult to resolve.	Hormonal deficiencies, illnesses Depression and anxiety Relationship dissatisfaction History of assault or abuse	Relationship counseling and sex education Therapy for psychological illnesses and abuse Behavioral exercises (e.g., sensate focus)
Compulsive sexual behavior. Constant sexual desire with pursuit of gratification, but an inability to have satisfying sexual interpersonal relationships.	Organic (e.g., disease or injury to the brain) Strong need for love but inability to relate	Lifestyle counseling or therapy Medications
Sexual aversion		
Extreme negative reaction to sexual activity. Repulsed by genitals (more often women).	Shame, fear, and anxiety History of abuse or assault	Medications Psychological counseling
Frequency of sexual activity and choice of behaviors. Partners' differences in timing, sex drive, and lifestyle demands, emotional needs, and activity preferences.	Perceived gender roles Lack of sex education Lack of trust	Identify and treat underlying causes Relationship counseling

Sources: American Psychiatric Association. (1994). Diagnostic and statistical manual of mental disorders (4th ed.). Washington, DC: Author; Kaplan, H. I., & Sadock, B. J. (1997). Synopsis of psychiatric: Behavioral sciences/clinical psychiatry (8th ed.). Baltimore: Williams & Wilkins; and Rathus, S. A., Nevid, J. S., & Fichner-Rathus, L. (1997). Human sexuality in a world of diversity. Boston: Allyn & Bacon.

TABLE 9.2
Female Sexual Dysfunction

Sexual Dysfunction	Possible Causes	Possible Treatment Strategies
Arousal disorders. Inadequate excitement and vaginal lubrication.	Diabetes Reduced estrogen levels Neurologic disorders (e.g., spinal cord injury) Anxiety or stress Narcotics, alcohol, medications Negative experiences, such as abuse	Medical intervention for physical causes Sexual counseling to reduce performance anxiety Relationship counseling
Orgasmic disorders (*anorgasmic or pre-orgasmic*). Difficulty or inability to achieve orgasm.	Most often psychological cause related to specific situations Guilt or anxiety Insufficient clitoral stimulation Often situational (e.g., orgasmic in masturbation but not during intercourse)	Counseling and education to counteract negative attitude toward sexual activity Self-exploration and massage Couple education on female sexual response Education and counseling on alternative sexual activities and use of devices such as vibrators

Dyspareunia. Painful intercourse or penetration of the vagina.	Most often inadequate vaginal lubrication Vaginal infection or sexually transmitted diseases Pelvic inflammatory disease, endometriosis, other diseases	Medical intervention for physical causes Use of artificial water-soluble lubricants Counseling for psychological causes (e.g., low self-esteem, anxiety) Education on sexual techniques (e.g., increased foreplay)
Vaginismus. Involuntary contractions of the pelvic muscles surrounding the outer third of the vaginal barrel.	Fear of vaginal penetration, often related to history of assault or abuse	Use of graduated plastic vaginal dilators Couples sexual activities with woman in control Intercourse with woman on top Counseling regarding prior abuse

Sources: American Psychiatric Association. (1994). Diagnostic and statistical manual of mental disorders (4th ed.). Washington, DC: Author; Kaplan, H. I., & Sadock, B. J. (1997). Synopsis of psychiatric: Behavioral sciences/clinical psychiatry (8th ed.). Baltimore: Williams & Wilkins; and Rathus, S. A., Nevid, J. S., & Fichner-Rathus, L. (1997). Human sexuality in a world of diversity. Boston: Allyn & Bacon.

TABLE 9.3
Male Sexual Dysfunction

Sexual Dysfunction	Possible Causes	Possible Treatment Strategies
Erectile dysfunction (impotence). Inability to achieve or maintain an erection of sufficient firmness to penetrate.	50% psychological. Diabetes (50% of all diabetic patients). Stress and fatigue. Low testosterone. Vascular problems. General illness. Use or abuse of narcotics, alcohol, and medications. Anxiety about sexual performance. Neurologic disorder.	Medical intervention for physical causes, such as medications, penile rings, vacuum pumps, penile injections, urethral suppositories, and surgical insertion of flexible or inflatable rods in the body of the penis. Psychotherapy aimed at decreasing anxiety so sexual response can occur normally. Treatment could include sensate focus.
Premature ejaculation. Inability to delay ejaculation for as long as desired.	Psychological causes Masturbating in secret, learned for immediate gratification. First sexual experience in less than ideal situation.	Goal of therapy is to train the man to focus his sensations. This focusing teaches him to anticipate orgasm and to gain control over the timing of his ejaculation.

Ejaculatory incompetence. Inability to ejaculate after penetration despite firm erection and sufficient arousal.	Anxiety. Physical causes, such as neurologic impairment, should be explored. Primarily psychological, anxiety related to penetration and ejaculation.	Two primary methods: Stop-go technique Squeeze techniques Focus on the psychological causes for the inhibition. Use a behavioral approach, such as sensate focus.
Dyspareunia. Recurrent or persistent genital pain occurring either before, during, or after penetration. Not very common.	Usually associated with an organic condition, such as herpes, prostatitis, or Peyronie's disease (curvature of penis caused by sclerotic plaques).	Medical intervention to address underlying organic causes.

Sources: American Psychiatric Association. (1994). Diagnostic and statistical manual of mental disorders (4th ed.). Washington, DC: Author; Kaplan, H. I., & Sadock, B. J. (1997). Synopsis of psychiatric: Behavioral sciences/clinical psychiatry. (8th ed.). Baltimore: Williams & Wilkins; and Rathus, S. A., Nevid, J. S., & Fichner-Rathus, L. (1997). Human sexuality in a world of diversity. Boston: Allyn & Bacon.

TABLE 9.4
Visible and Invisible Disabilities

Visible to Public	Invisible to Public
Multiple sclerosis	Heart disease
Spinal cord injury	Diabetes
Stroke	Mastectomy
Cerebral palsy	Ostomies
Amputations	Burns/scars/skin disorders
Head injuries	Hearing loss
Arthritis	Developmental disabilities
Blindness	Psychiatric illness
Burns/scars/skin disorders	Pain
Cancer	Cancer
Developmental disabilities	Chronic fatigue
Psychiatric illness	Epilepsy

wheelchair (a visible condition) versus meeting a woman who has a double mastectomy (an invisible condition). The person in the wheelchair does not have to inform any potential sexual partner that they have a disability, although he or she may later have to divulge other invisible problems (such as urinary devices) and clarify abilities (including sexual abilities). On the other hand, the woman who has had breast surgery has the difficult task of determining when and how to tell someone she is dating about her condition.

It is important not to assume that an invisible condition has less effect than a visible one on the person's social and sexual rehabilitation. It will, however, be different (Shipes & Lehr, 1980). The significance of any problem is unique to the individual living with it and should not be categorized by health professionals as a major or minor disability. Table 9.4 gives some examples of visible and invisible disabilities. Note that some appear in both lists, because the severity or location on the body may change the visibility to others and thus affect the individual differently.

A number of rehabilitation clients are elderly, so mention should be made here of some of the sexual concerns of older men and women. Interest in sexual activity and intimate relationships continues throughout life, however, there are a number of normal age-related physiologic changes that affect sexual response and self-esteem.

As men and women get older, most experience a general slowing of sexual response and a reduction in intensity of arousal and orgasm. In women, there is a decrease in vaginal lubrication and thinning of the vaginal lining that may lead to painful intercourse and possible tearing of the tissues. Orgasmic contractions are reduced, and resolution is quicker (McGracken, 1988; Thienhaus, 1988).

In men, erection is slower, less full, and disappears quickly after orgasm. The refractory period is longer, possibly as long as 12–24 hours.

Ejaculatory control is increased, but usually ejaculation is less powerful, and orgasm is less intense. Although fertility level is decreased, men do not become sterile (Laflin, 1990; McGracken, 1988; Thienhaus, 1988).

For many, the slowing down of their response provides an opportunity for closeness and pleasure, but for others, it is seen as a loss of their value as a partner. Discussion of these issues can help the individual or couple to accommodate to the changes.

For older individuals, social and psychologic concerns about sexuality are often related to their general decline in health, changes in body weight and physical appearance, or their loss of their partner. In addition, they are affected by the many common myths and the reproductive bias held by themselves and by society. These include the ideas that older people are no longer interested in sex; the only true and acceptable means of sex is through intercourse; institutionalized older adults should be segregated according to gender; privacy should be prohibited; and older people are physically unattractive and, therefore, sexually undesirable (Greengross & Greengross, 1989). Adult children of elderly individuals are often threatened by their widowed parent's interest in a new relationship and discourage such attachments. Clinicians should understand the physical changes and the psychological and social dynamics to provide information and support to their clients (Goldstein & Runyon, 1993).

Regardless of the age of the client or type of condition he or she presents, these areas of concern must be addressed in a routine manner with appropriate recording in the client's file.

Guidelines for Discussion of Sexual Health

A useful model for determining both the client's needs and the professional's level of skills in regard to provision of sexual health care is given by Annon (1976), who describes four levels: permission, limited information, specific suggestions, and intensive therapy (P-LI-SS-IT) (Table 9.5). All rehabilitation professionals should take the responsibility to apply their particular knowledge and skills to ensure they address at least the first level of intervention: permission. Levels two and three—limited information and specific suggestions—are also appropriate and within the professional expertise of most members of the rehabilitation team.

Interviewing and History Taking

Rehabilitation professionals may or may not be required to take a full sexual history as part of their role with clients; however, the following provides a framework for any interview regarding a client's sexuality.

Pomeroy et al. (1982) provide guidelines for history taking under three headings: relationship with the client, the format of the interview, and the content of the questions. Taking a history requires gathering information and not making judgments or providing solutions.

TABLE 9.5
P-LI-SS-IT Model for Sexual Counseling

Level	Explanation
Permission By bringing up the topic of sexuality, the practitioner validates sexuality as a legitimate health issue and gives the client permission to discuss sexual concerns now and later in the program.	Permission is needed by most clients. It provides them with a sounding board for their sexual concerns. Although many rehabilitation professionals may not feel confident discussing sexuality with their clients, most have adequate skills and knowledge to provide this level of service.
Limited information Practitioner should address specific sexual concerns and correct myths and misinformation.	Most health professionals' knowledge and training can be applied in a sexual context. The practitioner's primary role at this level is that of an educator. It is therefore his or her responsibility to acquire basic sexual information applicable to the area of practice. Many clients would benefit from this level.
Specific suggestions Involves taking a sexual history or profile. Definition of the problem. Course of the problem. Treatment of the problem. Ideas about causes and appropriate goals and treatment.	Fewer individuals qualified to provide this type of interaction, but fewer clients require such interaction. Counseling skills—as well as appropriate information and treatment skills—are necessary.
Intensive therapy Full history taken, specialized treatments.	Small clientele; requires special skills of sex therapist or other appropriate professionals.

Data from Annon, J. S. (1976). *Behavioral treatment of sexual problems: Brief therapy.* New York: Harper & Row.

Relationship. Treat the client as an equal and be nonjudgmental. Help the individual save face by "normalizing" the topic; that is, use your knowledge about the frequency and types of sexual behaviors found in society rather than your subjective views about right and wrong. The interviewer should be sensitive to the client's sense of timing in the discussion, but should take responsibility for the overall direction and progress of the interview. For example, know when to end long storytelling that may be used by the client to avoid discussion of specific issues.

Format. Have a systematic coverage of topics, starting with least sensitive subjects and progressing to more sensitive subjects. Avoid multiple questions and those that can be answered with yes or no. As sexuality is considered such a private subject, it may help the client if you use as little recording of the interview as possible.

Questioning. The interviewer may have his or her own concerns about the sensitive topic of sexuality and resort to general questions; however, it is important to be direct and not to use euphemisms. It is found that most clients respond more readily if you assume they have experienced a behavior or situation. That is, ask "When did you first . . ." rather than "Have you ever. . . ." Avoid suggesting answers, use appropriate words but avoid jargon, and cross-check answers for verification and inconsistencies. Close the interview by informing the client again about the purpose of the interview, reassure confidentiality, and provide the opportunity to come back to you in the future.

Sexual Health Record Keeping

Issues considered valid to the practice of each discipline are normally recorded in the client's main file and/or in the department's file. Until recently, little recording had been done regarding sexual issues, and few standardized forms have been developed by any health discipline.

To prompt rehabilitation professionals to include sexual issues in their client assessments and to validate such issues as part of their services, it is imperative that adequate recording methods be developed and used consistently (Fifield & Fifield, 1988). All clients old enough to comprehend the questions should be asked about sexual concerns. Language and the details of discussion should be tailored according to the professional's judgment, experience, and expertise and in regard to the perceived needs of the individual patient. However, exclusion of sexuality in a comprehensive assessment of a patient is inappropriate and based on judgments, such as, this person is too young or too old, too ill, single, or not sexually attractive. All people are sexual. Some may have concerns that they wish to discuss but are afraid to do so. You are responsible for bringing up this subject just as much as any other in your assessment and treatment of your clients.

Table 9.6 provides a basic template for rehabilitation professionals to use in their practice while conducting an initial sexual health interview.

TABLE 9.6
Sexual Health Care: Brief Initial Interview Record

Patient data:
Name: In/Out pt: Age:
Diagnosis: Other:

Note: Ask open-ended questions to encourage patients to give their interpretation of the situation. Validate their concerns and provide information throughout the interview.

Questions/Statements	Rationale
Opening statement	
Many people have sexual concerns related to their illness or disability, so I am going to ask you a few questions on that subject now. (Wait/respond to comments or questions.)	Shows importance of sexuality as part of rehabilitation
	Assertive
	Gives permission to discuss issue
	Validates that client is not alone
How has your illness/disability affected how you think of yourself as a man/woman/boy/girl?	Pertinent to self-esteem
	Need for introspection
	Open ended, a chance for them to describe
Are you sexually involved with a partner at present? (In the past?) With more than one partner? With men and women?	Pertinent to their health and sexual rehabilitation
	Makes no assumptions regarding activity, behavior, or orientation
	Permission to discuss current or future changes
Has your illness/disability affected your interest in sexual relationships and activities? Your ability to . . . be sexually aroused (how)? reach orgasm (how)? ejaculate (how)? choose positions for sexual activity (how)? participate in different sexual activities, such as masturbation, intercourse, oral sex (how)?	Specific, no euphemisms
	Follows the sexual response cycle
	Focuses on pleasure and reproduction
	Open-ended questions allow client to describe problem as he or she understands it

How long have you had difficulties? Have you had these difficulties before?	Describes course of problem
Are you able to discuss these concerns with your partner/someone in your family/friend?	Determining if the concern is pre- or postdisability Provides information regarding support system and openness to communication
Medications/alcohol/illicit drugs, may affect sexual function—tell me about your use of these.	Side effects need to be explored
Do you have any information on fertility and pregnancy, as well as on the importance of safe sex and prevention of disease? Would you like such information?	Relates to sexual health and contraception Preventive
Would you be interested in further discussion individually/with your partner/in patient group sessions?	Sets stage for sexual discussion/rehabilitation
Do you have questions you would like to ask me?	Gives the client some control and opportunity to bring up areas not addressed in the interview

Closing statement

Sexuality is an important part of all our lives. If you have any questions or concerns, ask to see me. If I do not have the information, I will try to find it for you.	Provides opportunity for them to come back when they are ready

The questions listed should be asked of all clients. However, practitioners are encouraged to add further questions pertinent to their client population and their own role in the provision of sexual health care.

Options and Alternatives

There are many strategies and techniques that can be suggested to clients to help enhance sexual functioning. It is not our intention to provide specific recipes for various illnesses and disabilities. It is crucial that the practitioner be client centered and identify each individual client's unique situation based on the client's assets and deficits, culture, and motivation.

One of the most important strategies a practitioner can use is to help the client become aware of the situation and to realize that sexual activity does not have to be terminated because of illness, disability, or aging. This may involve the reassessment of sexual activity and factors affecting it after the onset of an illness or disability. In rehabilitation services, there should be an open and caring environment that allows for sexuality discussion and education. This can be done by demonstrating a positive attitude toward sexuality and by including the topic in the normal assessment routines. Practitioners should demonstrate a nonjudgmental approach by using neutral tone and language. They should also be aware of limitations and know when and where to refer if they determine that more expertise is required. The P-LI-SS-IT model provides a mechanism to assist in making such decisions. Through open communication, being a good listener, and respecting clients' privacy and modesty, the practitioner will be able to validate clients' concerns. Clients should be encouraged to talk about any fears they may have about beginning or resuming sexual functioning. When discussing their altered body functions and sensations, including those in the genital area, it is important to emphasize the potential for positive, pleasurable experiences while at the same time acknowledging their disability. Although many sexual concerns relate directly to the limitations imposed by the individual's illness or disability, it is important to determine the onset of a problem. For example, a woman who has acquired a spinal injury and expresses no interest in having intercourse with her husband may have participated very little in this activity before the onset of her disability. Taking an adequate sexual history to differentiate dysfunctions that occurred after the illness/disability from those that occurred before is vital to successful counseling (Garner & Allen, 1988). The practitioner should discuss issues with both the client and his or her partner if possible.

When clients are first attempting to resume sexual activity, they may be anxious about various sexual issues, such as sexual abilities and performance, physical appearance, and whether their partner will find them attractive. Partners may also experience similar anxieties because of a lack of knowledge of the condition, fear of hurting the other person physically or emotionally, and coming to terms with their own reactions to changes in their partner's abilities and appearance. To decrease such anxiety, they should be encouraged to begin gradually, starting with cuddling, touching, and masturbation activities before resuming more complex or difficult sexual interactions, such as intercourse (Garner & Allen, 1988). It can be suggested that clients arrange for private times for exploration of their body and discussion with their partner to develop their understanding of their own sexual anatomy and response. For this purpose, a sensual awareness program, as we describe, can be used.

Sensual Awareness

Graded, progressive activities are used by rehabilitation professionals in most disciplines. This same approach can be used in sexual health interventions. The purpose of sensual awareness is to teach those with altered body functions that are due to illness or injury to learn or relearn sensual and sexual activities that feel pleasurable to themselves and their partners (Fifield & Fifield, 1986). Although it is based on Masters and Johnson's sensate focus regime, it does not use their highly structured schedule of specific activities that was designed to assist able-bodied couples to overcome difficulties in their sexual lives (Masters et al., 1982).

It is important that the couple is provided with privacy for this activity. Some rehabilitation facilities have private rooms or a suite where clients can practice their skills before returning home. However, it may be necessary to wait until the client is allowed to leave the facility for a few days or is discharged to fully use this regime. If it is acceptable to the clients, it is suggested that the exercises take place in a room with a comfortable temperature, in the nude, and on a bed of sufficient size. Some couples may wish to first explore less threatening areas of the body with some or all of their clothes on and later progress to nudity.

The objectives for the disabled person and their partner are to

1. Increase awareness of his/her own and partner's body sensations.
2. Learn to enjoy his/her own and other's body.
3. Develop greater satisfaction in physical experience together.
4. Enhance intimacy emotionally and physically.
5. Increase ability to talk openly about sexual thoughts and feelings.
6. Develop trust to talk openly about other options for sexual behaviors.

Activities for Sensual Awareness

Partners are instructed to take turns as giver and receiver:

- The giver applies various kinds of touch in all areas of the body (e.g., light caress, scratch, or firm pressure).

- The receiver gives feedback as sensations occur, pleasurable and nonpleasurable, including general body reactions as well as local sensations (e.g., shivers, goose bumps, and changes in blood pressure).

Awareness of all reactions is especially important for the disabled person so that he or she may learn to associate altered sensations with pleasurable experiences, but overall this should be a mutual experience without special focus on the person with the disability. It is important that the discussion is focused on what is happening at the time rather than making comparisons with predisability situations.

Touching and kissing are activities that are often described as foreplay, implying that they should lead to something else, namely intercourse or orgasm. Sensory awareness may or may not lead to climax as the couple chooses, but they should be encouraged to focus on the activities as a pleasurable and nongoal-directed learning experience.

Suggested Positions for Sensual Awareness Exercises

Suggested positions include:

- Lying on one's side, with pillows for support (this allows a disabled person to see and touch the partner without worrying about balance)
- Sitting supported by pillows or the head of the bed, partner back-first between legs
- Sitting, leaning forward, partner facing with legs over disabled person's legs to assist balance

Although sensual awareness is described here for couples, similar activities of self-exploration can be suggested to single clients. Such individuals may need assistance with positioning, removal of their clothes, and provision of assistive devices such as a hand mirror, before being left alone in the privacy of their own room.

In addition, the practitioner can assist with discussing positioning during sexual activity and evaluating the advantages and disadvantages of various positions. The primary goal is to help the client to be aware of and to experiment with different positions to increase function, comfort, and pleasure (Laflin, 1990).

Positioning for Heterosexual Intercourse

Depending on the individual's preferences and physical abilities, there are many possible positions for enjoying intercourse. The advantages and disadvantages of the most commonly used positions are described here (Rathus et al., 1997).

Male-Superior (Man-on-Top) Position

The male-superior position is often referred to as the *missionary position*. In this position, the partners face one another. The man lies above the woman, perhaps supporting himself on his hands and knees rather than applying his full weight against his partner. This position allows a couple to face one another so that kissing is easier. The woman may run her hands along her partner's body, stroking his buttocks and perhaps cupping a hand beneath his scrotum to increase stimulation as he reaches orgasm. This position makes it difficult for the man to caress his partner while simultaneously supporting himself with his hands. The position therefore may not be favored by women who enjoy having their partners provide manual clitoral stimulation during coitus. This position can be highly stimulating to the man, which can make it difficult for him to delay ejaculation. This position also limits the opportunity for the woman to control the angle, rate, and depth of penetration. It may thus be more difficult for her to attain the type of stimulation she may need to achieve orgasm, especially if she favors combining penile thrusting with manual clitoral stimulation. Finally, this position is not advisable during the late stages of pregnancy. At that time, the woman's distended abdomen would force the man to arch severely above her, lest he place undue pressure against her abdomen.

Female-Superior (Woman-on-Top) Position

In the female-superior position, the couple faces one another with the woman on top. The woman straddles the man from above, controlling the angle of penile entry and the depth of thrusting. Some women maintain a sitting position; others lie on top of their partners. Many women vary their position. With this position, the woman is psychologically—and to some degree, physically—in charge. She can move as rapidly or as slowly as she wishes with little effort, adjusting her body to vary the angle and depth of penetration. She can reach behind her to stroke her partner's scrotum, or lean down to kiss him. As in the male-superior position, kissing is relatively easy. In the female-superior position, the man may readily reach the woman's buttocks or clitoris to provide manual stimulation. Because of the increased stimulation and control of this position, it can facilitate orgasm in the woman. In contrast, this position tends to be less stimulating for the man, and it may help him to control ejaculation. For these reasons, this position is commonly used by couples who are learning to overcome sexual difficulties.

Lateral-Entry (Side-Entry) Position

In the lateral-entry position, the man and woman lie side by side, facing one another. This position allows each partner relatively free movement and easy access to the other. The side-by-side position, as well as changing positions, should be encouraged to decrease joint pressure. For clients with balance and perceptual deficits, lying on the side with pillows for support allows the client to see and touch the partner without worrying about balance.

Sitting Coital Positions

In the sitting coital positions, the man is usually sitting in a chair or on a bed, while the woman sits astride him and either faces toward or away from him. Unless the woman's weight is excessive, these positions can be very restful for both partners. This position can be useful for someone using a wheelchair, especially if he or she has difficulty transferring to a bed.

All of these positions describe heterosexual intercourse, but the same principles can be applied when discussing anal intercourse, use of dildos, or genital-to-genital contact with heterosexual, gay, or lesbian lovers.

Other Possibilities

It may be necessary to help clients to explore options other than sexual intercourse as forms of sexual expression and fulfillment. These may include masturbation, mutual masturbation, and oral-genital stimulation. Fellatio (oral stimulation of the male genitals) and cunnilingus (oral stimulation of the female genitals) are considered viable options by many individuals who choose to explore other forms of sexual expression or for whom intercourse may not be a realistic option.

When educating clients, it is first important to dispel any myths and misperceptions. For example, it may be necessary to reassure a client of the unlikelihood of another cardiac episode occurring during sexual activity (Hackett & Cassem, 1984). Clients should be informed about the possible effects of their illness or disability on sexual functioning. For example, a hemiplegic client may need to be told about the effects that perceptual or sensory deficits may have on their sexual functioning. Another area that needs to be addressed is medications. If clients are presently taking medications, they should be advised to consult their physician or pharmacist about possible medication side effects that could influence sexual functioning.

For clients who are experiencing pain and general discomfort, the practitioner should encourage them to seek a physician's guidance if pain occurs during sexual activity (Butler & Lewis, 1976). Advice about timing of medications, such as taking analgesics before sexual activity, may be appropriate. Another suggestion for pain is the use of a waterbed or pillows for increased comfort (Laflin, 1990) and the use of heat (heating pad, tub bath, shower, or paraffin wax) and relaxation techniques before sexual activity. Exercising is another strategy that may be used to decrease pain by increasing or maintaining range of motion and muscle strength and decreasing spasticity.

It is also the practitioner's responsibility to provide information on the availability of other devices and interventions that may aid sexual function and satisfaction. An example of this is encouraging the use of a vibrator if the hands are weak or uncoordinated. The vibrator can be adapted to strap onto the hand (Laflin, 1990). For clients with mobility issues, suggesting various assistive equipment such as grab bars or a trapeze bar can assist with positioning and movement during sexual activity. For clients who have poor physical endurance and fatigue easily, instructions should be given on basic energy conservation techniques, such as a rest before sexual activity. Placing full-length mirrors in treatment facilities and encouraging clients to do the same in their homes may assist them in reevaluating and maintaining their body image and self-esteem. Provision or recommendation of hand mirrors or other assistive devices for private use may be appropriate.

If the illness or injury has an effect on sexual arousal, the following suggestions may be helpful. If a women's vaginal lubrication is reduced and causing discomfort, the use of a water-soluble lubricant may be suggested. There are several methods to assist men with erectile difficulties, including medications, penile rings, vacuum pumps, penile injections, urethral suppositories, and surgical insertion of flexible or inflatable rods in the body of the penis. Clients and their partners should be informed of these possibilities and given the opportunity to discuss them with their physician or other appropriate professional.

Through application of their knowledge of body structure and function and their skills in teaching adaptation to illness and disability, rehabilitation professionals can help in identifying and overcoming specific limitations in sexual functioning through education, therapeutic strategies, and the use of equipment and devices. As stated earlier, there are many strategies and techniques. In using the various approaches described, the practitioner must examine each individual's specific situation and apply the various strategies as necessary to meet the client's needs.

Case Studies

The following scenarios illustrate possible sexual concerns that may be presented by clients during a sexual health assessment. This section is not intended to focus on solutions to client concerns but rather to demonstrate how to initiate the topic (permission), discuss specific issues (limited information), and collaborate with the client on dealing with their concerns (specific suggestions).

Case Study 1

Jennifer is a 29-year-old woman who indicates she had an onset of weakness from the trunk downward approximately 16 months before admission. She was diagnosed with multiple sclerosis. Since the onset of her symptoms, she has had several episodes of exacerbation and remission. She entered the rehabilitation center for evaluation and to gather information that would assist her in maintaining as much independence as possible.

Jennifer has normal range of motion in both upper and lower extremities. However, she has decreased strength, some incoordination, and tremors. She has urinary incontinence, mostly when lying down, and she uses intermittent self-catheterization. She cannot walk but can transfer from her wheelchair with assistance. She fatigues quickly, cannot tolerate heat, and finds cold weather helps her energy level.

Jennifer has been married for 9 years and has a 3-year-old daughter. She worked as a cashier at a local grocery store, but stopped work because of her illness. She has very few leisure pursuits and primarily spends her time with her husband and daughter.

Initial Sexual Health Assessment

Some of the concerns Jennifer has regarding sexuality are as follows:

She expresses concern about not fullfilling her role as a wife and mother. Specifically, she feels guilty regarding her lack of sexual activity and not meeting her husband's needs. She also reports having decreased sensation during intercourse. Before her diagnosis, she had orgasms regularly during intercourse; however, since her illness, she has been unable to achieve an orgasm during intercourse or masturbation.

Another major issue for her is poor tolerance and endurance for sexual activity. She reports being too tired to even consider having sex, and when she does, she finds she fatigues easily and is "wiped out" for the rest of the day. She wants to be able to discuss her concerns with her husband and requests some information to share with him. The option was given to her to include him in later sessions.

Jennifer expressed interest in information on the following areas, which were provided in subsequent sessions:

- The possibility of pregnancy and risks associated with it
- The risk of injury during sexual activity as a result of reduced sensation and lubrication
- Options for increasing pleasure, for example use of a vibrator and lubricants
- Energy conservation strategies
- Strategies for management of incontinence, e.g., limiting fluids and emptying the bladder before sexual activity

Case Study 2

Eric is a 24-year-old man who was burned in an apartment fire, which he evidently caused by falling asleep while smoking. He sustained approximately 30% second- and third-degree burns to his face, ears, nose, shoulders, chest, back, and arms, with the most severe burns on his hands and face. He has skin grafts to the back of his neck, arms, and hands, with amputation of the left index finger and right fifth finger. He has some contractures, especially in the shoulders, mildly limiting abduction bilaterally. In addition, he has flexion contractures of the elbows and some stiffness of the fingers of both hands. However, these do not greatly impede his general functioning.

Eric is single and lives alone. He completed high school and attended vocational school for instruction in data processing, but did not complete the course of study. For the previous 3 years, he was a mail carrier, and he is concerned that he will not be able to return to that occupation. Eric's previous pastimes included playing cards, watching TV, visiting with a friend next door, and going dancing with his many female friends. Since his injury, he has avoided social contact, and his primary leisure pursuits involve watching television.

Initial Sexual Health Assessment

The initial interview elicits very little response from Eric. Several days later, he approaches the staff member and asks to discuss some sexual concerns.

His appearance is his primary concern. He has not had a sexual relationship since his accident. He cannot see himself being involved in a sexual relationship in which someone would see him without his clothes.

Eric describes himself as having been quite adventurous in the past and was sexually active in a number of short-term relationships. Although Eric states that he fantasizes about past sexual relationships, he is afraid of rejection and tries not to think about it.

When asked, Eric reports having no difficulties with sexual response while masturbating. However, he expressed some general discomfort that is due to scarring in his hands. Use of a lubricant was suggested to reduce friction, and the option of a vibrator was introduced.

He has avoided discussing his sexual concerns with friends or family, and the sexual health assessment is the first time he had approached someone to discuss sexual issues. He was reassured that he was not alone in his concerns. Eric asked for any suggestions the staff member might have with regard to his concerns.

To increase his confidence and self-esteem, Eric was encouraged to increase his social contacts as opposed to looking for sexual partners immediately. In addition, it was suggested that he discuss some of his sexual concerns with a close friend he can trust. Further referral for counseling regarding his body image and self-worth was explored.

Conclusion

Being able to choose from several alternatives is a situation toward which most people strive. For example, people want freedom of choice to buy certain commodities, to select a certain job, to take one of several possible vacations, and to be able to interact with confidence with other people in a variety of situations and in a variety of ways. This freedom of choice, variety of behaviors, and control over one's life is equally important in the area of sexuality.

People with disabilities—both physical and mental—are encouraged to develop their general abilities to a level that provides them with choices. For example, people who are paralyzed in the legs learn how to transfer from a wheelchair to a variety of other objects—such as car, bed, toilet, and floor—to allow them choices and alternatives in mobility. Similarly, when assisting people who are mentally disabled, a variety of methods are stressed when teaching them self-care skills, vocational skills, and hobby interests, to promote motivation and increase their quality of life.

Physical and mental differences associated with various disabilities, as well as personal attitudes and values, may prohibit, change, or present difficulties with some sexual behaviors. It is important that individuals have alternative behaviors from which to choose if they wish to do so.

Attitudes concerning sexual behaviors are influenced by cultural, social, and religious traditions, as well as by many misconceptions and myths. Sexual behaviors acceptable to some are not acceptable to others. Providing accurate sexual information and teaching sexual skills to people with illnesses or disabilities gives them sexual alternatives. They may select behaviors and lifestyles compatible with their physical and mental abilities, value systems, and sexual desires.

To present such alternatives to their clients, helping professionals may first have to assess their own sexual attitudes and values and acquire necessary information. If the professional is able to communicate in a nonjudgmental manner, the client will learn to trust and will seek assistance.

All persons are sexual. Some have greater opportunity than others to express their sexuality in a positive manner.

References

American Psychiatric Association. (1994). Diagnostic and statistical manual of mental disorders (4th ed.). Washington, DC: Author.

Anderson, L. (1992). Physical disability and sexuality. The Canadian Journal of Human Sexuality, 1(4), 177–185.

Annon, J. S. (1976). Behavioral treatment of sexual problems: Brief therapy. New York: Harper & Row.

Butler, R., & Lewis, M. (1976). Sex after sixty: A guide for men and women for their later years. New York: Harper & Row.

Conine, T. A. (1984). Sexual rehabilitation: The roles of allied health professionals. In D. W. Kreuger (Ed.), Rehabilitation psychology: A comprehensive textbook. Rockville, MD: Aspen Systems Corp.

Dailey, D. (1984). Does renal failure mean sexual failure? The Renal Family, 6, 2–4.

Dailey, D. (1988). Understanding and helping the sexually unusual. In D. Dailey (Ed.), The sexually unusual (pp. 3–13). New York: Harrington Park Press.

Fifield, B., & Fifield, O. (1986). Spinal cord injury: Use of sensate focus. In Proceedings of the 14th Federal Conference of the Australian Association of Occupational Therapists (pp. 104–107). Brisbane, Australia: Australian Association of Occupational Therapy.

Fifield, B., & Fifield, O. (1988). Sexual health care: The need for standards. In Proceedings of the 16th World Congress of Rehabilitation International (pp. 460–464). Tokyo, Japan: World Congress of Rehabilitation International.

Garner, W., & Allen, H. (1988). Sexual rehabilitation and heart disease. Journal of Rehabilitation, 55, 69–73.

Goldstein, H., & Runyon, C. (1993). An occupational therapy education model to increase sensitivity about geriatric sexuality. Physical & Occupational Therapy in Geriatrics, 11(2), 57–76.

Greengross, W., & Greengross, S. (1989). Living, loving and aging. London: Age Concern.

Hackett, T. P., & Cassem, N. H. (1984). Psychological aspects of rehabilitation after myocardial infarction and coronary artery bypass surgery. In N. K. Wenger & H. Hellerstein (Eds.), Rehabilitation of the coronary patient (2nd ed.). New York: John Wiley & Sons.

Hawkins, R. O., Jr. (1998). Educating sexuality professionals to work with homoerotic and ambierotic people in counseling and therapy: A voice from the trenches. Journal of Sex Education and Therapy, 23(1), 48–54.

Hendrix, H. (1988). Getting the love you want. New York: H. Holt & Co.

Kaplan, H. I., & Sadock, B. J. (1997). Synopsis of psychiatric: Behavioral sciences/clinical psychiatry (8th ed.). Baltimore: Williams & Wilkins.

Kaplan, H. S. (1974). The new sex therapy. New York: Brunner Mazel.

Laflin, M. (1990). Sexuality and the elderly. In C. Lewis (Ed.), Aging: The healthcare challenge (2nd ed.) (pp. 330–355). Philadelphia: F. A. Davis Company.

Masters, W. H., & Johnson, V. E. (1966). Human sexual response. Boston: Little, Brown & Co.

Masters, W. H., Johnson, V E., & Kolodny, R. C. (1982). Human sexuality. Boston: Little, Brown & Co.

McGracken, A. L. (1988). Sexual practice by elders: The forgotten aspect of functional health. Journal of Gerontological Nursing, 14, 13–17.

Montagu, A. (1978). Touching: The human significance of the skin (2nd ed.). New York: Harper & Row.

Pomeroy, W. B., Slax, C. C., & Wheeler, C. C. (1982). Taking a sexual history: Interviewing and recording. New York: The Free Press.

Rathus, S. A., Nevid, J. S., & Fichner-Rathus, L. (1997). Human sexuality in a world of diversity. Boston: Allyn & Bacon.

Rodocker, M., & Bullard, D. (1981). Basic issues in sexual counseling of persons with physical disabilities. In D. Bullard & S. Knight (Eds.), Sexuality and physical disability (pp. 277–282). St. Louis: Mosby.

Rodrigues, G. P. (Ed.). (1989). Pocket criminal code. Toronto: Carswell.

Rozovsky, L. E., & Rozovsky, F. A. (1982). Legal sex. Toronto: Doubleday Canada Ltd.

Sandowski, C. L. (1989). Sexual concerns when disability or illness strikes. Springfield, IL: Charles C. Thomas.

Satir, V. (1972). People making. Palo Alto, CA: Science and Behavior Books, Inc.

Schnarch, D. M. (1997). Passionate marriage, New York: W. W. Norton & Co.

Shipes, E. A., & Lehr, S. T. (1980). Sexual counseling for ostomates. Springfield, IL: Charles C. Thomas.

Sternberg, R. J. (1988). The triangle of love: Intimacy, compassion, commitment. New York: Basic Books.

Thienaus, O. (1988). Practice overview of sexual function and advancing aging. Geriatrics, 43, 63–67.

World Health Organization. (1975). Education and treatment in human sexuality: The training of health professional (p. 6). Geneva: Author.

CHAPTER 10

Functional Assessment

Deanne Scoville Anderson

A Paradigm Shift in Health Care

Health care has undergone dramatic change since 1990. Amidst the change, rehabilitation has prospered. As hospitals have reduced the number of acute care beds, rehabilitation beds have increased (Keith, 1991). Outpatient and home health services continue to grow as well. The number of physical, occupational, and speech therapy practitioners continues to grow, along with the rehabilitation need.

For many years, rehabilitation professionals were educated in their clinical areas of expertise, with little awareness of the education and contribution of other professionals. However, technology has improved, quality of life and long-term disability have increased, and a larger population of aging individuals requires comprehensive rehabilitative care (Keith, 1991). With this in mind, the cost of expanded services and comprehensive care must be addressed.

Managed care and prospective payment systems aim to contain cost while maintaining quality of care. This changing model of health insurance has encouraged clinicians and health care organizations to address how care is delivered and by whom. It has reinforced the need for practitioners to work as a team to provide the most comprehensive, cost-effective services, with the best possible outcome (Evans, 1995).

Traditionally, therapy services have not been required to objectively qualify their outcomes (Landrum et al., 1995). Therapy service began with evaluation and ended when the patient reached the best possible level of independence. Time and cost were rarely considered. Each discipline evaluated the patient in a service-oriented manner, completing standardized and

---

Medical model

Assess/Diagnose ≡ Treat ≡ Wait for Result ≡ Discharge

Outcome-based model
Assess/Identify Skill Requirement for Success in the Discharge Setting ≡
Project Outcome ≡ Define Barriers ≡ Define Resources Available ≡ Manage
for Results

FIGURE 10.1. The medical model begins with assessment, and the clinicians wait
for results. Discharge is addressed at the later stage of treatment. Outcome-based
rehabilitation is proactive, addressing discharge on initial assessment of the client.
(Reprinted with permission from Landrum, P. K., Schmidt, N. D., & McLean, J. A.
[1995]. Outcome-oriented rehabilitation: Principles, strategies, and tools for effective program management [pp. 151]. Rockville, MD: Aspen Publishers. © 1995
Aspen Publishers, Inc.)

nonstandardized assessments. At best, the clinicians met and discussed the
patient's status, but more often, each discipline worked alone and addressed
individual goals with little overlap. Consideration of patient goals and the
intended outcome were addressed toward the middle or end of the treatment program. This was due, in part, to the rehabilitation delivery system
or medical model: treat the patient until they are better (Figure 10.1).

Cost containment and comprehensive services have advanced the
rehabilitation profession toward outcome-oriented rehabilitation. Identification of the intended outcome of the service provided—as well as justified—the need for each involved service. In essence, the identification of
the outcome justified the rehabilitation professional's existence.

Rehabilitation professionals appear to have accepted the model of
comprehensive care with greater enthusiasm than the medical community
of physicians. It has been very difficult for physicians to relinquish responsibilities or allow other professionals to carry out common procedures that
they once completed independently (Begun & Lippincott, 1987). However,
the comprehensive team is essential to treating the whole person. Restoration of function in decreased physical, psychological, social, and vocational
skills requires all disciplines to be involved (Keith, 1991). Each discipline
provides a distinct, but complementary role in client treatment and outcome (Begun & Lippincott, 1987; Landrum et al., 1995).

As the treatment team has evolved, so has the role of the patient and
family. Health care cost containment has enhanced the role of the family
in identifying the expected outcome of a client's care. The clinician must
now address the family early in the treatment process to identify the prior
level of function, amount of assistance, and family resources available in

caring for the client (Begun & Lippincott, 1987). The information then becomes part of the assessment and treatment planning process.

However, as an increasing aged population is living longer, there are several implications for family care. The family unit may include an elderly parent and elderly child. This can limit the family resources or amount of assistance that a child is able to provide to his or her parent. Also, the extended family has evolved to a nuclear family. Many clients have strong family units, but they live thousands of miles away. The implication is a greater need for independence or increased reliance on the health care system for solutions.

Transitional living, intermediate care, assisted living, and expanded home health care are examples of the growing solutions to care for the disabled. In all of the identified areas, a client's functional skills in activities of daily living (ADLs), mobility, and safety are the primary considerations for placement in the appropriate setting (see Case Study 1) (Keith, 1991). The specific activities addressed with the client in Case Study 1 are listed here. If the expected outcome for this client is assisted living, what are the most important functional areas to address? And what level of function would the client need to reach in each area to reside at home, in an assisted-living situation, or in a long-term care facility?

- Bathing, dressing, grooming
- Toileting—skill and continence
- Mobility
- Medication management
- Ability to make basic wants/needs known
- Safety and carryover with all of the above tasks

Consideration is taken for level of assistance, amount of verbal and tactile cues, and assistive devices required. Thus, a person's ability to live in a specific setting depends almost entirely on his or her ability to carry out functional tasks.

Functional assessment is the starting point for the functional outcome. It seems clear that comprehensive care and function-based evaluation provides the necessary information to establish a treatment plan that will lead to a client's ability or inability to function in an identified environment (Landrum et al., 1995).

What Is Function?

Function, as defined by the Random House dictionary, is "the kind of action or activity proper to a person, thing or institution; the purpose for which something is designed or exists; role" (Random House, 1987). To assess function, one must understand its meaning. Historically, occupational therapists have identified function as a client's ability to perform daily tasks related to ADLs and instrumental activities of daily living (IADLs), work, and leisure. Assessment by the occupational therapist includes data collection related to the daily life activities that are important to the individual. For example, the life roles and functional tasks that are important to a college student may be very different from the roles and tasks that are important to the same student's grandparent. Independence in driving, daily social activity, and employment may be the functional tasks that are most important for the college student and his or her personal satisfaction. However, the grandparent may be retired and enjoy the company of only a close group of friends who live within the same senior housing complex. Thus, independence and functional assessment may differ for each person. This is due to age, gender, personality, and the situational context.

Clinical Perspective

Physical therapists have routinely identified a patient's status based on assessment in areas of strength, range of motion (ROM), and gait pattern. Documentation of improvement has been based on incremental changes in a muscle grade or increased ROM of a joint. In the past, this process had been sufficient in justification of continuing therapy services (Cornely & Coffman, 1998). However, with the onset of managed care and changes in the American Medicare system, the focus of reimbursement is on functional outcomes (Keith, 1991). Therefore, health care professionals are beginning to recognize the need to identify functional performance measurements that will sustain them into the twenty-first century. This will mean a change in not only how to assess, but also what to assess, and how to treat the patient. The focus is now on individual function and function within the community.

Historically, the speech and language pathologist has used structured, standardized testing to assess the cognitive and language skills of the client. The outcome would reflect a numeric score or percentage versus a functional representation of cognitive or language skills. Documentation of a change in comprehension may be reflected as 50% to 60% accuracy in auditory comprehension at a sentence level. Although very important, it has been more difficult for the lay person and the reimbursement source to translate the relevance to daily function.

What is the context of a client's life? At a vision conference presented by occupational therapist Mary Warren, she described that the clinician is merely an act in the play of the client's life. As a therapist, one is not expected to change the course of the play or the outcome, but to assist the client to the next act. Therefore, it is important to identify what *function* is to the client. Think for a minute of what it means to you to be "functional." Identify where you are in life. Think about what was important to your independence 5 years ago, what is important now, and how this may change in 5 years. Once the therapist has an understanding of what it means to be functional in his or her own environment, he or she can then look into the client's environment and begin to understand and assess function.

Difficulty may arise as each member of the team attempts to define his or her role in assessment. For years, rehabilitation professionals have used standard assessment and documented their findings accordingly. Figure 10.2 represents a clear delineation between occupational, physical, and speech therapy. The areas assessed are distinct to each discipline, and goals are written accordingly. For example, if the client is noted to have 20 degrees of limited shoulder flexion by goniometric measurement, the goal is then to increase shoulder flexion by 20 degrees. If the client is a major league pitcher or enjoys tennis as a form of recreation, then the 20 degrees of shoulder flexion is a functional deficit and must be addressed. In the example, assessment by functional measures—as opposed to standard goniometry—may not identify a deficit in shoulder flexion. In another example, if on standard assessment a client reveals comprehension of single words, the goal may be to increase comprehension to phrase-length material. In this instance, the standardized assessment may have been a repetitive task with little meaning to the client. Therefore, comprehension was notably limited. Functional assessment, which occurs in the context of a restaurant with questions related to food, may reveal that the client has greater comprehension skills.

As health care progresses toward functional assessment, standardized assessment becomes more of the exception instead of the rule. The assessments that 10 years ago identified specialization of a discipline are now fading. The question becomes "What do I assess, and how?" Until recently, specialization has maintained the boundaries and clarified the differences between disciplines (Keith, 1991). As functional assessment has become more prevalent, therapists begin to overlap in their assessment procedures and treatment activities. For some, it is difficult to accept this change. However, as Keith (1991) notes, "Challenges to customary forms of treatment are difficult for professionals because such forms are built on long-standing traditions of practice and belief. History has shown that change is inevitable."

Rehabilitation and health care are constantly changing. Therefore, the professional must understand the similarities and differences among the disciplines and respect each other's role in functional assessment:

- *Occupational therapists* bring an understanding of the whole person in relation to physical, psychological, and cognitive skills. Assessment relates to work, play, and self-care. In general, assessment has been based on standardized techniques, observation of tasks, and interviews.
- *Physical therapists* provide a strong knowledge of the physical skills necessary for mobility, including balance and gait. Their

Physical Therapy Initial Evaluation

| Right | | | Left | |
PROM	AROM	Motion	PROM	AROM
		Scapular Elevation		
		Depression		
		Protraction		
		Retraction		
		Shoulder flexion		
		Extension		
		Abduction		
		External rotation		
		Internal rotation		
		Elbow flexion		
		Extension		
		Supination		
		Pronation		

Physical Therapy Clinical Skill Assessment

Lower body	WFLs	IMP	Comments
Lower-extremity Strength			
Coordination			
Sensation			
Endurance			
Edema			
Balance			
Pain			
Tone			
Posture			

Occupational Therapy Evaluation

Pinch	Right	Left
Lateral	lbs.	lbs.
Pincer	lbs.	lbs.
3-Jaw chuck	lbs.	lbs.
Grasp	lbs.	lbs.
	lbs.	lbs.
Sensation	A=absent I=impaired INT=intact	Comments
Light touch		
Deep pressure		
Temp./pain		
Dull		
Localization		
Proprioception		
Stereognosis		

FIGURE 10.2. Excerpts from discipline-specific evaluation tools. (AROM = active

---

Speech Therapy Assessment

Current diet: _____

Results of bedside swallow evaluation: _____

❒ Refer for modified barium swallow

❒ Oral phase/Pharyngeal phase (Circle) Dysphagia

Summary of cognitive and communication assessment findings:

Standard assessments utilized:　　❒ Boston Naming Test
　　　　　　　　　　　　　　　　　❒ Minnesota Test for Differential Diagnosis
　　　　　　　　　　　　　　　　　　 of Aphasia
　　　　　　　　　　　　　　　　　❒ Boston Diagnostic Aphasia Examination
　　　　　　　　　　　　　　　　　❒ Rivermead Behavioral Memory Test
　　　　　　　　　　　　　　　　　❒ Other:_____

FIGURE 10.2. *continued.* range of motion; IMP = impaired; PROM = passive range of motion; WFLs = within functional limits.)

assessment focuses on standardized techniques, observation, and mobility in daily life.

- *Speech therapists* provide an understanding of language (comprehension and use) and cognitive skills as they relate to the client's ability to communicate and function in daily life.

All three disciplines are important in understanding the complexities of the human body after injury or onset of disease. Therefore, each should respect the role of the other and learn from the knowledge and expertise of the subsequent discipline.

Components of Functional Assessment

Client-Centered Interview

Chart review or medical history is the logical place to begin when initiating the evaluation process. Oftentimes a client's chart may list numerous diagnoses, past medical history, and psychosocial issues, although on standard evaluation procedures, the patient appears to be functioning at a high level. However, the opposite may occur, and a patient with a fairly benign medical history may, on evaluation, have notable deficits in functioning. In either case, unless the therapist has an adequate awareness of the patient's personal history and life roles, the initial assessment is incomplete.

On more than one occasion, a therapist may evaluate a patient with a complex history, and on ADL and mobility assessment find that he or she requires significant assistance for self-care (e.g., bathing, dressing, grooming) and transfer activities. Therefore, the goals would be to increase functional independence in the area of self-care and mobility. However, on further interview of the client or primary caregiver, it becomes apparent that the client has required assistance for these tasks for an extended period of time. Thus, the goals for treatment are not as relevant as once thought, and the treatment plan changes dramatically.

A significant amount of information may be obtained by client interview. However, the client may not be an accurate historian or may be physically unable to participate in the interview process because of fatigue or communication deficits. In this case, the significant other, or a primary caregiver, should be contacted to verify and provide information. In some instances, a case manager is present in the organization to obtain necessary information. However, most often it is the rehabilitation therapist who interacts with the client directly and gathers the most pertinent and accurate data.

Basic client interview should include open-ended questions, and address topics such as "What activities are important to you?" "Describe a typical day," and "What relevance do certain activities have in your daily life?" (Landrum et al., 1995). Once the client begins to describe a typical day, other questions may be generated, such as "Are you currently enrolled in an education program?" or "Do you drive a car or use public transportation?" This provides information regarding physical mobility needs and cognitive skills necessary for daily function of the client. For instance, if the client reports the need to use city transit, he or she must

- Be aware of the schedule.
- Manage a morning routine to catch the bus on time.
- Ambulate or have a means of mobility to access the transit.
- Generate alternative solutions if he or she misses the bus.

Use of public transportation also implies that the client must have sufficient communication to ride city transit and the cognitive skills to be aware of the route and the appropriate bus line and adequately manage the money or tokens necessary to ride the transit.

The information gathering described is the part of functional assessment that provides the therapist with a means to the end or an outcome. If the therapist is aware of the client's functional level before disability, then it provides for a more efficient and accurate assessment of the client (Figure 10.3). During an interpersonal exchange, the client is able to provide information that informs the clinician of client preference regarding care. This also allows for communication of information that is vital to diagnostic and

Health and Medical Management

Diagnosis_____Onset _____

MD_____

Past/present medical history_____

See MD history and physical for detailed information

Client interview

	Previous functional level (A=Assist, I=Independent, D=Dependent)	Assistance provided by:
Toileting	_____	_____
Wash/dress	_____	_____
Meal prep	_____	_____
Household gait	_____	_____
Stairs/steps	_____	_____
Community gait	_____	_____
Driving	_____	_____
Shopping	_____	_____
Other	_____	_____

Equipment used at home:_____

Previous home services:_____

Previous rehab:_____

Prior vocational status: ❐ Disabled ❐ Retired ❐ Currently employed
❐ Part time ❐ Full time
vocation:_____

Level of education:_____

Language barrier: ❐ Yes ❐ No   Interpreter needed: ❐ Yes ❐ No

Support system:

Lives: ❐ Alone ❐ With spouse ❐ With other:_____

Primary support:_____Works: ❐ FT ❐ PT

Drives: ❐ Yes ❐ No

Able to provide physical assist: ❐ Yes ❐ No

Concerns/limitations:_____

Other support:_____

Home environment:

Steps to enter: ❐ Yes ❐ No How many?_____ Railing: ❐ Yes ❐ No

Bedroom on_____floor

Ability to be more accessible?_____

Bathroom on _____floor

FIGURE 10.3. This form illustrates information that may be obtained from the client/caregiver interview. Questions are generated to provide accurate information and documentation. (Adapted with permission from Gaylord Hospital, Wallingford, Connecticut.)

Funding:
  Managed: ☐ Yes ☐ No
  Case manager:_____
  Preferred providers: Y   N _____
Anticipated discharge outcome:
Client goals for discharge:_____
  ☐ Home ☐ Alone ☐ w/Family or significant other ☐ w/Home services as
                                                              necessary
  ☐ transfer to extended care facility ☐ skilled nursing facility ☐ transitional living
  ☐ other_____

FIGURE 10.3. *continued*

treatment modalities (Cornely & Coffman, 1998). This holds true for the physician as well. If, on interview, you determine that the client required assistance for ADLs before his or her current admission to the facility, then the occupational therapist may not address ADLs, unless level of assistance has declined. In some cases, assessment may only focus on the use of adaptive techniques or the caregiver's skill level in providing assistance to the client. Similarly, if the client reports use of an assistive device for ambulation before the current episode of illness, then the goal is to return to the prior functional level of gait with the appropriate assistive device.

Hence, the client-centered interview is the beginning of a good functional outcome. It provides the clinician with knowledge of who the client is and what the context of his or her life is. It also allows the therapist to identify which functional assessment—standard or nonstandard—is most appropriate in identifying the patient's level of function for return to daily living. The focus of health care is quality and efficiency. Some clinicians feel this cannot be done. They interpret quality to mean lengthy rote assessment and standardized evaluation procedures. Although relevant, much of the same information may be gathered by client interview and functional assessment.

Discipline Contributions

Each discipline brings a knowledge base specific to its area of expertise. Not all disciplines are necessary in assessment of a client's disability; however, when appropriate, input from a speech and language pathologist, physical therapist, and occupational therapist is comprehensive and benefits the client. Physical therapy is the best understood and most used therapeutic intervention of these three rehabilitative services. Rehabilitative

Case Study 1

A client, 40 years of age, who recently experienced a stroke, reports that it is important for her to complete her own laundry (which is located in the basement of her home), prepare light meals (hot and cold), and speak with her siblings on the phone, several of whom live in the next state.

Based on client report, identification of three tasks in this patient's life have been revealed as important to daily function: meal preparation, home management, and effective communication. Therefore, as a therapist you may decide to assess each task individually or identify the skills necessary to complete each task, then evaluate each skill.

settings include pediatric, geriatric, inpatient, outpatient, and home care services. Physical therapists, in general, provide assessment of balance, gait, ROM, strength, and all areas of movement dysfunction.

Occupational therapy is often the second-most used in the physical rehabilitation setting. Focus of evaluation and treatment is on functional skill in daily tasks. This includes ADLs, home management, upper-body function, cognition, and visual skills related to daily living.

Speech therapy is the least utilized of services. This is due in large part to the specialization of speech and language pathology in which evaluation and treatment focus on the following areas: speech, language, comprehension, cognition, and social aspects of communication and swallowing disorders (www.asha.org). Also, speech therapy may be the least understood by the medical profession in relation to their scope of practice.

Functional assessment begins with knowledge of the tasks that are important to the client. As discussed earlier, this can be obtained by interpersonal communication with the client or the client's family.

Activity Analysis

Because our discussion focuses on functional assessment, you may, in fact, assess both the task and the components of each task. However, before assessment or evaluation, the therapist must do an activity analysis. Activity analysis has long been used by occupational therapy to "understand an activity and its explicit components; that is, the aspects of the activity which are evident and will be present regardless of the context, the therapeutic goals, or the frame of reference within which the activity is to be used" (Hopkins & Tiffany, 1988). For the therapist in training, activity analysis assists in development of problem solving and clinical reasoning skills. This occurs through actual written analysis of the activity and each component part. As a clinician gains more experience, activity analysis occurs without a written protocol or format. It is second nature. It is what

TABLE 10.1
Basic Steps of Functional Tasks

Laundry	*Phone Conversation*	*Peanut Butter/Jelly Sandwich Preparation*
Gather laundry	Obtain phone book	Obtain bread, peanut butter,
Sort laundry	Locate number	jelly, knife, and plate
Transport to washer/dryer	Recall phone number	Open bread and containers
Load washer	Dial phone	Place bread on plate
Add detergent	Converse on phone	Pick up knife
Turn washer on	Hang up phone	Place knife in jar and remove
Remove clothes	Recall conversation	Spread jelly on bread
Place in dryer		Spread peanut butter on bread
Turn on dryer		Place bread slices together
Remove dried clothing		Eat sandwich
Fold clothing		
Return to drawers		

evaluation and treatment are based on—the performance skills and their component parts that are necessary to complete the task. Table 10.1 visually identifies the steps of the three tasks. The laundry task, if broken down into each subskill required, would encompass the three disciplines of occupational therapy, physical therapy, and speech and language pathology. For example, the task requires, but is not limited to, upper- and lower-body strength, gross and fine motor coordination, high-level cognitive skills of organization and categorization, short-term memory, and sequencing.

Are there other skills that may be required to complete the task? Review the phone conversation and simple meal preparation task and identify what physical, cognitive, and visual skills may be necessary to complete each task. It may be "easy" to identify the skills, but more difficult to identify which discipline is responsible for assessment of the tasks.

As clinicians, the performance area assessed has always been defined by discipline. Typically, the physical therapist assesses the lower body for gait, balance, ROM, and strength. Occupational therapy assesses upper-body strength, ROM, coordination, and ADLs. Speech and language pathology assesses language, comprehension, cognition, and dysphagia. However, as prospective payment systems and managed care have emerged, the need for less specialized assessment and greater focus on the actual task has occurred. This causes role blurring and turf wars. However, the confident therapist is able to look beyond this and respect each discipline for its area of expertise and knowledge. If this occurs, each clinician may decide to assess the client together, still addressing areas of function with which they are familiar. The end result is a comprehensive assessment of the client's function, as well as development of improved communication and mutual respect among team members. In the end, the client benefits from the comprehensive commitment of the health care team to the goal of rehabilitation: improvement or prevention of disability (Christiansen, 1993). Thus, interdisciplinary teams have become more prevalent, and documentation of assessment procedures has begun to focus on functional area versus discipline specificity (Figure 10.4).

Health care organizations are also focusing on the outcomes of their services as a whole versus each component part. This is a paradigm shift for health care in the United States. Canadian and British health care systems reveal a less fragmented health care system with less specialization (Grumbach & Bodenheimer, 1995). National health care has a more generalized approach. This parallels changes in the delivery of rehabilitative care by occupational therapy, physical therapy, and speech and language pathology practitioners. Rehabilitation is moving away from specialized evaluation toward functional, general assessment. This is not true for all areas of rehabilitation; however, physical dysfunction in home health, outpatient, inpatient, and subacute care is less specialized and more integrated. Often, professionals forget that their position in the larger professional community is complemented by those who surround and support their efforts (Christiansen, 1993). Although functional assessment is a challenge to customary evaluation and treatment measures, it is inevitable. Rehabilitation professionals must have the ability to monitor and influence the direction of this change (Keith, 1991).

Assessment of Function

It is important to remember that functional assessment is client centered and not discipline specific. Therefore, as discussed earlier, the initial part of the assessment is identification of who the client is and what his or her specific roles are in daily life. This occurs through the interpersonal exchange and interview. You may wish to develop your own written interview (see Figure 10.3). When developing the initial part of the assessment, it is important to first ask yourself what questions, if posed to you, would describe what your roles are in daily life and what tasks are important to you on a daily basis? Also, how would you identify your current skill level in completing each task? Once you are able to understand the purpose of the interview and how to ask the "right" questions, you will be more efficient and concise in the interview process.

It is also essential to identify if the client is able to communicate and provide accurate information. Is the client a good historian? The clinician may need to address family members for a more accurate initial assessment of the client's functional skills before illness or injury. Also, the knowledge of the speech and language pathologist may be essential if the client has had a stroke or traumatic brain injury that has caused cognitive or language dysfunction.

Cognition/Communication

Cognition:	WFL	IMP	Comments	Initials
Attention				
Memory				
Functional problem solving				
Reasoning				
Executive functions				
Safety ❑ Requires supervision ❑ Can dial 911	Orientation ❑ Person ❑ Place ❑ Time ❑ Reason for hospitalization			

Comments:_____

_____

_____

Cognition/Communication

Communication:	WFL	IMP	Comments	Initials
Intelligibility				
Follows 1 2 3 4				
Step commands				
Follows: ❑ Basic questions ❑ Moderate length questions ❑ Multiunit Y/N questions				
Follows: ❑ Familiar conversation ❑ Unfamiliar				
Expresses basic wants/needs				
Functional reading tasks				
Biographical information				
Functional writing				
Other				

❑ Requires further assessment of cognitive deficits

❑ Hearing evaluation recommended/completed

❑ Requires further assessment of language deficits

Comments:_____

_____

_____

FIGURE 10.4. This form provides a comprehensive functional assessment, including the areas addressed in a comprehensive evaluation. (CL MGMT = clothing management; IMP = impaired; LE = lower extremity; OT = occupational therapist;

Initials	Signature	Initials	Signature

Self-care

ADL	NA	7	6	5	4	3	2	1	Comments
Feeding									❏ With adaptive equipment
UE wash									❏ Bed ❏ W/C ❏ Shower
LE wash									❏ Bed ❏ W/C ❏ Shower
UE dress									❏ Bed ❏ W/C
LE dress (pants)									❏ Bed ❏ W/C
LE dress (shoes/socks)									❏ Bed ❏ W/C
LE brace/ prosthesis									❏ Bed ❏ W/C
Grooming									❏ Bed ❏ W/C
Bathroom transfers									
Toilet transfer									❏ Ambulate w/out device ❏ Ambulate w/device ❏ Stand pivot ❏ Sliding board
Tub transfer									❏ Ambulate w/out device ❏ Ambulate w/device ❏ Stand pivot ❏ Sliding board
Clothing management									
Hygiene									
Other									

Comments:_____
_____
_____

FIGURE 10.4. *continued.* PT = physical therapist; PTA = prior to admission; SB = sliding board; SLP = speech language pathologist; SP = stand pivot; UE = upper extremity; W/C = wheelchair; WFL = within functional limit.) (Adapted with permission from Gaylord Hospital, Wallingford, Connecticut.)

Functional Mobility

Mobility	NA	7	6	5	4	3	2	1	Comments
Bed mobility									
Lateral transfers									❏ With adaptive device ❏ Stand pivot ❏ Sliding board
Car transfers									❏ With adaptive device ❏ Stand pivot ❏ Sliding board
Floor transfers									❏ Bed ❏ W/C
LE dress (pants)									❏ Bed ❏ W/C
W/C mobility									❏ Bed ❏ W/C
W/C management									❏ Bed ❏ W/C
Gait on level									❏ With adaptive device ❏ Without adaptive device
Gait on elevations									❏ With adaptive device ❏ Without adaptive device
Other									

Comments:_____

_____

_____

Score explanation   **7** Independent   **6** Independent w/equipment, extra time or safety considerations   **5** Supervision and/or cues   **4** Minimal assist   **3** Moderate assist   **2** Maximal assist   **1** Dependent

PT _____   Date _____

OT _____   Date _____

SLP _____   Date _____

❏ Home management   ❏ WFL _____

❏ Obtaining prepared items from the refrigerator

❏ Simple cold meal prep

❏ Other_____

❏ Simple hot meal prep

Kitchen safety: ❏ Supervision   ❏ Cues   ❏ Minimal assist
                  ❏ Moderate assist
                  ❏ Maximal assist   ❏ Unsafe for kitchen activities

FIGURE 10.4. *continued*

❐ Money management_____
❐ Light Housekeeping:_____
❐ Driving PTA   ❐ Not an active driver
❐ Retired   ❐ Working PTA:_____

Comments:_____
_____
_____

Treatment/Care Plan

Long-term goals	Short-term goals
Cognition/Communication	
___Oriented X _____ ___ Self-transport to therapy ___ Self-scheduling ___ Use of compensatory strategies for visual/ cognitive deficits during_____ ___Attend to functional task for_____ with/without cues in a quiet/busy environment. ___Recall daily events with/without strategies (memory book/daily planner). ___Generate solutions to daily tasks with safety awareness with/without assistance ___Functional cognition for daily ADL/ mobility/home management.	
ADLs	
___UE Wash___UE Dress ___Grooming ___LE Wash___LE Dress ___Hygiene ❐ bed level ❐ sinkside ❐ shower	
Mobility	

___Toilet transfers SP SB   Amb w/ device
                                          Amb w/out device
___Tub transfers   SP SB   Amb w/ device
                                          Amb w/out device
___CL MGMT ___Hygeine
___Bed mobility
___W/C to/from bed SP SB   Amb w/ device
                                          Amb w/out device
___W/C to/from car SP SB   Amb w/ device
                                          Amb w/out device
___Gait _____FT. w/device w/out device
___Elevtions _____W/C mobility	

FIGURE 10.4. *continued*

Long-term goals	Short-term goals
Other	
___Family training completed in ADL/toilet transfers/ambulation/stairs/car transfers. mobility/home management. Discharge and equipment needs _____ _____	

Initials___Signature_____Initials___Signature_____

FIGURE 10.4. *continued*

Once the initial interview/history of the client is determined, the clinician identifies what functional assessment is necessary and where to begin. Functional assessment may be broken down into several areas, depending on the client's cultural background, roles, occupation, and prior level of function. However, for the purpose of this chapter, we focus on assessment of basic life skills and functional abilities (Table 10.2).

Specific skill areas (such as vision, cognition, strength, ROM, and sensation) are not addressed in Figure 10.4, as they are inherent skills required to carry out each of the identified tasks. A physical therapist may argue that it is necessary to first measure ROM with a goniometer and strength via manual muscle testing before requesting the patient to stand or ambulate. However, it is possible to ambulate with limitations in ROM and strength, and this can be observed during the actual task, without formal goniometric measurement of joint motion. The same is true for cognition during meal preparation. The ability for the client to attend and shift attention between each item, sequence the task, recall each step, and show adequate safety awareness are all cognitive skills observed during a meal preparation task. The skills that are often evaluated independently may be observed in the context of the patient's involvement in the task.

Contextual Observation

Along with physical ability or level of assistance required, further observation of the client identifies the need for cueing or adaptive techniques during task completion. This provides a more accurate portrait of the client. ADL, mobility, and cognitive assessment may be completed by direct observation of patient participation in the task. It is important to assess the client in the context in which they are most familiar.

TABLE 10.2
Assessment of Basic Life Skills and Functional Abilities

Daily living activities: Dressing, hygiene, grooming, toilet use, eating, activity
    planning or scheduling, home care or management, meal planning and preparation
Communication skills: Interaction with others, whether related to spoken or
    written communication or some adaptive communication procedures
Physical mobility: Bed mobility, wheelchair mobility, walking, and community
    access
Vocational/leisure activities: Preparation for employment, preparation for school,
    vocational or other leisure-related activities

- *Example 1: ADL assessment.* Client has taken showers for 50 years
  and has never taken a sponge bath seated at a sink. The most accurate assessment occurs with the client in the shower.
- *Example 2: Home management assessment.* A client is asked to
  prepare a meal. The clinic has a microwave and stovetop. The client
  has never used a microwave oven. The microwave is not incorporated into the assessment. It may be addressed later if it appears to
  be a better treatment alternative for the client's outcome.
- *Example 3: Short-term memory assessment.* A client reads the
  newspaper daily. Initially, he questions the need for speech and
  occupational therapy intervention. The therapist would like to
  understand how well the client understands what he has read and
  how well he carries over the information. Assessment should focus
  on reading the daily newspaper (which is relevant to the client) and
  reflecting this information back to the clinician.

As stated earlier, many standardized functional assessments limit the
need for specific evaluation of performance areas, such as muscle strength
or short-term memory. Function is the outcome; therefore, it should be the
initial measurement as well.

Common Language

A clinician should not rely on one assessment alone. Often several assessments—standardized and nonstandardized—are required to completely
understand the client's status. Also, the importance of team communication before, during, and after assessment cannot be underestimated. This
provides greater understanding of the client and the goals and provides
greater continuity of care (Keith, 1991).

    As clinicians begin to work more closely together, it reinforces the need
for universal terminology. It is important for clinicians to qualify a client's
status in similar terms and to clearly understand each term (Table 10.3).

TABLE 10.3
Functional Assessment and Impairment Terminology

A client who is *independent* requires no cues. A client who requires *supervision* to *maximal assistance* (numbers 2–7) may require cueing that is visual, verbal, or tactile in nature.

Independent: Client is consistently able to perform skill safely with no one present.

Supervision: Client requires someone within arm's reach as a precaution; low probability of client having a problem requiring assistance.

Close guarding: Person assisting is positioned as if to assist, with hands raised but not touching client; full attention on client; fair probability of client requiring assistance.

Contact guarding: Therapist positioned as with close guarding, with hands on client but not giving any assistance; high probability of patient requiring assistance.

Minimum assistance: Client is able to complete majority of activity without assistance; completes 75% of the task without assistance, and therapist provides 25% of the total assistance.

Moderate assistance: Client is able to complete part of the activity without assistance; completes 50% of the task without assistance, and therapist provides 50% of the total assistance.

Maximal assistance: Client is unable to complete the activity without a majority of assistance from the therapist; client completes 25% of the task without assistance, and the therapist provides 75% of the total assistance.

Dependent: Client is unable to complete the activity without complete assistance from the therapist.

Source: Adapted from Guccioni, A. (1994). Functional assessment. In S. P. O'Sullivan & T. Schmitz (Eds.), <u>Physical rehabilitation assessment and treatment</u> (3rd ed.) (197). Philadelphia: F. A. Davis.

Many facilities choose to incorporate outcome-based evaluation measurements in their assessments as well. The most widely recognized and accepted measurement is the Functional Independence Measure (FIM). The Uniform Data System identifies 18 FIMs that have proven to be important in terms of long-term success of rehabilitation. The areas of self-care, bowel and bladder control, mobility (bed and transfers), locomotion (community/residential), communication, and social cognition are rated using a 7-point scale. Originally, the scale was designed to provide a score after a summation of all 18 items. However, subsequent research has revealed that the items represent two category constructs: motor skills and cognition. The FIM is used by rehabilitation facilities to compare their performance with other similar facilities on an ongoing basis (Fisher, 1993; Fisher et al., 1995). Most often, FIM scores are observed and rated by the trained therapist at admission (initial assessment) and discharge (Fisher et al., 1995). In facilities where the FIM is used, functional data must be collected on admission. The information is more precise if it is gathered by clinicians with expertise in the assessment of each area. The rehabilitation therapist is most successful in identifying the FIM score in conjunction with support staff. However, initially the functional data must be collected, and it becomes more precise if it begins with the client's initial evaluation and is rated on a similar scale as the FIM (see Figure 10.4).

Efforts to use functional assessment are often viewed by clinicians as nonstandardized and thus an invalid approach to evaluation. However, there are a number of standardized assessments that do relate to function and may satisfy the clinician or reimbursement source that identifies standardization as necessary for accurate, reliable information.

A standardized assessment has established and tested norms. An assessment that is reliable "measures a phenomenon dependably, time after time, accurately, predictably and without variation. Instruments should have strong inter-rater reliability, or agreement among multiple observers of the same event" (Guccioni, 1994). In an effort to use functional assessments with the greatest degree of accuracy, scoring criteria must be clear, mutually exclusive, and strictly applied to each situation. Each therapist must undergo periodic review of testing procedures. Validity of an assessment is multifaceted. It attempts to identify if the assessment truly measures the attribute that it is expected to measure. Also, it identifies the quality of the assessment based on appropriate application and how the data is interpreted (Guccioni, 1994).

Standard assessment is often not a consideration at the payer level. Because rehabilitative therapy is a reimbursable service, the payer is interested in the outcome of the patient's treatment. If initial evaluation occurs and the anticipated outcome is good, the payer expects that the money is well spent. The payer may be interested in an evaluative measure that may predict outcome and relates to the patient's functional skills. In this case, standardized functional assessment may be used. However, more often, it is strictly based on functional tasks. The payer is more likely to understand and accept responsibility for payment of a service that will "increase balance and locomotion as it relates to the client's ability to ascend and descend the ten stairs to attend work daily" versus "increase balance to Good (G) and increase ambulation to 200 feet with an assistive device." Therefore, the clinician must identify assessments that meet the client, payer, and clinician needs. Time required for assessment and documentation must also be considered.

Table 10.4 reviews standardized functional assessments, including the physical performance test (Figure 10.5).

Implementation: How to Make It Work

An acute rehabilitation treatment setting is more conducive to organized comprehensive treatment, but the clients are removed from their own envi-

TABLE 10.4
Standardized Functional Assessments

Assessment	Type	Description	Features
Assessment of Motor and Process Skills (AMPS)[a]	Structured tasks	Assessment of ADL and IADL. Clients are rated on 15 motor-skill items and 20 process-skill items after observation in performance of two or three IADL tasks. Client chooses an IADL task that is familiar out of a field of 50.	Client choice. Used to predict future performance.
Kohlman Evaluation of Living Skills (KELS)	Structured interview with tasks	Assessment of ADL and IADL skills, such as in self-care, safety and health, money management, transportation, telephone work, and leisure activity.	Clear directions for observation, recording, and implications for community living. Easy to administer and score.
Rivermead Behavioral Memory Test (RBMT)	Structured interview with tasks	Assessment of adult and geriatric cognitive skills—specifically attention, orientation, and memory. Assessment of daily routine tasks that require visual and auditory memory.	Designed to determine a person's ability to function in basic living skills. Clear directions for observation and recording, four parallel versions. Easy to administer and score in a half-hour session.
Physical Performance Test (PPT)[b]	Structured with tasks	Assessment of nine items, which include writing, simulation of eating, lifting and removing items, locomotion, and stair climbing. Task assessment involves balance, coordination, strength, and endurance (see Figure 10.5).	Identifies a client's deficits in ADL and IADL. Useful for documentation of progress. Easy to administer and score in a brief period of time.
Berg Balance Scale[c]	Structured with tasks	Adult and geriatric assessment within 14 items, scored on a 5-point scale. Detection of balance impairment and pro-	Easy to administer in most environments with little equipment.

Assessment	Method	Description	Administration
		gress over time. Also used to predict falls, evaluate outcomes of intervention, and identify clients who will benefit from formal therapy.	Easy to administer and score.
Behavioral Assessment of Dysexecutive Syndrome (BADS)	Structured with tasks	Assessment of adults with cognitive dysfunction in the areas of planning, organization, decision making, and judgment. Activities include map reading, time estimation, and mile following.	
Test of Everyday Attention (TEA)	Structured interview with tasks	Assessment of adults with cardiovascular accident, traumatic brain injury and Alzheimer's disease. Test of attention based on everyday tasks. Written and auditory testing occurs with familiar tasks. Tasks include a map search, auditory and visual elevator tasks, telephone directory search, and lottery activity.	Easy to administer and score, with three parallel versions.
Communicative Abilities in Daily Living (CADL)[d]	Structured interview using pictures and photographs to describe various everyday contextual situations	Assessment of functional communication skills in aphasic adults. Incorporates daily language activities to assess a client's functional adequacy versus degree of aphasic involvement. The test simulates communication in daily situations (e.g., using the telephone, shopping).	Easy to administer in 45 minutes to 1 hour. Communication effectiveness is rated on a scale of 0–2.

ADL = activities of daily living; IADL = instrumental activities of daily living.

[a]Fisher, A. G. (1993). The assessment of IADL motor skills: An application of man-faceted rosch analysis. American Journal of Occupational Therapy, 47(4), 319–329.

[b]Brown, M. (1998). The physical performance test for the assessment of frailty. Geri Notes, 5(4), 7–9.

[c]Berg, K. (1998). The Berg balance scale. Geri Notes, 5(4), 12–14.

[d]Holland, A. L. (1980). Communicative Abilities in Daily Living. Austin, Texas: Pro-Ed.

Physical Therapy Assessment
Physical Performance Test　　　(PPT)
Date _____/_____/_____
　　　　M　　　　D　　　　Y
Test # _____
Tester _____　　　　　　　　　Subject (Last)_____(First)_____

1. Book lift 　　To score..........If time is	≤2 sec = 4 2.1-4 sec = 3 4.1-6 sec = 2 >6 sec = 1 Unable = 99.9	Trial 1____ ____ ____ Trial 2____ ____ ____
2. Lab coat 　　To score..........If time is	≤10 sec = 4 10.1 – 15 sec = 3 15.1 – 20 sec = 2 >20 sec = 1 Unable = 99.9	Trial 1____ ____ ____ Trial 2____ ____ ____
3. Pick up nickel 　　To score..........If time is	≤2 sec = 4 2.1-4 sec = 3 4.1-6 sec = 2 >6 sec = 1 Unable = 99.9	Trial 1____ ____ ____ Trial 2____ ____ ____
4. 50-foot walk 　　To score..........If time is	≤15 sec = 4 15.1-20 sec = 3 20.1-25 sec = 2 >25 sec = 1 Unable = 99	Trial 1____ ____ ____ Trial 2____ ____ ____
5. Climb one flight 　　To score ....If time is	≤5 sec = 4 5.1-10 sec = 3 10.1-15 sec = 2 >15 sec = 1 Unable = 99.9	Trial 1____ ____ ____ Trial 2____ ____ ____
6. Chair rise 　　To score........If time is	≤11 sec = 4 11.1-13.9 = 3 14-16.9 = 2 >17 sec = 1 Unable = 99.9	Trial 1____ ____ ____ Trial 2____ ____ ____
7. Climb 4 flights 　　To score........If time is	4 flights = 4 3 flights = 3 2 flights = 2 1 flight = 1 Unable = 0	Score____ ____ ____

8. Turn 360 degrees in the direction of choice.　　　　　　　　　Discontinuous score 1 ____75
　　To score... Discontinuous steps = 0, Continuous step = 2　　　Unsteady score 2 ____76
　　　　　　Unsteady = 0, Steady = 2

9. Standing balance

To score........	Full tandem	Semitandem	Side-by-side	
4	10s	10s	10s	Side-by-side_____
3	3-9s	10s	10s	
2	0-2s	10s	10s	Semitandem_____
1	Unable	0-9s	10s	
0	Unable	0-9s	0-9s	Full tandem_____

FIGURE 10.5.　Physical therapy assessment: Physical performance test (PPT).
[Reprinted with permission from Brown, M. [1998]. The physical performance test
for the assessment of frailty. Geri Notes, 5[4], 7–9.]

ronments. Conversely, home health care delivery is more fragmented, but the client performs in a familiar environment. Each rehabilitation setting has its limitations, therefore, the clinician must recognize the differences and account for this during assessment. Also, the clinician must attempt to relate the assessment task to real life. This is much easier to carry out in the home. Essentially, acute rehabilitation focuses on skill acquisition, whereas home care takes it a step further, to skill application (Landrum et al., 1995).

Skill application occurs through functional tasks. The client who has learned to express his or her basic needs in the clinic is able to apply the skill at home with the caregiver when requesting a drink of water. The client who ambulated with physical therapy 5 days per week for 2 weeks in acute care returns home to apply the skill while ambulating to and from the bathroom or out to the mailbox to get the morning paper. The skills that were acquired initially are done so to encourage a greater functional outcome. Therefore, it is always important to begin with the end in mind. Initiate assessment with functionally based assessments, as their purpose is to identify deficit areas that affect the functional outcome. This also provides the client with greater insight into his or her deficits and the impact on daily living.

The functional outcome is identified by all clinicians and caregivers and drives the process of rehabilitation for the client. In the service-based model, clinicians work toward their own goals, sometimes criticizing other clinicians for their lack of awareness of "what the patient really needs." For example, the physical therapist may not recognize that the client's visual deficits are affecting balance and mobility, or the occupational therapist may not realize that the client's lack of understanding is due to a language deficit, not poor motivation.

Providing outcome-oriented rehabilitation not only requires function-based assessment and treatment, it also requires teamwork. The disciplines identify more clearly their role in attaining the outcome versus which discipline will address which task. Physical, speech, and occupational therapy work toward the same goals, which are client centered and not discipline specific (Landrum et al., 1995).

Documentation

As health care has begun to make the paradigm shift toward function and outcome-oriented rehabilitation, the most frequently asked question is "How do I document what has occurred?" There are several factors to consider in documentation. The documentation of a client's care must incorporate the following:

- Clear, concise, and objective information
- Functional status, level of assistance, cues, strategies, or equipment necessary to carry out a task

Case Study 2

Mrs. J, a client who has experienced a stroke, is admitted at 9 a.m. to the rehabilitation facility. The therapists, who were anticipating her arrival the previous day, have scheduled her interdisciplinary evaluation from 1–2 p.m. The occupational therapist, physical therapist, and speech and language pathologist gather the interdisciplinary evaluation forms and arrive in the clinic treatment area.

As the speech therapist and physical therapist relate verbally to the occupational therapist the medical history and pertinent data, the clinician documents the information on the appropriate evaluation form. At the same time, an aide transports the client to the clinic. The assessment begins as each clinician works with the client, the uninvolved clinician(s) asking questions of the client and documenting status as it is observed. Finally, the clinicians discuss their findings with the client and establish goals for treatment and the anticipated outcome. The goals are documented, and all clinicians sign the evaluation and place it in the client's record.

- Payer-specific data (e.g., meet Medicare or health maintenance organization requirements)
- Client-centered information

Information that is gathered and dispersed to other team members ensures that everyone begins with the same information. It also reduces the time and redundancy of asking a client the same question numerous times (Landrum et al., 1995). The most cost-effective and time-efficient process of gathering data and completing documentation is to assess the client together (Keith, 1991). Two or three clinicians can divide the documentation tasks and comprehensively assess the client.

Federal agencies often have more stringent guidelines for documentation and sometimes require each discipline to provide its own form. However, this does not limit the clinicians' ability to assess the client together. Many rehabilitative agencies and home health providers use one evaluation with signatures of each clinician at the end of the document. Other organizations require initials in each area that a specific discipline has assessed (see Figure 10.4).

Functional Goal Writing

Managed care, Medicare, and private insurance companies all look to the rehabilitation clinician to provide information that states the client's cur-

Case Study 3

Initial evaluation results: Client is a 75-year-old man who underwent total hip arthroplasty 5 days ago. He currently requires

- Moderate assistance for ADLs.
- Minimal assistance for transfers and ambulation.
- Supervision for safety with cues for carryover of new learning.

Expected outcome: Independent for ADLs, mobility in household distances, and safe within home environment.

Goals:
1a. Client will show increased upper-extremity strength to Good + (G+), or
1b. Client will don/doff shirt overhead with supervision.
2a. Client will recall hip precautions on request of the therapist, or
2b. Client will carryover hip precautions with minimal verbal cues during bed mobility, transfers, and home management tasks.
3a. Client will transfer sit to stand and to wheelchair with supervision, or
3b. Client will transfer out of bed to chair for breakfast daily with supervision.

rent status and what it will be at the conclusion of service delivery. In other words, what is the client's current function, and what is the anticipated functional outcome? The information and documentation to support the outcome should reflect tasks and activities that relate to the outcome. Identify the most *functional* treatment goals and activities that support the following case example.

The outlined goals could have been written by more than one discipline. It is important to understand the guidelines of the organization in which you practice and expectations of the payer as they relate to documentation. Frequently, the documentation that the rehabilitation clinician provides is viewed and interpreted by a nurse, social worker, or other rehabilitative clinician. Because function is universally understood, it is more likely that the payer or reimbursement agent will authorize care that they understand and can place meaning on.

Therefore, when writing goals—long term or short term—relate the task to function. The following are examples of functional goals related to specific performance areas. Documentation across disciplines must be objective and measurable to provide information regarding a change in function.

Activities of Daily Living

1. Client will retain and use (visual, verbal, tactile) information to complete daily medication routine.
2. Client will use a written checklist to sequence morning routine of (bathing, dressing, grooming) with minimal (verbal, tactile) cues daily.
3. Client will complete morning ADLs with minimal assistance daily.
4. Client will express the need for (breakfast, medication) to the appropriate (staff, caregiver) daily with minimal (verbal, tactile, visual) cueing.
5. Client will initiate 10 functional words related to eating or dressing during morning care.
6. Client will provide a yes-no response consistently when interacting with (therapy staff, nursing) 75% of the time.
7. Client will safely manage or tolerate intake of puree foods (with/without) supervision.
8. Client will complete meal preparation with (supervision, cues, assistance) while ambulating safely in the kitchen.
9. Client will don/doff lower-extremity prosthesis independently using (written instruction, picture cards).
10. Client will demonstrate the ability to follow conversation in a group treatment and interact with other members when answering related questions.

Mobility

1. Client will safely (transfer, ambulate, propel wheelchair) to toilet daily.
2. Client will lift objects off the floor to 5-foot-high shelves while consistently carrying out proper lifting techniques.
3. Client will (ambulate, propel wheelchair) household distances (bedroom, bathroom, kitchen) to carry out daily home management.
4. Client will direct caregivers in techniques and positioning in (bed, wheelchair) to prevent pressure sores.
5. Client will safely negotiate 10 stairs with one railing to enter and exit home.
6. Client will transfer out of bed to chair daily to consume meals.
7. Client will negotiate curbs with (cane, wheelchair, walker) and cross street safely.
8. Client will improve ambulation to the bathroom from minimal assistance to supervision.
9. Client will engage in (tennis, jogging, golfing) with no reports of knee pain after 60 minutes of play.
10. Client will carry out energy conservation techniques while ambulating community distances with minimal cues.

Cognition/Communication

1. Client will use (single word responses, picture board) to express basic daily needs.
2. Client will demonstrate the ability to use the phone in a simulated emergency situation by accurately using (visual, auditory) strategies.
3. Client will initiate one-word responses during conversation with caregiver.
4. Client will use (memory notebook, daily planner) to recall schedule of therapies and attend each activity on time.
5. Client will identify solutions to problems that arise during daily home management group by verbally providing this information.
6. Client will divide attention between two items cooking on the stove with minimal cues to remain on the task.
7. Client will identify and gather all items necessary to complete a specified leisure activity.
8. Client will safely cross the street using the crosswalk and appropriate strategies in a low-traffic area.
9. Client will identify the areas of a specified task that were difficult and strategies to limit difficulty (e.g., quiet environment, ask for assistance, increase structure).
10. Client will recall home telephone number and address during group activity 75% of the time.

Whether you are formulating a goal or identifying the outcome, it must be client centered. Consideration for cultural, family, and client perspective as well as function should be made in developing long-term goals.

Future Trends

Changing payer sources and prospective payment systems have shifted the focus from standard, service-oriented assessment to functional, outcome-oriented health care (Landrum et al., 1995). Therefore, it is important for health care providers to clearly understand their roles and the clinical knowledge and expertise they bring to the clinic. While it is necessary to be educated in specific clinical areas (e.g., gait analysis, manual muscle test (MMT), dysphagia), it is even more important to understand the skill application to real-life situations. This has been a difficult area for clinicians and academic institutions to address.

For many years, advanced education has maintained a focus on theory, measurement, and skill acquisition. As this method is service oriented, the paradigm shift toward function and context is less definitive. Thus, many institutions find it difficult to educate students with functional orientation to the theories or measurement tools they are learning.

The challenge continues as clinicians and educators attempt to identify the appropriate tools and provide education in the use of those tools for patient-centered care (Christiansen, 1993). Historically, the exclusion of standard assessment measures has received criticism (Landrum et al., 1995). Although functional assessments are available, there continues to be a greater portion of specific skill-based assessments than standardized functional assessments (Fisher et al., 1995). This has been a major limitation for academic coordinators as well as practicing clinicians. Rehabilitation professionals must continue to develop and improve standard functional assessment measures. Ongoing research and education in function will continue to justify the need for skilled services. Function in daily living is the desired result of rehabilitation.

Case Study 4

H.L. is a 65-year-old man admitted to a subacute rehabilitation center after a transient ischemic attack (TIA) and brief acute hospital stay.

Prior medical history: Significant for mild memory deficits and prior TIA.

Social history: Before admission, client lived with his significant other. He drove daily and enjoyed many different leisure activities. He managed his own medications and spent periods of time by himself. Currently the client's status is as follows:

Activities of daily living

- Bathing and dressing with moderate assistance
- Grooming with supervision and verbal cues
- Toileting with contact guard/minimal assistance to ambulate to and from the bathroom, transfer on and off toilet, and manage clothing and hygiene
- Dependent medication management

Mobility

- Bed mobility; requires minimal assistance
- Transfers in and out of bed to chair, contact guard/minimal assistance
- Ambulates 100 feet with a rolling walker with minimal assistance
- Stair management, maximal assistance

Cognition/Communication

- Difficulty expressing basic needs due to confusion and poor short-term memory
- Unable to carryover and recall the names of the nurses or therapists on a daily basis
- Mild agitation when asked to do activities such as walking in the hallway or participating in tasks with unfamiliar staff

Based on the information provided, answer the following questions:

1. Identify which rehabilitation therapists should be involved in this client's assessment.
2. How was the information regarding client's living situation obtained? Is there any other information in the social history that has not been provided that may be important to obtain before evaluation?
3. What standardized assessments, discussed in this chapter, would be appropriate to use in assessing this client? Identify why each assessment was chosen. Identify which clinician(s) should administer each assessment.
4. List five functional goals for this client to reach on discharge. Based on the five goals, list five functional tasks that the client will engage in during therapy.

Case Study 5

B.K. is a 45-year-old man admitted to an acute care hospital after experiencing a severe pontine hemorrhage. The client was placed on a ventilator and was unable to physically move all four extremities. The client was able to move his eyes superiorly and inferiorly and was observed to have minimal tongue movement. He was subsequently placed on a feeding tube. After 3 months, B.K. was admitted to an acute rehabilitation center.

Social history: Before admission, client lived at home with his wife. He worked full-time in the computer field. Client drove, attended church weekly, and was involved in the community.

On admission to the rehabilitation center, the client's status was unchanged. Answer the following questions based on the information provided.

1. Is a client interview appropriate? Who will carry it out and how?
2. Identify five areas that you will evaluate with this client.
3. Identify the importance of involving physical, occupational, and speech therapy in the initial assessment.
4. Based on the information provided and the client's limited physical function, identify three activities that the client will participate in during therapy.
5. Explain the importance of the knowledge of the client's social history and function in relation to evaluation and treatment planning.

Based on the information provided, answer the following questions:

1. Identify the advantages and disadvantages of using functional assessment.
2. Identify what each discipline may evaluate individually and as part of a team with the following patients:

   - A 70-year-old man who experienced a subdural hemorrhage as the result of a fall
   - A 25-year-old woman who experienced a C7 spinal cord injury
   - An 85-year-old man who has early Alzheimer's dementia

3. Formulate a list of questions that if asked would provide a window to your daily function. Identify the physical, visual, cognitive, and communicative skills necessary to engage in this daily function.
4. Make a chart identifying the functional assessment, purpose, functional performance areas assessed, and discipline(s) responsible for administration.

References

Begun, J., & Lippincott, R. (1987). The origins and resolution of interoccupational conflict. Work and Occupation, 14(3), 368–386.

Christiansen, C. (1993). Continuing challenges of functional assessment in rehabilitation: Recommended changes. American Journal of Occupational Therapy, 47(3), 258–259.

Cornely, H. Z., & Coffman, A. C. (1998). Letter from the guest editors. Geri Notes, 5(4), 4.

Evans, R. (1995). Healthy populations or healthy institutions: The dilemma of health care management. Journal of Health Administration Education, 12(3), 453–472.

Fisher, W. P., Harvey, R. F., Taylor, P., & Kilgore, K. M. (1995). Rehabits: A common language of functional assessment. Archives of Physical Medicine and Rehabilitation, 76, 113–122.

Grumbach, K., & Bodenheimer, T. (1995). The organization of health care. JAMA, 273(2), 160–167.

Guccioni, A. (1994). Functional assessment. In S. P. O'Sullivan & T. Schmitz (Eds.), Physical rehabilitation assessment and treatment (3rd ed.) (193–205). Philadelphia: F. A. Davis.

Hopkins, H. L., & Tiffany, E. G. (1988). Occupational therapy base in activity. In H. L. Hopkins & H. D. Smith (Eds), Willard and Spackman's occupational therapy (7th ed.) (93–95). Philadelphia: J. B. Lippincott.

Keith, R. A. (1991). The comprehensive treatment team in rehabilitation. Archives of Physical Medicine and Rehabilitation, 72, 269–274.

Landrum, P. K., Schmidt, N. D., & McLean, J. A. (1995). Outcome-oriented rehabilitation: Principles, strategies, and tools for effective program management (pp. 147–157). Rockville, MD: Aspen Publishers.

The Random House Dictionary of the English Language, Unabridged. (1987). (p. 775). Toronto: Hearst.

CHAPTER 11

Rehabilitation Ergonomics

Shrawan Kumar

This chapter introduces ergonomics to the undergraduate and puts it in perspective in relation to the field of rehabilitation. In this chapter, I define and describe ergonomics and build an argument for its relevance in the field. Furthermore, I give an account of the parallelism between the fields of rehabilitation and ergonomics by comparing their histories, philosophies, and goals, as well as by outlining their differences. Finally, I describe some applications of rehabilitation ergonomics and elucidate its uses in the field, thereby demonstrating its need in the field of rehabilitation.

What Is Ergonomics?

The term *ergonomics* is derived from Greek words *erg* (meaning work) and *nomos* (meaning natural laws). It was coined by Murrell (1949), who defined ergonomics as "the study of natural laws governing work." In the traditional sense, if the context is not work, then content is not ergonomics.

Ergonomics deals with person-work interface in the working environment. Therefore, all those factors that may affect the person during the course of work—and thereby affect the work as well—are studied in ergonomics. These factors may be anthropometric; physiologic; kinesiologic; biomechanical; work design; workplace layout; or environmental factors affecting comfort, health, safety, and productivity of the worker. One may, therefore, recognize that ergonomics is multidisciplinary—and at many times interdisciplinary—science. Each of the contributing disciplines exists as an independent discipline in its own right.

Temperature may affect a person in an identical way whether loung-ing at home or working at the office. Only the latter is an ergonomic con-cern. The application of traditional ergonomics is limited to work-relevant interface design. If the application is unrelated to work, it is dealt with by one of the other relevant disciplines. However, the principles of ergonom-ics, which serve to enhance and optimize interfaces, have progressively been applied to environments, products, and facilities that are not found within the strict boundaries of work. Thus, home, leisure, and recreational objects and surroundings have also been significantly affected by these principles to improve the interface/design in order to enhance the compati-bility with their human users.

Although ergonomics affects every man, woman, and child each day of their lives, the discipline continues to remain on the sidelines. The primary reason for this is that ergonomics is a modifier rather than a causal factor. Whatever one does, one can do with or without ergonom-ics. This breeds a sense of indifference toward this science of subtle effects. One can get by without ergonomics, but they would do much better with it. In fact, in a rehabilitation context, the impact of ergonom-ics can be more effective in some cases compared with management devoid of ergonomics.

It may be pertinent to introduce the term *human factors* to avoid confusion in further reading. The birth and evolution of the terms *human factors* and *ergonomics* have taken place in parallel on the two sides of the Atlantic Ocean. The military role that the United States played in World War II was largely aerial. The factors that could optimize the functions of U.S. Air Force personnel were largely cognitive, hence the field took on the name *human factors*. In Europe, the involvement of military personnel was on ground, thus demanding physical and physiologic variables. The discipline, therefore, was named *ergonomics*. There is a continuing debate whether the field is *ergonomics* or *human factors*. In recent years, there has been progressive convergence of views, and these terms are beginning to be used interchangeably.

Why Ergonomics in Rehabilitation?

Rehabilitation professionals are involved in restoration of function with their clients. Frequently, physical methods are used when therapists try to maximize the impaired function, although not always. Depending on the nature and severity of impairment, age and motivation of the patient, and the techniques available, the therapists choose their strategy and execute it. Frequent assessment of the outcome measure(s) provides the therapist with evaluative feedback. This sequence of events is repeated by every therapist in treating each patient. In many treatment regimes, there are two components: the treatment and the training of the patient. In both aspects, ergonomics can play a significant role. I will discuss this role after explaining the concept, uses, and limitations of ergonomics.

Rehabilitation and Ergonomics

Parallelism between rehabilitation and ergonomics appears counterintuitive to professionals of each discipline. However, the theoretical underpinnings of both disciplines, to a large extent, are identical. Until recent times, both disciplines have coexisted with little interaction between them. Professionals of either discipline have considered the other to be unrelated and remote. The circumstances of development, the location of application, and the diversity of clientele tended to accentuate the alienation one from the other. The origins of these two disciplines were motivated by very different human needs. However, considerable likeness in the philosophy, evolution and evolutionary struggles, era of development, technology employed, contributing disciplines, and practice is obvious. The relationship between these two sciences has drawn increasing attention.

Origin

The same period in human history and the same events precipitated the birth, development, and application of both rehabilitation and ergonomics. The specific courses these two disciplines followed were, of necessity, different because of dissimilar immediate needs of the clients and different training and focus of the providers. Hence, each of them are described separately.

Rehabilitation

Before World War I, disability was not considered a medical or social problem in the United States (Gritzer & Arluke, 1985). Such a situation was due to a combination of no demand for expensive medical care and the lack of financial ability of the disabled to pay for lengthy treatment. However, just before World War I, the issue of permanent disability caused by industrial accidents received some attention. Several states in the United States passed workmen's compensation laws, providing medical services and financial aid for the disabled (Mock, 1917). With the outbreak of World War I, the number of permanently disabled grew rapidly. By May 1919, approximately 123,000 disabled soldiers returned to the United States. Heavy casualties in Europe also forced those nations to develop medical and rehabilitation services. Therefore, because of necessity, the profession of rehabilitation emerged and gained support.

During those early years, rehabilitation was primarily staffed by orthopedic surgeons and nurses. However, the orthopedic surgeons trained and employed physiotherapy aides to help them deliver the physical part of the treatment. These physiotherapy aides have since evolved into 4-year professionally trained physical therapists. Although occupational therapy has its roots outside World War I, the war brought it into the rehabilitation fold. The wartime territorial struggle over vocational rehabilitation resulted in occupational therapists proclaiming that "vocational training or education per se is not a form of occupational therapy, but when given to re-establish function, to give a more normal view of life, it may well be classed as a form of occupational therapy" (American Occupational Therapy Association, 1918). Finally, the specialty of speech therapy, although created as a separate occupation in the 1920s, joined rehabilitation after World War II. The ties of speech therapy with rehabilitation are not as strong as physical and occupational therapy.

Ergonomics

An inception of ergonomics can be traced back to hominoids making simple tools and shelter. The improvement to these, occurring in discrete steps in advancement of technology, were incorporated in subsequent products. However, no conscious attention was paid to ergonomics. It was later necessitated by the industrial revolution and accelerated by two World Wars.

An interest in the relationship between man and his working environment became unmistakably clear during World War I. The productivity of ammunition factories became critical to the war effort. The production pressure and schedule in Great Britain resulted in worker's health problems and necessitated the formation of the Health Committee in 1915, which was renamed the Industrial Health Research Board in 1929. It was not recognized until the second World War that some of the newly developed military equipment could not be operated safely or effectively. This started a conscious effort to design tools, machines, and tasks for people, rather than to expect workers to adapt to them. Under such urgency, diverse research activity was undertaken with one goal in mind: to achieve military superiority. The wars thus provided impetus to initiate, pressure to evolve, and purpose to focus.

Such a scenario set the stage for the birth of the science of ergonomics. In fact, the ongoing activity of professionals involved in this field and their desire to continue to collaborate resulted in formal adoption of the term *ergonomics* in 1950 (Edholm & Murrell, 1973). This term had been proposed by Professor Murrell in 1949. According to Christensen (1976), the growth of ergonomics took place in three phases: (1) the age of machines, (2) the power evolution, and (3) machines for the mind.

Philosophy

Rehabilitation

Rehabilitation is concerned with restoration of physical and psychosocial functions. This involves enhancement and optimization of the residual

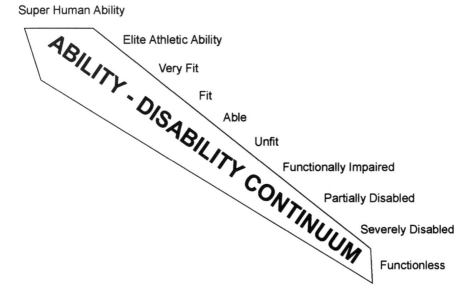

Super Human Ability

Elite Athletic Ability

Very Fit

Fit

Able

Unfit

Functionally Impaired

Partially Disabled

Severely Disabled

Functionless

FIGURE 11.1. Scale of functioning. (Reprinted with permission from Kumar, S. [1989]. Rehabilitation and ergonomics: Complementary disciplines. <u>Canadian Journal of Rehabilitation</u>, 3[2], 101.)

human faculties. Where normalcy cannot be restored or recovery has not reached a functional level, a technologic intervention is to bring the environment to the patient, such as with augmentative devices. Philosophically, one may argue that most people are disabled to some extent on the continuum scale of "super-able" to "functionless" in one or more of the multitude of functions they perform (Figure 11.1). The evidence of such a disability can also be provided in various assistive devices that the able-bodied use in the multitude of functions they perform in their activities of daily living. Nevertheless, the complement of faculties with which most people are born is considered to be the reference point. A decrement from this natural endowment—congenital or a result of disease activity or accident—is considered a functional impairment that necessitates rehabilitation intervention. A physical impairment may lead to psychological maladjustment and social problems. Therefore, rehabilitation is concerned with complete reintegration of the disabled individual into the mainstream of society.

Ergonomics

Philosophically, ergonomics emphasizes two aspects: (1) the worker and (2) the work, with the former being given priority. Within the discipline, it is recognized that the worker is responsible for productivity. A healthy,

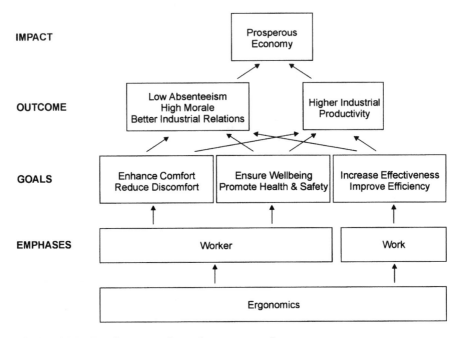

FIGURE 11.2. Emphases, goals, and outcomes of ergonomics.

comfortable, well-adjusted worker with high morale is optimally productive. In addition, when the job is fitted to the worker, production is optimized. The two aspects contribute to better industrial relations and productivity. Thus, the complementary nature of these emphases enhances their effectiveness (Figure 11.2).

Goals

Rehabilitation

The primary goal of rehabilitation is to remedy impairment and disability and restore function. This will overcome the handicap and rehabilitate the person. Rehabilitation strives to liberate a person from both physical and psychosocial limitations. However, it is more desirable to avoid the need for rehabilitation. Thus, health promotion and disability prevention is another important goal.

Even with the best efforts of health promotion, diseases and accidents occur. Given this, arresting deformity and dysfunction becomes an urgent need. Arresting dysfunction can be followed with functional restoration in an effort to reach the premorbid functional level. When, for a number of possible reasons, full recovery becomes unfeasible, patient's training for adaptation to the disability is attempted. If functional deficiencies remain, augmentative devices are used to compensate for residual deficits. Finally, to overcome any psychosocial impediments, counseling and information on support groups and social/government agencies are provided. In summary, the goals of rehabilitation include: (1) restore function, (2) promote health, (3) arrest deformity and dysfunction, (4) train patients, (5) implement augmentative devices, and (6) counsel patients. Based on these goals and the strategies used to achieve them, Kumar (1989) defined rehabilitation as follows: "Rehabilitation is a science of systematic multidimensional study of disordered human neuropsychosocial and/or musculoskeletal function(s) and its (their) remediation by physicochemical and/or psychosocial means."

Ergonomics

Ergonomics has three discrete goals: (1) comfort of the worker, (2) well-being of the worker, and (3) efficiency and effectiveness on the job. Maintenance of comfort of the worker on the job reduces impediments to higher productivity and boosts morale. Reduction or elimination of hazards from the workplace ensures promotion of health on a long-term basis. Together, these optimize productivity, enhance worker morale, encourage employee's loyalty, and reduce labor turnover, therefore, leading to good labor relations. All of these factors collectively increase efficiency and effectiveness of the industrial operations on the shop floor. This goal is further achieved by job design, workspace layout, and appropriate worker training. Thus, ergonomics recognizes the need to harness all human faculties—perceptual, cognitive, and motor—at a heightened level to sustain optimal function.

For many years, the study of all these factors did not fall within the expertise of any given existing discipline. Instead, studies were addressing the diverse aspects of human performance. Thus, to encompass all variables in a cohesive definition, ergonomics (or human factors) has been defined as the science that studies the natural laws governing human work. The merit of this definition is that it encompasses all physical, perceptual, and cognitive factors without giving superiority to any one aspect. It is accepted that this field of study addresses the issues at the human-work interface.

Parallelism

The foregoing review of the origin, philosophies, and goals of the two disciplines indicates significant commonality between these two sciences. The central goal for both is to enable, enhance, and optimize human function. The context and clientele may, however, be different.

TABLE 11.1
Goals of Rehabilitation and Ergonomics Compared

Rehabilitation	*Ergonomics*
Health promotion	Ensure comfort
Disability prevention	Maintain well-being
Dysfunction prevention	Worker safety
Relieve pain	Avoid pain
Functional restoration	Achieve effectiveness
Skill development	Training
Deficit compensation by augmentative devices	Enhance efficiency by job design
Environmental adaptation	Workplace layout
Social adjustment through counseling	Industrial relations

Rehabilitation is concerned with disability prevention, restoration of function, and deficit compensation among patients who have lost some of their previous faculties. Ergonomics, on the other hand, is driving to increase efficiency and effectiveness by tapping the maximum possible from the existent resources of a normal person. The adaptation and adjustments are made in the environment for human-work interface to optimize human capability. The central goal for both rehabilitation and eregonomics, nonetheless, is to enhance and optimize human function in different regions of the disability/ability scale. Because of the scale difference, the populations for whom these goals are geared are different, therefore creating an impression of exaggerated divergence.

The relationship between the goals of these two disciplines are summarized in Table 11.1. It is evident that these two disciplines have shared goals. Rehabilitation generally seems to be content with functional independence, activities of daily living being the most significant measure. For ergonomics, though, industrial production and accident prevention are important measures.

Because both ergonomics and rehabilitation are goal-oriented disciplines, their approaches remain open and flexible to ensure the success of the final objective. Both have drawn their relevant concepts from the same established basic and applied sciences and integrated them in an appropriate manner to achieve the desired effects. Therefore, both these sciences are inherently multidisciplinary. Each one has received generous contributions from the physical sciences, life sciences, behavioral sciences, anthropometry, biomechanics, and kinesiology. Thus, identical goals, reliance on the same constituent disciplines, and working toward enhancing and optimizing human function ties these two disciplines closely.

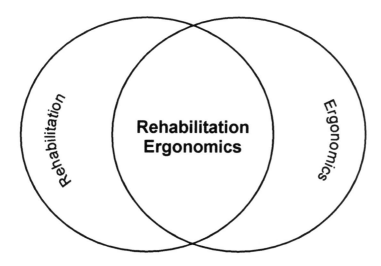

FIGURE 11.3. Overlap and commonality between rehabilitation and ergonomics. (Adapted from Kumar, S. [1992]. Rehabilitation: An ergonomic dimension. International Journal of Industrial Ergonomics, 9[2], 97–108.)

Various ergonomic concepts and practices interweave through the rehabilitation fabric insensibly. However, a more structured but integrated approach may enhance the effectiveness of rehabilitation. In many cases, a lack of application of, or regard for, ergonomics may precipitate injury and necessitate rehabilitation. The relationship between these two sciences is intimate, although not commonly recognized.

A more representative relationship between these two sciences is depicted in Figure 11.3.

Divergence

Despite large overlap and significant complementarity between rehabilitation and ergonomics, it is misleading not to indicate the essential differences. In addition to the context and clientele, the differences between these two sciences lie in the specific body of knowledge that may be described and differentiated as clinical and basic. In addition, practitioners and researchers in ergonomics work toward adjusting and optimizing factors *external* to the workers to enhance comfort, well-being, effectiveness, and efficiency of operation. Rehabilitation practitioners and researchers, on the other hand, work mainly toward enhancing factors *internal* to the patients for restoration of function. However, effort is also made to compensate for residual dysfunction by external factors, such as augmentative

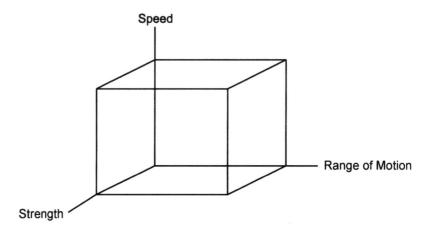

FIGURE 11.4. Functional capacity boundary. (Adapted from Kumar, S. [1989]. Rehabilitation and ergonomics: Complementary disciplines. <u>Canadian Journal of Rehabilitation, 3</u>[2], 99–111.)

devices. Such activities are mostly undertaken by prosthetists or orthotists and rehabilitation/clinical engineers. Of necessity, ergonomics is practiced with people supposedly of "normal" functional capacity in an industrial productive environment. Rehabilitation, on the other hand, is practiced in hospitals with people with impairment or disability.

Complementary Role of Ergonomics

Impairment may be defined as a perturbation that adversely affects function, thereby leading to disability. An individual with a disability who performs a multitude of activities may have decrement in one or more of the variables. To continue to perform normally, one has to have normal kinematics, kinetics, range of motion, strength, endurance, perception, cognition, motor coordination, mobility, and no pain. Decrement in one may significantly affect the performance scores in others. Therefore, activities of daily living—as well as vocational tasks—have to be rated for multidimensional parameters, including all variables that are used. If in a given activity only strength of the body member is needed, it can be measured and reported. If the strength is required to be exerted through a range of motion, both criteria need to be tested. For the activity in question, if a certain speed is necessary, it also has to be assessed. Thus, the boundary in Figure 11.4 represents the functional capacity of the worker for this given task based on the tests conducted.

One must recognize, however, that these are not the only variables that affect human performance. The combination of strength, range of motion, and speed characterize some of the physical demands of activities performed once. The frequency of operation and the duration of work shift must be considered for vocational rehabilitation. Muscle tone determines the endurance, and cardiopulmonary fitness determines the aerobic capacity. Dexterity and precision of the operation are other physical variables that need to be accounted for. It is obvious, therefore, that even in the physical domain, the task requirements become multidimensional. Similar multidimensional requirements in social and psychological domains are also essential ingredients for work worthiness of any person undergoing rehabilitation. In the final assessment, the patient has to be tested for all these aspects. The decision to return a given worker to work depends on the demands of the task. By overlapping the requirements of the task on the pool of resources that an individual has, one can clearly see the suitability of the patient to the task being considered (Figure 11.5).

For final assessment, the patient has to be quantitatively tested on all affected relevant variables. The decision of further treatment, training, or returning to work significantly depends on the job demand. It is only through a quantitative overlap of the patient's physical and psychosocial capacity over the job requirement that an ergonomically trained rehabilitation professional is able to determine the short fall and select a strategy to manage. This hypothetical task requires a great deal of speed, precision, dexterity, perception, cognition, and fast reaction time. Given these criteria, the hypothetical patient has deficiencies and is at the time of assessment unsuitable to be sent back to his job. A similar deficiency, hence incompatibility, could be found in the physical domain. Under these two sets of conditions, different decisions are made for divergently different rehabilitation strategies. Furthermore, a comparison of patients with normative data on all these scales helps determine quantitative functional impairment or disability. To achieve this, a systematic study of the physical demands on the job and work site must be performed. Included in this analysis should be work postures, tool use, material handling, environmental factors, and work pacing. This information must then be compared with work methods or work-site modifications.

Based on the previously conducted job analysis, job/job site modification may be implemented, if necessary, to enhance workers' ability to function. The modifications made should be individual specific to ensure an optimum worker-work fit. Such a modification may be augmented by necessary education of the employee and the employer in the ergonomic and related issues of the given case.

Application

Functional restoration is the final outcome of rehabilitation. The effectiveness and efficiency of the process is an ergonomic concern. In ergonomic

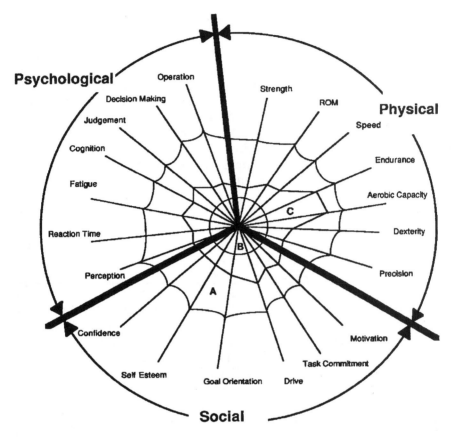

FIGURE 11.5. A hypothetical example showing the comparison of task demand and pool of resources available. (Reprinted with permission from Kumar, S. [1989]. Rehabilitation and ergonomics: Complementary disciplines. <u>Canadian Journal of Rehabilitation, 3</u>[2], 109.)

terms, the process of rehabilitation involves two interfaces: first, the interface between therapist and the patient, which has a bearing on the effectiveness of the treatment, and second, the interface between the patient and his or her surrounding environment, which determines the quality of rehabilitation. Both these interfaces interact in determining the final outcome of the functional restoration of the patient. Although the components of rehabilitation ergonomics are multifarious, they either affect the therapist-patient interface or the patient-environment interface. It is only through a thoughtful and careful application and execution that we may overcome the barriers for a significant segment of our population and make a positive contribution toward the health and well-being of the society and economy. Figure 11.6 represents the theoretical framework of rehabilita-

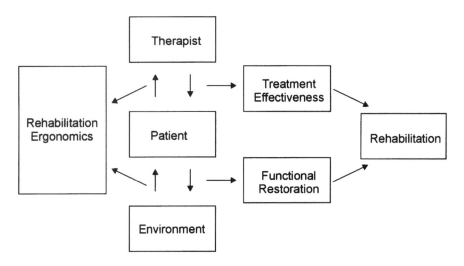

FIGURE 11.6. A theoretical model of rehabilitation and rehabilitation ergonomics. (Adapted from Kumar, S. [1995]. Rehabilitation ergonomics: Rationale, means and justification. <u>Proceedings of the IEA World Conference,</u> 84–89.)

tion ergonomics and Figure 11.7 elucidates the components of rehabilitation ergonomics.

Therapist-Patient Interface

In any rehabilitation treatment, intense therapist-patient interaction occurs in two domains: psychological and physical. The knowledge, biases, and expectations of the therapist may have a significant impact on the final functional outcome of the patient's rehabilitation. These may shape the patient's expectation, motivation, and compliance. Basmajian (1975), Peat (1981), and Harkappa et al. (1991) have all reported that psychosocial factors may have a significant impact on the treatment outcome. To ascertain if such biases do exist among therapists, Simmonds and Kumar (1995) tested a set of 69 physical therapists. These were divided into three groups, and each group was asked to watch a videotape of assessment of a low back pain patient. Each group received the same videotape to view, but they were given either no accompanying history, or a brief history of the patient containing his worker's compensation status, or a brief history of the problem without worker's compensation association. These therapists were required to make prognoses based on the physical assessment shown on the videotape. The therapists made similar physical assessments, but their prognoses for the patients were significantly different across the information groups. The workers' compensation status had a negative effect on the outcome in patients, even with the same patient having the same impair-

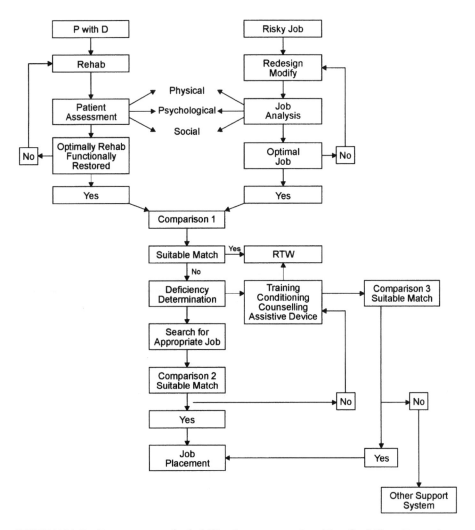

FIGURE 11.7. Components of rehabilitation ergonomics. (D = disability; P = patient; RTW = return to work.)

ment. On the other hand, the non–workers' compensation status was considered positive by therapists in prognosis of recovery. Such knowledge biased the opinions and expectations of therapists. A preventive ergonomic intervention in the psychological domain at the therapist-patient interface may have a significant impact on the outcome.

At the physical level, over and above the validity of the technique, the efficiency and the accuracy of treatment is of paramount importance for an effective treatment. The point is illustrated by two examples. First, physical medicine and physical therapy are delivered through physical medium.

Therefore, an accurate location of a physical landmark is essential. These are invariably determined by the technique of palpation before delivering the treatment. An identification of the landmark through palpation has been considered accurate and objective (Grieve, 1981; Lee, 1989). This prevalent belief has generally gone unchallenged, despite the lack of objective evidence. To test this assumption, Burton et al. (1990) tested reliability of repeated identification of palpable landmarks. They used an invisible marking pen and measured the distance between consecutive marks for spinal levels S2, L4, and D12. Although the distances between the consecutive marks varied, they remained within 5 mm for S2 and L4, and 10 mm for D12 landmarks within raters. Between raters, however, for D12, this distance was 35 mm. Thus, within raters, these palpation results were considered repeatable and reliable for bony landmarks "easy-to-palpate from surface."

In a second study, Simmonds and Kumar (1993) investigated the reliability of palpability of (1) the anterior border of lateral collateral ligament at the level of the knee joint, (2) the spinous process of L4, (3) the posterior-superior iliac spine, and (4) the transverse process of L4. Experienced therapists were asked to mark each structure with an invisible ink and repeat the process after lapse of some time. Whereas the palpation of L4 was done accurately, all others were not accurate. The level of inaccuracy increased with the depth of the tissue. It is conceivable that a poor reliability of many clinical tests may be due to errors associated with palpation. Thus, standardization of this procedure to enhance accuracy at this interface is of vital importance for the optimal outcome.

The next stage of effective treatment depends on the delivery of an appropriate dose of a valid treatment. One of the common treatment modalities for low back pain is spinal mobilization. Four grades of mobilization and their needs have been advocated in the literature. Therapists commonly administer spinal mobilization subjectively, assessing the grade of the treatment they administer. The accuracy of such an assessment needs to be established. Therefore, Simmonds et al. (1995) quantified the forces exerted on the displacements produced by the vertebral body during mobilization of a spinal model. On an electromechanical one-segment spinal model (Kumar, 1995), ten experienced therapists performed four grades of mobilization at three different levels of joint stiffness: low, medium, and high. The mean peak force values recorded were lowest in the least-stiff condition across all grades of mobilization. For medium- and high-stiffness conditions, the exerted force values were similar. The peak displacement for each grade of mobilization for low, medium, and high levels of stiffness did not vary significantly. The results show that there is a significant difference in force exerted that is due to the stiffness of the spine as well as the grade of mobilization. However, there is a large range of intertherapist variability. The force exerted by different therapists varied between 7 to roughly 400 times, whereas the displacement produced varied between 12 to 110 times.

The value of any treatment depends on the delivery of a valid treatment in a consistently standardized manner. The degree of variability encountered among seasoned therapists may be a reason for concern. It is essential to standardize treatment. This can be assisted through the medium of ergonomics. Enhancing this consistency may optimize the outcome of rehabilitation.

Patient-Environment Interface

There is considerable value in objective and realistic assessment of a patient's performance and a profile of the tasks to be performed. Such matching for determination of deficits, as previously advocated in this chapter, is essential to focus the rehabilitation attempts for optimizing the rehabilitation outcome. The means of successful implementation of the objectives of rehabilitation ergonomics lie in the development of methodology and databases, and the interpretation and integration of these databases. The methodology may be adapted from the existing ergonomic literature. Using the literature, relevant databases need to be created to develop norms or ranges of samples of interests. These databases then need to be integrated for appropriate use—in this case, design or modification.

The Need for Rehabilitation Ergonomics

The United Nations disability statistics database reported a disability spread from lowest of 0.2% in Peru to highest of 21% in Austria (United Nations, 1990). We also have to recognize the ever-increasing number of senior citizens in the aging population. Statistics Canada (1990) reported that a significant proportion of the population with disability requires help from family, friends, volunteers, or paid caregivers. Almost one-half of all disabled people require assistance with heavy household work, and one-fourth need assistance with daily housework. Cost is anticipated to be significant. Many able-bodied people have to spend their time assisting people with disability. The cost of this time, along with the cost of a paid health care worker, can be significant. It may be useful to point out that the largest cost is not in medical care but in maintenance, attendant care, nursing home care, and home care expenses, in addition to loss of productivity because of inability to work.

Environment modification and assistive devices may offer disabled people a chance to decrease these costs and be productive members of the society. An emphasis on maintenance continues to be a primary strategy in managing disability. In the United States, 3,000 times more money is spent on maintenance than what is spent on development of methodology that would allow self-care for the disabled (McNeal, 1982). Self-care allows self-fulfillment—in part, a sense of self-worth—and also feeds the economy.

The calculation of LeBlanc and Lefier (1982) provides a strong economic justification. They reported that every dollar spent on assistive devices produced an elevenfold return. In conclusion, given the size and significance of the population with disability, the rationale of extensive application of rehabilitation ergonomics is not only economically viable, but profitable. Given the additional benefits of self-worth and actualization of people with disability, the development and application of rehabilitation ergonomics is not only desirable but becomes the strategy of choice.

Summary

Traditional ergonomics is defined as the study of natural laws governing work. It is also concerned with the person-work interface. However, the field has grown to incorporate interfaces between environment, products, and humans at home, leisure, and recreation as well. Due to its goal of enhancing and optimizing role, ergonomics is important for rehabilitation. Consequently, the subfield of rehabilitation ergonomics developed.

The tangible origin of both rehabilitation and ergonomics has been traced to World War II. The philosophies and goals of both fields have been shown to have significant dissimilarities as well (e.g., clientele). However, using principles of ergonomics, the practice of rehabilitation can benefit by enhancing targeted treatment delivery. Use of ergonomic principles can also benefit the recipient of rehabilitation in negotiating the environment or handling property-designed products.

References

American Occupational Therapy Association. (1918). Proceedings of the Second Annual Meeting American Occupational Therapy Association. Then and Now.

Basmajian, J. V. (1975). Research or retrench: The rehabilitation professions challenged. Physical Therapy, 55(6), 607–610.

Burton, K., Edwards, V. A., & Sykes, D. A. (1990). "Invisible" skin marking for testing palpatory reliability. Journal of Manual Medicine, 5, 27–29.

Christensen, J. M. (1976). Ergonomics: Where have we been and where are we going? Proceedings of the 6th Congress of the International Ergonomics Association, July 11–16.

Edholm, O. G., & Murrell, K. H. F. (1973). The Ergonomics Research Society: A history 1949–1970, Ergonomics, 1(1), 6–39.

Grieve, G. P. (1981). Common vertebral joint problems. Edinburgh, Scotland: Churchill Livingstone.

Gritzer, G., & Arluke, A. (1985). The making of rehabilitation: A political economy of medical specialization, 1890–1980. Berkeley: University of California Press.

Harkapaa, K., Jarvikoski, A., Mellin, G., Hurri, H., & Luoma, J. (1991). Health locus of control beliefs and psychological distress as predictors for treatment outcome in low back pain patients: Results of a three-month follow-up of a controlled intervention study. Pain, 46, 35–41.

Kumar, S. (1989). Rehabilitation and ergonomics: Complimentary disciplines. Canadian Journal of Rehabilitation, 3(2), 99–111.

Kumar, S. (Inventor). (1995). Therapeutic Spinal Mobilizer, U.S. Patent.

LeBlanc, M., & Leifer, L. (1982). Environmental control and robotic manipulation aids. Engineering in Medicine and Biology, 16–22.

Lee, D. (1989). The pelvic girdle. Edinburgh, Scotland: Churchill Livingstone, 15–91.

McNeal, D. R. (1982). Applying technology to help the disabled. Engineering in Medicine and Biology, 15–16.

Mock, H. (1917). Industrial medicine and surgery: The neo specialty. Journal of the American Medical Association, 68, 1.

Murrell, K. H. F. (1949). Cited in Edholm, O. G., & Murrell, K. H. F. (1973). The Ergonomics Research Society: A history 1949–1970. Ergonomics, 1, 6–39.

Peat, M. (1981). Physiotherapy: Art or science? Physiotherapy Canada, 33(3), 170–176.

Simmonds, M., & Kumar, S. (1993). Location of body structure by palpation: Reliability study. International Journal of Industrial Ergonomics, 11, 145–151.

Simmonds, M., & Kumar, S. (1996). Does knowledge of a patient's workers compensation status influence clinical judgments? Journal of Occupational Rehabilitation, 6(2), 93–107.

Simmonds, M., Kumar, S., & Lechelt, E. (1995). Use of a spinal model to quantify the forces and motion that occur during therapists' tests of spinal motion. Physical Therapy, 75(3), 212–222.

Statistics Canada. (1990). The health and activity limitation survey: Highlights: Disabled persons in Canada. Catalogue number, 82-602, Ottawa.

United Nations. (1990). Disability statistics compendium. Series Y:4, New York: Department of International Economic and Social Affairs Statistical Office.

CHAPTER 12

Vocational Rehabilitation and Work Hardening

Muriel Westmorland

Vocational Rehabilitation: A Definition

Vocational rehabilitation is a multidisciplinary process. Berkowitz (1990) defines vocational rehabilitation as "the array of services designed to facilitate and ease the return to work." In a recent Association of Workers' Compensation Boards of Canada publication (1998), it is defined as a "goal oriented process which involves a sequence of services that are designed to help disabled people pursue their optimal vocational adjustment." The origin of the words *vocational* and *rehabilitation* suggests that the activity has something to do with the vocation or occupation in a person's life, and rehabilitation is understood as a process that an individual may go through as a result of an illness or injury (Ontario Ministry of Health, 1996). Isernhagen (1995) calls work injury management and prevention a multidisciplinary effort, primarily because many professions are usually involved in the rehabilitation process (e.g., physiotherapist, occupational therapist, vocational rehabilitation specialist, social worker, physician, psychologist, chiropractor, kinesiologist).

Over the years, the body of knowledge related to vocational rehabilitation has been enriched by those who practice in the field. If you are a psychologist, in all likelihood your focus will be on vocational attributes, such as cognitive function and work behaviors. If you are a kinesiologist, you may place more emphasis on the normal body mechanics required to carry out a job. If you are a chiropractor, you may use a particular assessment related to the vocational issues the client presents. If you are an occupational therapist in Canada, you may use the Canadian Occupational Performance Model (Canadian Association of Occupational Therapists, 1997) coupled with the person-environment-occupation model (Law et al., 1996), which emphasizes the importance of the "fit" between the person (patient, client, consumer) and his or her environment (in this case, the work environment). If you are a physiotherapist, you may approach the process of vocational rehabilitation from a functional perspective—in other words, the functional components of the job that cannot be met, such as walking, standing, climbing, lifting, and sitting. Social workers may also be involved in vocational rehabilitation. Depending on their background and experience, they may work with clients in a counseling role or, in some cases, as the workplace liaison.

The legal profession is also a player in the area of vocational rehabilitation. This perspective is usually directed by the rights of the client in the context of the particular legislation that provides services—e.g., auto insurance legislation and general litigation (Isernhagen, 1995).

Review of the Literature

It is important to note that the term *vocational rehabilitation* is not used by all professionals in this field. Some call the process *work rehabilitation* (Isernhagen, 1995) or *occupational rehabilitation* (Shervington & Balla, 1996). Countries, such as Canada and the United States, vary in what they include as vocational rehabilitation services. Perron and McKay (1997) describe vocational rehabilitation services as learning job skills for a new occupation or job modifications to assist the employee's return to work. They consider services such as case management, acute care rehabilitation, and work hardening separate from vocational rehabilitation. A recent report from the Association of Workers' Compensation Boards of Canada (AWCBC) defines vocational rehabilitation services as assessment services, counseling, education, job placement, job accommodation, and other services (AWCBC, 1998). Nevertheless, in spite of these differences, there is no contest in terms of what vocational rehabilitation is and what it involves. While the process components may appear to be labeled differently, there are congruent themes. These generally fall under the process stages or steps of assessment, development of a plan, implementation, and evaluation.

Assessment

Authors in this field agree that it is necessary to assess or gather baseline data related to the person with a disability and his or her ability to perform vocational tasks (AWCBC, 1998). Shervington and Balla (1996) emphasize that standardized testing is essential and that these objective tests should reflect "criterion-referenced and industrially accepted standards." Strong and Westmorland (1995) and Rumrill et al. (1998) suggest that mixing situational and standardized assessments provides a more holistic approach that takes into consideration the client's perspective and provides an opportunity to observe a variety of job-related characteristics unique to that individual.

Physical ability is not the only variable to be assessed. Assessment of cognition and behavior is equally important. Moglowsky and Rumrill (1996) stress the need for a holistic approach to assessment and emphasize the use of situational assessments that "consider the ecologic milieu in which the person lives." This is also integral to the model of person-environment fit (Law, 1996), which will be discussed later in this chapter.

Babineau (1998), writing about brain-injured clients, refers to McCue's outline of what is typical vocational rehabilitation and notes that the initial assessment step is the interview with the client, family, and previous employer. The objective here is to establish the "client's perceptions of his injury, obstacles he must overcome, vocational goals and any discrepancies between the client's perception of problems and the family's perceptions and observations" (McCue, 1994). Inherent in this statement is the importance of involving the client in the assessment process. Baum and Law (1996) also identify the importance of working with the client or patient. They state that "In a client-centered approach, clients and therapists work together to define the nature of the occupational performance problem, the focus and need for intervention and preferred outcomes of therapy." They argue that the clients know themselves best and can, therefore, contribute realistically to the assessment process.

Koch et al. (1998) provide a rationale for why client involvement (as defined) is so important and cite key principles such as holism; rights, dignity, and worth of individuals; commitment to promotion of ability; and participation and personal ownership of the rehabilitation process.

Functional assessment is considered an integral component of the initial vocational rehabilitation data-gathering process. This is described in Chapter 11.

Strong and Westmorland (1995) provide a framework for the assessment process that consists of seven components: (1) the evaluation of client (vocational) performance in the form of the interview; (2) observation of performance; (3) disability self-reports; (4) pain drawings or pain ratings; (5) identification and documentation of nonorganic signs; (6) psychopathology screening and personality tests; and (7) functional assessments/testing and work simulations.

Bellini et al. (1998) stress that there is a need for improvements in how rehabilitation counselors (substitute vocational rehabilitation practitioners) use assessment data to determine the vocational rehabilitation

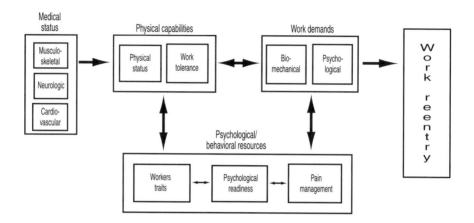

FIGURE 12.1. Multiple factors potentially affecting return to work after occupational musculoskeletal injury/illness. (Reprinted with permission from Feuerstein, M. [1991]. A multidisciplinary approach to the prevention, evaluation and management of work disability. <u>Journal of Occupational Rehabilitation,</u> 1[1], 5–12.)

plan. They note that the wide array of diagnostic categories that vocational rehabilitation clients present provides a major challenge, and that every effort must be made to not only use standardized data when possible but also to use consistent protocols. At the end of the assessment, the vocational rehabilitation professionals should be able to identify inconsistencies in performance (based on the results of the assessment tests/observations/simulations), explore the reasons for those inconsistencies, and then formulate conclusions.

Development of a Plan

Talo et al. (1996) propose that the plan be cost effective; that it be made specifically for the individual and "devised by a comprehensive (bio-psychosocial) team"; and that the basis for any plan should be "theory based . . . and clinically validated."

Feuerstein (1991) proposes a conceptual framework for factors that affect the return to work of individuals with musculoskeletal injury/disease and emphasized the importance of considering multiple factors (Figure 12.1).

Shervington & Balla (1996) advocate a "productivity practice model" that starts with standardized testing, moves through simulated work to job analysis and job task sampling, and ends with a work trial (Figure 12.2).

Shervington emphasizes the importance of using the particular occupational classification system available in the practitioner's country—e.g.,

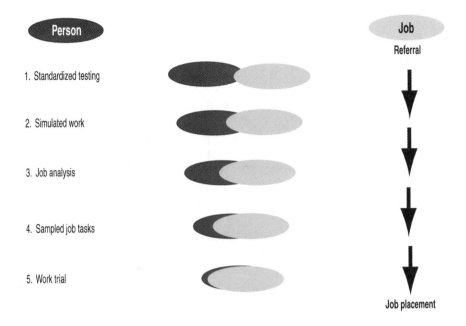

FIGURE 12.2. Productivity practice model. (Reprinted from Shervington, J. & Balla, J. [1996]. Workability mark III: Functional assessment of workplace capabilities. Work, 7, 191–202, with permission of Elsevier Science.)

in Canada, the National Occupational Classification (1993). In other words, use data available regarding the range of job classifications, and match that to your assessment of the client.

Law et al. (1996) have developed the person-environment-occupational model, which emphasizes that the "fit" between these three constructs is not only important, but that it varies depending on where the individual is in his or her development (Figure 12.3).

These models have not yet been well validated, but they can be used as frameworks for the development and evaluation of a vocational rehabilitation plan. The advantage of vocational rehabilitation professionals adopting a particular model is that not only can data be collected and compared, but consistent protocols can also be developed. The latter is an important issue that vocational rehabilitation professionals need to address.

No plan can and should be developed without consideration of the specific vocational rehabilitation context (e.g., Workers' Compensation Board, auto insurance, litigation case, long-term disability, short-term disability, specialist referral, or family physician referral). Each of these situations has legislative and other implications that may dictate elements that

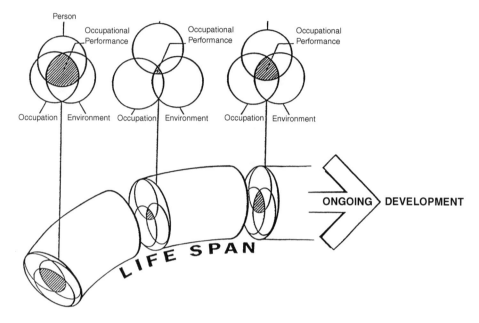

FIGURE 12.3. Depiction of the person-environment-occupational model of occupational performance across the life span, illustrating hypothetical changes in occupational performance at three different points in time. (Reprinted with permission from Law, M., Cooper, B., Strong, S., Stewart, S., Rigby, P., & Letts, L. [1996]. The person-environment-occupational model: A transactive approach to occupational performance. <u>Canadian Journal of Occupational Therapy, 63,</u> 15.)

must be considered. This is critical to the formulation of any plan. It is also critical that the patient or client plays a major role in the development of the vocational rehabilitation plan. The AWCBC document (1998) emphasizes the importance of the development of an individualized plan in discussion with the client. Moglowsky & Rumrill (1996) add the importance of considering independent living needs as well as hygiene, money management, and living accommodation (when planning for clients with psychiatric problems).

The involvement of employers and unions in the development of the plan is also referred to in the literature (Rumrill et al., 1998). Legislation over the past 2 years, both in Canada and the United States, has placed more responsibility on the employer to be a full participant in the vocational rehabilitation process (AWCBC, 1998). Rumrill et al. (1998) cites a study by McMahon et al. (1993) that rates linkages between the vocational rehabilitation professionals and employers as important to employers in the United States. In Canada, there is a growing move by many corporate employers to hire their own in-house trained disability management personnel rather than hire vocational rehabilitation "experts." This was endorsed at a 1998 Canadian National Workplace Equity Symposium for Persons with Disabilities (Human Resources Development Canada, 1998), where the key elements of successful employment of persons with disabilities were identified as "collaborative environment(s)," autonomy, and skill development.

Gardner and Campanella (1997) propose that the approach to program planning for persons enrolled in vocational rehabilitation programs needs to change. They stress that the client's personal goals must be taken into consideration and that those goals may well go beyond the narrower work or employment focus. In other words, work activities (based on employment tasks) usually meet other needs that clients may have, such as meeting other people, providing income to sustain them in their daily lives, and giving them an improved sense of self-worth. If we support this notion, then those who practice vocational rehabilitation need to be acutely aware of the place that work or employment has on their client's lives and develop each program with suitable goals and objectives that helps the client to meet those needs.

Implementation of the Plan

How plans are implemented or carried out is very important, yet there is little rigorous evidence to guide us in terms of frameworks that work well and facilitate the achievement of vocational rehabilitation goals. In the allied health professional literature, the term *intervention* is used, which reflects the more "medical" or "treatment" approach. A Canadian Association of Occupational Therapy (CAOT, 1988) position paper on work-related therapy suggests that the goal of the intervention process should be to "increase the fit between the demands of the job and the client's skills, ability, aptitudes and interests." It includes as part of the process ergonomic interventions and adaptations to the environment (e.g., raised or lowered surfaces, lifting devices). Before implementing the plan, it is important to consider three integral components: the model or framework used to develop the plan, the context or site where the plan is carried out, and staff roles and functions.

Implementation components (AWCBC, 1998) frequently include but are not limited to

- Work site assessment.
- Work hardening.
- Career- or job-related testing.
- Simulated work experience.
- Vocational retraining.
- Modified work trial.

- Work site modifications.
- Job-seeking advice or placement.

Implementation of Context/Site

Some of the implementation components could be carried out anywhere, such as in a specialized vocational rehabilitation unit/agency, a community worksite, or a personnel/employment facility.

Hallam and Leach (1997) describe how the vocational rehabilitation model uses the approach of "train, then place." They also list the benefits and disadvantages of this approach. The benefits of the train-then-place method include

- Staff working in a rehabilitation center may be able to supervise more than one client at one time.
- Clients' vocational aspirations and potential are not limited to one type of occupation.
- A sheltered environment allows for clients to deal with salient symptoms at a reasonable pace.

The disadvantages of the train-then-place method include

- The skills taught may not be relevant to the jobs available in the market.
- Clients may have difficulty transferring their new skills outside of the workshop.
- The closed and segregated aspect of the workshop may cause low expectations in both the clients and staff.
- The segregation of people with mental health problems is not good for changing the prejudices or stereotypes held by the public.

Some employers provide a comprehensive vocational rehabilitation service in house or on site so that the minute an employee has to deal with work-related issues that are affected by accident, disease, or other trauma, they can provide a fast response. Rumrill et al. (1998) discuss the importance of in-house management approaches and list relevant responsibilities of the rehabilitation professional. These range from contacting employees after an injury or illness and arranging modified duties to identification of assessment programs, development of a return-to-work plan, providing reports, training coworkers and supervisors, and evaluating the efficacy of disability management services.

Perron and McKay (1997) list the positive aspects of these types of programs:

- Early medical intervention
- Reduced lost work time

- Convenience for worker
- Accessibility of professional consultations
- Support for ongoing warm-up and stretches prevention program
- Timely work site inspections, job modifications, and worker education
- Increased employee self-esteem and satisfaction in gainful employment
- Increased employee ownership of their responsibilities in the work re-entry process

Perron and McKay (1997) describe the benefits when rehabilitation professionals and employers work together, no matter what the context. They outline what each brings to the process. The vocational rehabilitation professional brings knowledge about

- Medical literature.
- Human anatomy and physiology.
- Healing processes and successful treatments.
- Medical or rehabilitation protocols and procedures.
- Community contacts and relationships.
- Availability of other health care resources.
- Teaching resources.
- Local hot lines or information centers that deal with injury-prevention materials or questions.

The employer provides knowledge about

- Corporate/plant operations and procedures.
- Production/assembly processes.
- Practical application of safety programs.
- Industrial hygiene experience.
- Company resources.
- Other business contacts/referrals.
- Work site culture.
- Union-management relationships.
- Job descriptions and role delineation.

Employers may also treat persons with disabilities in a more integrated fashion, according to a recent study by Trach et al. (1998). Their study of employers looked at the kinds of workplace supports that were in place for all employees (e.g., availability of human resource counseling, flexible work schedules). They found that the majority of employers hiring persons with disabilities did not set up special additional supports in the workplace. Instead, they tended to use the ones already available to all employees. In contrast, the study found that sheltered workshops tended to identify supports that were in excess of what the workplace would tend to provide (e.g., extended counseling; major workplace modifications; and, in some cases, total restructuring of the job description). The authors thought that these "supports" were not as reasonable or reflective of the real world of work. These findings would tend to suggest that the employer views an employee as an employee whether disabled or not. By contrast, the sheltered workshop attitude toward employment supports may well be perpetuating the culture of disability as those who are "not able," therefore needing more supports. The latter has an important message for all vocational rehabilitation practitioners: the workplace culture is not the vocational rehabilitation agency or sheltered workshop culture, but rather a business where the job needs to be carried out and may need various workplace supports to make that happen.

Implementation of Staff Roles and Functions

The implementation of any plan requires the staff to move it toward goals and objectives. Some vocational rehabilitation programs favor a case management approach, whereas others work as teams, with each team member playing a role in the implementation process.

Using a case manager is one model. A case manager is either part of the established vocational rehabilitation team (from any professional background) or purchased from a company/agency. Case management is defined as "simultaneous co-ordination" and "a structured approach to planning" (AWCBC, 1998). The Worker's Safety and Insurance Board—formerly the Workers' Compensation Board—in Ontario has employed nurse case managers to fulfill this role.

Rumrill et al. (1998) suggest that the rehabilitation counselor is the professional who co-ordinates the disability management plan. His or her role would be identical to a case manager in some jurisdictions. Rumrill et al. comment that opportunities for vocational rehabilitation professionals are "at an all time high" in the United States. This may be because many work site disability management programs are employing these professionals to co-ordinate their programs. Canada is currently exploring the development of standards for disability management training courses and national certification of disability managers.

It is important to note that unions are playing an increasing role in the implementation of workplace rehabilitation, and some large unionized companies may have their own rehabilitation coordinators (e.g., United Steelworkers). These individuals frequently follow up on sick or injured employees and provide support over the phone, through visits, or at the work site.

How a vocational rehabilitation plan is implemented may have a positive or negative effect on the person with the disability. The literature points to the importance of using a model to guide the plan and to listen to the client while developing a customized plan to meet the client's needs. The link between vocational rehabilitation and the employer base cannot be overemphasized. No matter whether the work site is the agency or the employer or both, it is essential that vocational rehabilitation staff solve problems with the reality of the workplace in mind.

Work Hardening

Work hardening is one component of the vocational rehabilitation implementation process. Smith (1986) defines work hardening as "a restorative and reconditioning treatment process (that) must incorporate the goals of expeditious and physically appropriate return to employment." It is usually person or client specific. Isernhagen (1991) agrees that job tasks relevant to the client's current or former job must be part of a work hardening program. The Commission on Accreditation of Rehabilitation Facilities (CARF) provided the following definition of work hardening in 1988 (Ogden-Niemeyer & Jacobs, 1989):

> It is interdisciplinary in nature, involves the use of conditioning tasks that are graded to progressively improve the biomechanical, neuromuscular, cardiovascular, metabolic, and psychosocial functions of the client in conjunction with real or simulated work activities. Work hardening provides a transition between acute care and return to work, while addressing the issues of productivity, safety, physical tolerances, and worker behaviors. Work hardening is a highly structured, goal-oriented, individualized treatment program designed to maximize the individual's ability to work.

Many work hardening programs use a multistation approach, in which clients move through several work stations and carry out a variety of physical and functional tasks for a specific length of time. Work simulation is usually part of this process, and clients are encouraged to practice safe postures or movements and to avoid risk. Work behaviors are usually monitored, such as focusing on the task, punctuality, and ability to follow and understand instructions (Strong & Westmorland, 1995).

In recent years, the site of work hardening programs has moved from rehabilitation centers to work sites (Cooper et al., 1997), with the critical component being work simulation. Once simulation has been successfully carried out, then the client is placed in a modified work situation anywhere from 1 to 6 weeks (Cooper et al., 1997). Careful monitoring should accompany this period to evaluate whether the client is meeting work hardening goals. In Cooper et al.'s example of nurses, the client is also "closely monitored for the first month" (Cooper et al., 1997). The results of this particular research (N = 7) are very positive, however, the authors caution that the results probably cannot be generalized, given the small number and specific population. Six months after this carefully graded and monitored work hardening program, all nurses were able to complete an 8-hour work day. The authors contend that the data appear to "support the concept of maintaining individuals with back injury in the workplace by providing early intervention, on-site work hardening and the opportunity for modified work."

Isernhagen (1995) emphasizes the importance of objective information provided by properly trained and certified or licensed professionals. This is particularly important because inappropriate grading activities could set the client back considerably and or prolong his or her symptoms. Vocational rehabilitation practitioners carrying out work hardening programs need to be able to refer (if necessary) to appropriate team members (e.g., social worker, psychologist) when problems arise.

Ideally, vocational rehabilitation practitioners should familiarize themselves with the wide range and complexity of paid occupations and, when possible, carry out site visits to expose their senses to the work environments (smells, physical layout and structure, types of equipment used). Factors that may be critical can frequently be left out of a client's job description. For example, a client states that his job involves checking levels of fat in vats or tanks and topping up from holding tanks. This happens in one area, with a limited amount of walking. However, there is another part of the job: once a week, the client has to climb up several flights of stairs outside in all types of weather to check on the holding tanks and to open valves associated with the flow to the vats. This activity could make a significant difference as to whether this particular client could, in fact, return to work. Having an accurate grasp of the workplace reality can mean the difference between a successful or unsuccessful work hardening program.

More than 26 years ago, I successfully established a creative work hardening program (although it was not known by that name in those days) at McMaster University Medical Centre, Hamilton, Ontario. Real work sites were negotiated across 45 settings in the Medical Centre and the university at large. The effect of "real work" experiences had a positive impact on the clients. They were much more motivated than they otherwise might have been. However, establishing this was not easy. Discussions regarding liability and insurance coverage had to take place, and guidelines related to accountability and responsibility issues between the therapists and the supervisors had to be developed. The effect that the presence of other employees had on the clients was notable. Not only did clients feel better about themselves, but their fellow workers provided normalizing experiences without this being deliberately factored into the work hardening program plan (e.g., taking clients to coffee or lunch, celebrating client birthdays, assisting with the occasional work task, and providing overall support). Not only did this program affect the clients, it also provided a major opportunity to educate the employees and supervisors. Not all were supportive—some were mired in concerns regarding liability or had values that made it difficult for them to work with psychiatric patients. Others embraced the idea with enthusiasm, particularly in the animal quarters (the area that looked after animals required for research studies), which proved to be a very therapeutic placement for clients, given that animals give affection without judgment. The placement in the animal quarters provided many a client with increased feelings of self-worth as well as providing an opportunity to increase the ability to match workplace standards. Work hardening programs vary in length and may be as short as 1–2 weeks or as long as 3–4 months (Pratt & Jacobs, 1997).

Evaluation

The importance of evaluating the vocational rehabilitation process cannot be overemphasized. Using a theoretical framework based on vocational rehabilitation theory or theory related to work or occupation can and should guide this process. No longer is it good enough to go with experience or your gut feeling about a client or work situation and how successful you think his or her program is. Clients are much more knowledgeable about their rights to safe and appropriate employment. Governments and financial institutions are cautious about what they will fund and are asking for programs that are based on evidence of reliable outcomes. Vocational rehabilitation programs can be costly, and the payers need to be reassured that they are not wasting their money on programs that show no evidence of positive vocational rehabilitation outcomes.

Talo et al. (1996) propose a model based on biopsychosocial constructs. Superimposed on that is the World Health Organization classification of impairment, disability, and handicap (Figure 12.4). This model is one framework for approaching evaluation in that it diagrammatically articulates the matrix of principles that need to be considered in the assessment and implementation process of rehabilitation in general. Talo et al. take the biopsychosocial components of an individual along one axis and intersect those with the impairment, disability, and handicap outcomes along the other axis. In other words, one could develop an evaluation process based on the change outcomes that have occurred at the biopsychosocial levels and whether they have significantly affected the individual's degree of impairment, disability, or handicap.

Given that the theoretical basis of vocational rehabilitation is challenging, with so many different professionally based values, specific professional theory, and approaches, it is important that programs establish evaluation benchmarks at the outset. There is an abundance of social theory related to the individual and society, and one of the most important connections an individual has with society is through his or her occupation. Work is said to be (Stuckey, 1997)

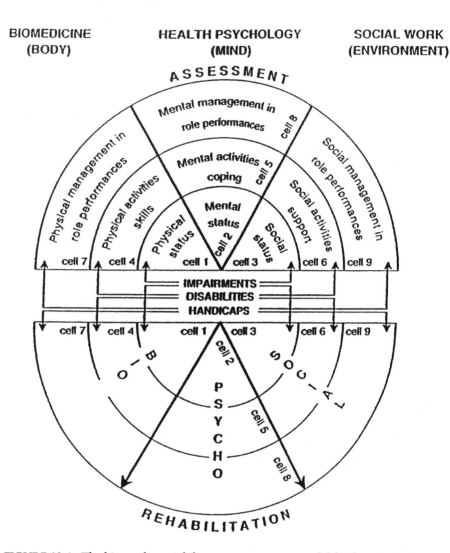

FIGURE 12.4. The biopsychosocial disease consequence model for functioning, assessment, and rehabilitation. (Reprinted with permission from Talo, S., Rytokoski, U., Hamalinen, A., & Kallio, V. [1996]. The biopsychosocial disease consequence model in rehabilitation: Model development in the Finnish work hardening programme for chronic pain. International Journal of Rehabilitation Research, 19, 93–109.)

- An expression of human purpose.
- The basis of social life.
- A provider of a sense of identity and status.
- A source of self-respect and meaning.
- A means to enable people to offer a product or service that is necessary or helpful to their social environment.

- Added value to the human condition.
- A necessary part of earning a living.

Gardner and Campanella (1997) postulate that evaluation of work program outcomes must consider whether the client is "successfully integrated into the work environment." The notion of *successful* is important, and the authors point out that people do work to meet their own goals. In other words, vocational rehabilitation evaluation programs and protocols must consider whether client goals have been met. The evaluation principles should include whether the program has contributed to overall client goals (increased opportunity to make friends, feeling better about themselves, financially more self-sufficient). Traditionally, many vocational rehabilitation programs have considered goals to be met if the client returned to work. This is no longer the only evaluation benchmark. Partridge (1996) stresses the importance of "the need for more research and promotion of vocational assessments and outcome measures" in order that vocational rehabilitation programs can include those components that lead to "successful outcomes."

McMaster School of Rehabilitation Science researchers have adopted the program logic model (Letts et al., 1993) as part of a workbook that has been designed to assist occupational therapists in the evaluation of occupational therapy programs (Figure 12.5). The model helps programs to work through the evaluation process by using a diagrammatic model. The program is described in terms of what it does and also what the end products or outcomes are. Main components have to be described first, followed by objectives that show what those components are supposed to do. Then, outcomes are identified with their specific objectives, which indicate what the expected change might be. Arrows are arranged so that the elements are linked. This forms the "logical" steps of the program. The usefulness of this framework is that it provides those who are evaluating the program with some important steps to follow.

Ideally, the program logic model should be used at the beginning of a new program as a framework that guides program development as well as program evaluation. The logic process encourages participants to think about goals or targets and identifiable outcomes. It can be used in a number of ways and in some situations has been a useful tool for maintaining quality assurance goals.

Emerging Themes

Over the past 5–10 years, several themes have emerged with respect to the areas of vocational rehabilitation and work hardening. Contributing factors have been legislative changes (Workers' Compensation Board, auto insurance legislation), gains made by injured workers and union lobby groups, the shift in vocational responsibility to employers, recognition of work as a

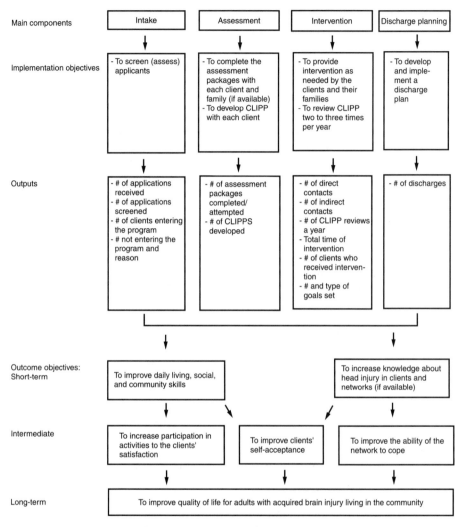

FIGURE 12.5. HICAP program logic model. (CLIPPS = client initial program plans, HICAP = Head Inform Community Adjustment Programme.) (Reprinted with permission from Letts, L., & Dunal, L. [1995]. Tackling evaluation: Applying a programme logic model to community rehabilitation for adults with brain injury. Canadian Journal of Occupational Therapy, 62, 272.)

determinant of health, impact of injury/disability on employer and employee costs, and the concern about evidence-based outcomes. Some of these changes have been loud and clear (e.g., legislation). Others have accrued more slowly (e.g., stronger voices of unions and disabled advocacy groups). The latter has affected or will affect the role of the vocational rehabilitation professional. In some quarters, the vocational rehabilitation professional is seen as self-serving (e.g., they charge high fees and demand immediate changes to the work environment). Unions have become very knowledgeable about the vocational rehabilitation process, and some unions have developed excellent return-to-work guidelines (e.g., United Steelworkers).

Simultaneously, large companies and some crown corporations in Canada see the advantage of training their own in-house human resources staff because they know the specific work environment and occupational roles as well as the organizational culture. Some staff would already be members of the company's joint worker/management health and safety committee, which is a very important body in issues related to return to work of persons with disabilities. Workplace-based vocational rehabilitation departments need to be cognizant of issues such as conflict of interest and bias, given that they do not provide these services at arm's length. Dispute resolution systems need to be established to deal with such issues and to ensure that the employee is dealt with in a fair and unbiased manner.

Terms such as *disability management* (in the workplace) are now becoming more common, and one example is the innovative educational program called the Disability Management Coordinator Certificate Program, developed by the National Institute of Disability Management and Research (NIDMAR, 1998) in Port Alberni, British Columbia. This program provides human resources staff and others with a 6-week certificate course in how to manage employees with disabilities in the workplace. It has strong support from unions, employees with disabilities, and human resources representatives. Disability management, according to Millington & Strauser (1998), has three major components: interdisciplinary team format, proactive intervention, and early intervention/return to work.

Despite the differences that may occur within the vocational rehabilitation process from province to province or state to state, it is vital that the practitioner stay abreast of these important themes in order that he or she can provide clients with the most comprehensive, valid, and reliable process possible.

Conclusion

This chapter provides only a limited overview of the complexity of the vocational rehabilitation process and the important component of work hardening. The fact that vocational rehabilitation is more than one specific intervention cannot be overemphasized.

The population health literature—in particular, the *Wealth and Health, Health and Wealth* report published by the Ontario Premier's Council on Health, Well-Being and Social Justice (1994)—identifies factors that determine health. Unemployment and underemployment are associated with poorer health. Being employed enables a person to survive (e.g., provision of food, clothing, and housing). Unemployment has a significant impact on health, quality of life, and community participation. There is also evidence that a lack of work activity can cause a deterioration in those with mental disorders.

This knowledge about determinants of health underscores the importance of vocational rehabilitation programs that are client focused, comprehensive, and relevant. The client must be a major partner in this process, and programs should be able to tailor their approaches to the unique needs of each client.

It is important that vocational rehabilitation programs have a multidisciplinary team that can assess the complexity of work skills and make the program relevant to current employment expectations. Employers (current or potential) need to be an integral part of planning implementation and evaluation. Vocational rehabilitation professionals need to work in partnership with the employer community.

There is a major need for well-documented evidence about frameworks, models, or protocols that will provide evidence of successful vocational rehabilitation strategies. There are exciting opportunities here for collaborative multidisciplinary research that will not only add to our body of knowledge, but could also influence government policy and legislation regarding return to work for persons with disabilities as well as accreditation standards for those working in the field.

Program evaluation must be built into the vocational rehabilitation framework with clear goals and objectives and mechanisms for evaluating those. This information needs to be written up in appropriate journals and presented at conferences so that the body of evidence will increase. Governments are also examining the cost-effectiveness of programs and are becoming more sophisticated in approach as they determine who will be funded and who will not.

There is much to be done in the field of vocational rehabilitation as we move this important field forward into the twenty-first century.

Suggestions for Student Study

1. What are the four stages of vocational rehabilitation?

   Answers

   - Assessment
   - Development of a plan
   - Implementation
   - Evaluation

2. Discuss what might be included in a vocational rehabilitation assessment.

   Answers

   - Physical factors (standing, walking, lifting, carrying)
   - Cognitive factors (ability to read and understand, memory, following through on instructions)
   - Psychological factors (attention, concentration, attitudes)
   - Environmental factors (previous work environment—hot, dry, dusty, noisy, busy, quiet, involved equipment handling)
   - Social/family (single income earner supporting family, spouse is unable to work and needs care)

3. Develop a vocational rehabilitation plan for the following cases:

   Case Study 1

   Leila had arrived in Canada from Lebanon 6 months ago. She was planning on bringing her mother over once she had secured a job as a nurse's aide (she had worked in this field in Lebanon). Leila was offered a job as a nurse's aide 1 month ago. The weekend before she was due to start, she was hit by a car at an intersection. She suffered bruising to her lower back and right arm (she is right-handed). Leila was referred to your vocational rehabilitation practice by an auto insurance company that has asked you to assess her and develop a vocational rehabilitation plan.

   Answer

   You will need to consider Leila's physical status, the effect of the accident on her self-confidence, and the status of her new job. She has a mother who is waiting to come over and stay with her daughter, and this will also need to be addressed. Consider ethnic issues, attitude toward disability, and involvement of family. How long will Leila have to remain in rehabilitation to resume her usual functional independence?

Case Study 2

Max is a 40-year-old father of three children (ages 10, 14, and 20). All are living at home. Max's wife is working at a variety store part time. Max is an auto mechanic who has injured his lower back on the job (he lifted a car panel). He has been experiencing numbness and pain down his left buttock and into his foot and is unable to reach forward more than 10 degrees at the waist. He is currently off work on Workers' Compensation Benefits. As the vocational rehabilitation case manager hired by the Board in your province, you are asked to assess his suitability to return to work and if necessary develop a work hardening program.

Answer

You will need to consider Max's physical/functional status and gather data on the physical demands of his job as an auto mechanic. You will need to determine if he can return to work given his present physical status and develop a plan to improve his function. You will also need to check with the employer regarding whether modified duties are available.

Case Study 3

Elizabeth is a 28-year-old who has been diagnosed with bipolar affective disorder. Three years ago, she found that could not continue to work in a local bakery and has been on medication and at home ever since. She is getting restless and would really like to get a job. She is exploring alternative therapies at the present time. She has contacted a local employment agency that posts job opportunities for persons with disabilities, and you are the vocational rehabilitation counselor assigned to develop a plan for Elizabeth.

Answer

You will need to consider if Elizabeth is functionally ready for employment given her psychiatric illness. How might you do that? Assessment from a psychiatrist? Referral to a functional assessment program? Does Elizabeth want to return to her former job? Can she handle it? Is there a possibility of a work placement before finalizing a permanent position? What are the funding implications (i.e., will she get paid, or is this a work trial)? Would you suggest other programs that might help Elizabeth meet her own vocational goals?

Acknowledgments

The author acknowledges the contributions of student Natalie Quick, who assisted with the literature search and compilation of the chapter; and Julianna Durham, manager of vocational services at the Hamilton Health Sciences Corporation, who reviewed the chapter. Grateful thanks are also extended to Dr. Ed Gibson (formerly occupational health physician at Dofasco) for his insightful editorial comments.

References

Association of Workers' Compensation Boards of Canada. (1998). Vocational rehabilitation and workers' compensation. AWCBC, pp. 15, 17, 34, 54, 99, 100.

Babineau, J. (1998). The value of early placement in a supported employment program for individuals with traumatic brain injury. Work, 10, 137–146.

Baum, C., & Law, M. (1996). Occupational therapy practice: Focusing on occupational performance. American Journal of Occupational Therapy, 51(4), 227–287.

Bellini, J., Bolton, B., & Neath, J. (1998). Rehabilitation counselors' assessments of applicants' functional limitations as predictors of rehabilitation services provided. Rehabilitation Counseling Bulletin, 41(4), 242–259.

Berkovitz, M. (1990). Returning injured workers to employment: An international perspective (p. 21). Geneva: International Labour Office. Canadian Association of Occupational Therapists. (1988). Position paper on Canadian occupational therapist's role in work related therapy. Canadian Journal of Occupational Therapy, 55(4), 2–4.

Canadian Association of Occupational Therapists. (1997). Enabling occupation: An occupational therapy perspective. Ottawa, Ontario, Canada: CAOT Publications.

Cooper, J. E., Tate, R., & Yassi, A. (1997). Work hardening in an early return to work program for nurses with back injury. Work, 8, 149–156.

Feuerstein, M. (1991). A multidisciplinary approach to the prevention, evaluation and management of work disability. Journal of Occupational Rehabilitation, 1(1), 5–12.

Gardner, J., & Campanella, T. (1997). Challenging tradition: Measuring quality as outcomes for people. In J. Pratt & K. Jacobs (Eds.), Work practice: International perspectives. Oxford: Butterworth–Heinemann.

Hallam, R., & Leach, J. (1997). Work programmes to enhance psychosocial performance components. In J. Pratt & K. Jacobs (Eds.), Work practice: International perspectives (pp. 126–144). Oxford: Butterworth–Heinemann.

Human Resources Development Canada. (1998). National Workplace Equity Symposium for Persons with Disabilities (p. 45). Ottawa, Canada.

Isernhagen, S. (1991). Physical therapy and occupational rehabilitation. Journal of Occupational Rehabilitation, 1(2), 71–82.

Isernhagen, S. J. (1995). The comprehensive guide to work injury management (p. 557). Gaithersburg, MD: Aspen Publishers Inc.

Koch, L. C., Williams, C. L., & Rumrill P. D. Jr. (1998). Increasing client involvement in vocational rehabilitation: An expectations-based approach to assessment and planning. Work, 10, 211–221.

Law, M., Cooper, B., Strong, S., Stewart, S., Rigby, P., & Letts, L. (1996). The person-environment-occupational model: A transactive approach to occupational performance. Canadian Journal of Occupational Therapy, 63, 9–23.

Letts, L., Fraser, B., Finlayson, M., & Walls, J. (1993). For the health of it!: Occupational therapy in a health promotion framework. Ottawa, Ontario, Canada: CAOT Publications ACE.

McCue, M. (1994). Attaining employment goals through vocational rehabilitation. The National Head Injury Foundation TBI Challenge! Vol. 2, p. 4–10.

McMahon, B. T., Dancer, S., & Jaet, D. N. C. (1993). Providers of technical assistance and employers: Myths, concerns, and compliance behaviors related to the Americans with Disabilities Act. Journal National Association of Professional Private Sector, 8, 53–66.

Millington, M. J., & Strauser, D. R. (1998). Planning strategies in disability management. Work, 10, 261–270.

Moglowsky, N., & Rumrill, P. D. Jr. (1996). Schizophrenia: Strategies for rehabilitation professionals. Work, 7, 21–29.

National occupational classification. (1993). Ottawa, Ontario, Canada: Ministry of Supply and Services.

National Institute of Disability Management and Research. (1998). Disability Management Coordinator Training Program. Port Alberni, B.C.

Ogden-Niemeyer, L., & Jacobs, K. (1989). Work hardening: State of the art. Thorofare, NJ: SLACK, Inc.

Ontario Ministry of Health. (1996). Future directions for rehabilitation. Toronto, Ontario, Canada: Health Strategies Group, Government Publications.

Partridge, T. M. (1996). An investigation into the vocational rehabilitation practices provided by brain injury services throughout the United Kingdom. Work, 7, 63–72.

Perron, J., & McKay, M. (1997). Current models and trends in work practice service delivery. In J. Pratt & K. Jacobs (Eds.), Work practice: International perspectives (pp. 39–68). Oxford: Butterworth–Heinemann.

Premier's Council on Health, Well-Being, and Social Justice. (1994). Wealth and health, health and wealth. Toronto, Ontario, Canada: Ontario Ministry of Health.

Rumrill, P. D., Koch, L. C., & Harris, J. (1998). Future trends in assessment and planning: Priorities for vocational rehabilitation in the 21st century. Work, 10, 271–278.

Shervington, J., Balla, J. (1996). Work ability mark III: Functional assessment of workplace capabilities. Work, 7, 191–202.

Smith, P. (1986). Work hardening guidelines for occupational therapists (p. 272). Rockville, MD: American Association of Occupational Therapists.

Strong, S., & Westmorland, M. (1995). <u>Measurement of effort: Work function unit, McMaster University.</u> Unpublished report.

Stuckey, R. (1997). The nature of work and work patterns. In J. Pratt & K. Jacobs (Eds.), <u>Work practice: International perspectives</u> (pp. 4–5). Oxford: Butterworth–Heinemann.

Talo, S., Rytokoski, U., Hamalinen, A., & Kallio, V. (1996). The biopsychosocial disease consequence model in rehabilitation: Model development in the Finnish work hardening programme for chronic pain. <u>International Journal of Rehabilitation Research, 19,</u> 93–109.

Trach, J. E., Beatty, S. E., & Shelden, D. L. (1998). Employers' and service providers' perspectives regarding natural supports in the work environment. <u>Rehabilitation Counseling Bulletin, 41</u>(4), 293–312.

CHAPTER 13

Supervision of Service Delivery in the Rehabilitation Disciplines

Paul Hagler

This chapter provides a practical, organizational framework on which reha-bilitation professionals can arrange their existing knowledge, experiences, and beliefs regarding the clinical supervisory process. This organizational structure is designed to serve administrators, program managers, clinical educators, and clinical professionals in occupational therapy, physical ther-apy, speech-language pathology, and nursing as a beacon to guide them as they navigate the sometimes foggy milieu of the clinical supervisory process.

Very few clinical professionals receive what might be termed *adequate* exposure to supervisory theory during their formal education. For the most part, clinicians become supervisors of students simply by working for a year or so and then being asked by a practicum or fieldwork placements coordina-tor to take a student. Clinicians become supervisors of other clinicians sim-ply by working long enough in one setting to have a thorough knowledge of the workings of the facility. After agreeing to serve as a clinical supervisor in either capacity, most supervisors implement the supervisory process in ways that directly reflect how they were supervised. Supervisors try to treat their supervisees the way they wish they had been treated, and they try to avoid treating their supervisees in ways they found objectionable. In short, no one taught us how to supervise, so we cast about in the fog in the best way we know how. Evidently, we are supposed to know how, because academic pro-grams don't routinely offer course work in the area of clinical supervision, professional associations don't seem to expect it, and employers don't usually fund continuing education opportunities for clinicians who suddenly find themselves in management positions.

The assumption that we should know how to supervise as a function of having worked for awhile as clinicians is, of course, nonsense. There is a great deal to know about good clinical supervision, what it looks like, and how to do it, and working as a clinical professional for 1 year doesn't provide us with that knowledge. This chapter serves as a good starting point. Most of the information provided on the following pages is a synthesis of theory and research from the health sciences disciplines and even some from business management. It saves the reader a lot of time by bringing it all together in one place, and it provides a template with which to structure the entire process the next time the reader is in the position of being a clinical supervisor.

Each of the rehabilitation professions has built up its own jargon around the supervisory process. For example, the nursing profession often refers to the registered nurse who assumes the responsibility of role model, teacher, counselor, and resource for a baccalaureate nursing student as a *preceptor* and to the student nurse as a *preceptee* (Barrett & Myrick, 1998). Thus, an arranged practical experience in a clinical setting with an immediately available resource is sometimes called a *preceptorship* (Barrett & Myrick, 1998). Pharmacy uses this terminology as well. What is referred to as a *preceptorship* in nursing and pharmacy is called a *fieldwork placement* in occupational therapy and a *practicum assignment* in audiology, physical therapy, and speech-language pathology. Arranged, full-time, practical assignments of longer duration tend to be called *internships* or *externships*, and the distinction between these two terms usually depends on how close the host facility is to the student's academic program. Similarly, the rehabilitation disciplines have developed preferences with regard to the label they use for the nonprofessionals who provide clinical assistance under the supervision of audiologists, nurses, occupational therapists, physical therapists, and speech-language pathologists. The most common labels include *aide*, *assistant*, and *support worker*. Most rehabilitation professionals acknowledge the appropriateness of the term *clients* when referring to the individuals and their families who are being served, unless those people are actually *patients* in a hospital or some other medical facility. There is a growing preference for the term *client*, because it implies less passivity and more partnership with caregivers.

In the following pages, I tend to use the term *practicum* when referring to arranged practical experiences for students. The term *supervisor* is used when referring to the individual who monitors and provides feedback on the work of others, except in examples specific to nursing. The term *supervisee* is used when referring to the individuals whose clinical work is being monitored, except in examples in which students are the supervisees. Students are usually called *students*. The labels *patient* and *client* are used interchangeably, and sometimes they are joined with a slash as a reminder that they mean essentially the same thing in this discussion of the clinical supervisory process.

Need for Supervision

Let's begin by discussing why clinical supervision is so important. If one tries to distill the raison d'être for the rehabilitation disciplines into one phrase, it probably would be "to provide high-quality specialized health care services not otherwise available." Few, if any, health care professionals are capable of functioning completely independently. We rely on one another for formal and informal consultations, because we cannot possibly keep track of all the tests, forms, protocols, interventions, rules, and information sources that are essential to the delivery of good health care, even when our own discipline is the sole service provider. When the services of multiple disciplines are required, our reliance on others intensifies. When one considers the limited independence of even the most technically competent clinician combined with the usual frailties of the human organism, it becomes clear that clinical professionals need others to organize, facilitate, educate, monitor, and question what they do. The individuals who perform these functions are supervisors, and their work—clinical supervision—is crucial to the operation of the health care system. Good clinical supervision ensures quality service delivery, accurate record keeping, fiscal responsibility, a secure and comfortable working environment, and general accountability. Good clinical supervision, applied to students, optimizes the teaching/learning experience to create the next generation of clinical professionals.

It is noteworthy that only "good" clinical supervision does these things. Bad supervision actually has deleterious effects on each of these aspects of an otherwise smoothly functioning health care setting. Clinical supervision affects professionals, students, support staff, patients or clients, and even their families. Simply put, supervision affects people, so it's worth doing well.

Goal of Supervision

The ultimate goal of the supervisory process is defined by the supervisee's long-term needs. For example, Anderson (1988) described the goal of the supervisory process with students as being the creation of independent, self-supervising new professionals. Obviously, that is not the goal with all supervisees. Some supervisees are already independent, self-supervising professionals, and other supervisees, such as assistants, should not aspire to independence. Thus, the goal of the supervisory process differs slightly according to the type of person being supervised.

There are four types of supervisees: (1) professionals (occupational therapists, physical therapists, speech-language pathologists, and nurses), (2) students (future professionals), (3) assistants (also referred to as support workers), and (4) assistant students (future assistants or support workers). The goal of supervision with regard to professionals is to ensure that health care services are delivered in ways that are consistent with the mandate of the employment facility. The goal of supervision with regard to assistants is to form a collaborative partnership. A collaborative partnership is one that (1) enables the assistant to continually refine skills and increase independence without ever exceeding a carefully circumscribed scope of practice, and (2) enables the professional to increase the amount of time spent in clinical activities requiring higher levels of education and experience. Of course, the overarching goal with an assistant/professional partnership is to structure service delivery and supervisory routines in such a way as to provide more patient/client care at a reduced cost. Thus far, no one has carried out a cost/benefit analysis to find out if more care can be offered at reduced cost and, if so, how many assistants one professional can supervise without passing the point of diminishing returns. The goal with assistant students is to prepare them to assume as many of the responsibilities typically assigned to assistants in their area of practice as possible so that, when employed, they can hit the ground running.

An important distinction should be made at this point. The goals of the supervisory process with each of the four types of supervisees represent the ultimate or final objectives. They are holistic in that they refer to the long-term objective. They define where the process is taking the supervisee at the end of a series of clinical experiences. This is even true of employed professionals and assistants insofar as they, too, change employment settings and program assignments within a setting and, therefore, require supervisory input to bring them up to speed. The final goals of the supervisory process may be very different from the purpose of a specific supervisory encounter. A specific supervisory encounter, for example, might have as its objective the planning of a particular patient's or client's therapy session or the resolution of an interpersonal problem between the supervisor and the supervisee. Supervisors must be aware of both types of goals to know how to supervise.

Knowing where one is headed has a lot to do with how quickly one gets there. For example, the supervisor who is instructing a newly employed professional in the intricacies of institutional record keeping or giving a performance appraisal does most of the talking and uses lots of information-loaded declaratives. On the other hand, the supervisor who is teaching a physiotherapy student how to independently analyze the last treatment session to revise her strategies for the next session needs, more than anything else, to be a good listener. Only occasionally will that supervisor interject with information-loaded declaratives, choosing instead to offer thoughtful, leading questions to steer the student's process of self-analysis. Later in this chapter, I return to the topic of how to plan specific supervisory encounters. Understanding the differences between goals of the process and goals of the moment and keeping them both in mind goes a long way toward ensuring that supervision is effective.

Impact of Assistants and Students on Service Delivery

The impact of assistants and students on service delivery is a topic that stimulates lively discussion among clinical professionals and administrators. Clinical educators often express paradoxically different opinions regarding the impact that students have on service delivery. Some assert, with heartfelt passion, that students are basically a nuisance. Student clinicians, they say, are a serious drain on staff time and, for the most part, interfere with client care. For some of these clinical educators, their strong convictions have led them to discontinue their participation in the clinical education process. However, others say, with equal verve, that students are an exciting addition to their work routine and that when students are present, their program is able to provide more service. They love having students and often report warm and productive therapeutic relationships between students and their clients. Obviously, both conditions could be true, but one thing seems clear: more research is needed to better understand these conflicting accounts of the same activity.

Similarly, discrepant arguments surround the use of assistants or support workers in the rehabilitation disciplines. Some clinical professionals perceive assistants to be a threat, not only to their jobs but to their professions. The paradox is that on the one hand, professionals portray assistants as a threat, and on the other hand, suggest that most assistants are not adequately trained to assume significant portions of their responsibilities and that assistants require so much monitoring that there is no gain in amount of service. Between 1991 and 1993, a Canada-wide study of the role, use, and supervision of support workers in the rehabilitation disciplines was conducted. It was the only national-scale study of these important issues. That 3-year project culminated in a report about the current status of the training, use, and supervision of support workers in audiology, occupational therapy, physical therapy, and speech-language pathology and included a feasibility study in nursing (Hagler et al., 1993). The report also contained recommendations for the future training, use, and supervision of support workers in those same professions. Findings regarding the impact of assistants on service delivery were compiled from supplementary analyses of two subsets of the data from that national study. Findings indicated that professionals perceived themselves to be able to offer more services with assistants than without them in audiology (Hagler et al., 1995a) and speech-language pathology (Hagler et al., 1995b). Unfortunately, those findings were based only on respondents' perceptions or estimates of amount of service with and without assistants. No actual client service records, such as workload measurement system data, were accessed for those reports. Again, it becomes clear that more research is needed to better understand the complex issues surrounding the impact of this category of workers on amount and quality of patient care.

These debates strike at the very heart of the supervisory process, because they ask the question, "Are we better off with them or without them?" If the answer is that we are better off without them, then clinical education programs for students may need to be extensively restructured, perhaps even supervised in other, more controlled settings. Likewise, the currently expanding use of assistants in delivery of health care services would need to be curtailed or at least restructured. It is curious that relatively little research has focused on trying to find answers to these fundamental questions. Although very little information exists with regard to the impact of assistants, there is some limited but persuasive evidence to suggest that students are more an asset than a liability.

Cost-Benefit Studies of Students' Impact on Service Delivery

Many of the studies that relate to the impact of practicum students on service delivery have been conducted in the United States with a focus on cost-benefit analyses, emphasizing the monetary impact of students on facilities that generate revenue from procedural charges (Hammersberg, 1982; Leiken, 1983; Leiken et al., 1983; Lopopolo, 1984; Porter & Kincaid, 1977). Historically, in Canada, health care institutions have been funded primarily by the individual provinces with complicated preservice grants, rather than by revenue for services rendered. Therefore, cost-benefit studies have, until recently, been less common among Canadian health care facilities. Hammersberg (1982) used survey instruments completed by supervisors and staff members of six allied health programs. The surveys required the subjects to estimate the amount of time given to the education of students, the cost of supplies, and the contribution of students to the performance of the daily workload. The survey responses were averaged, and the results indicated that the costs of having students outweighed the contribution the students provided. Findings from studies pertaining to clinical education for physical therapy students have suggested that financial benefits, rather than financial liabilities, accrue for institutions (Leiken, 1983; Lopopolo, 1984; Porter & Kincaid, 1977). Financial benefits also were reported for physical therapy, occupational therapy, and radiologic technology students by Leiken et al. (1983).

In summary, findings from cost-benefit studies have been conducted in various disciplines and have resulted in contradictory conclusions regarding the impact of students on operational costs. It is possible that these inconsistent findings may relate to differences in educational or institutional practices across disciplines. Of course, studies that reduce cost-benefit to a dollar value do not consider the many positive qualitative effects students have on their training facilities. Students are often reported to be challenging and stimulating to their supervisors and other members of their departments. They bring youthful enthusiasm and new ideas with them to their practicum sites, and their presence is often an opportunity for practicum institutions to screen potential future employees (Cebulski & Sojkowski, 1988; Halonen et al., 1976; Leiken, 1983).

Productivity Studies

The most persuasive research using productivity in terms of patient service as a dependent variable has been done in physical therapy. The amount of patient/client service in physical therapy was investigated in acute care hospital environments by Bristow and Hagler (1994, 1997), Cebulski and Sojkowski (1988), Ladyshewsky (1995), and Ladyshewsky et al. (1994). Cebulski and Sojkowski (1988) found that the clinical instructor–student pairs in the study were more productive than were the same clinical instructors without students. Bristow and Hagler (1994) examined the productivity of physical therapy students during clinical placements and assessed the impact of supervision on professional staff time. Their results indicated that staff members' patient-related service decreased during periods of supervision, but the direct patient care provided by students was greater than the therapists' supervision time. Bristow and Hagler (1997) extended their 1994 study by comparing the amount of service provided by individual staff with no student assignments with the amount of service provided by the same staff in combination with their students. That investigation supported their earlier findings by indicating clinical placements had positive effects on service delivery. Results indicated that the number of patients seen per day significantly increased with students present. Ladyshewsky et al. (1994) examined the impact of physical therapy student placements on outpatient service productivity. They concluded that factors of staffing level, length of waiting list per full-time equivalent staff, caseload mix, and meeting time—not student factors—had the greatest influence on outpatient service productivity. Ladyshewsky (1995) studied productivity using a collaborative clinical education model in the acute inpatient clinical setting. The findings demonstrated that students increased productivity levels while using the collaborative model.

The main concern of productivity research has been to investigate how students affect patient care, but some productivity studies have considered other variables. Bristow and Hagler (1994, 1997), for example, used physical therapy service areas as an independent variable to see if productivity differed among them in an acute care hospital when students were present. No service areas demonstrated a significant reduction in amount of service as a function of having students on site, and the net effect across service areas was a significant increase in client attendance per worked day when students were present. Cebulski and Sojkowski (1988) indicated that length of internship may affect productivity. They also attempted to explain lower productivity levels from certain supervisor-student pairs by relating it to student/supervisor weaknesses, such as short internships, student performance problems, and supervisors' non–work-related personal difficulties. Their study described the supervisor subjects as being chosen from various levels of personnel and did not describe the student educational level. Other studies (Bristow & Hagler, 1994; Bristow & Hagler, 1997; Ladyshewsky, 1995; Ladyshewsky et al., 1994) have attempted to control for students' educational level and practicum experience by matching student subjects to achieve sameness across comparison groups in terms of these variables.

Some persuasive findings from two, small N-studies in speech-language pathology now exist. Hancock and Hagler (1997, 1998) studied the effects of practicum students on service delivery. The 1997 study was a retrospective pilot project that did little more than establish that student subjects, who were in their final full-time practicum placements, were not a service delivery liability in one rehabilitation hospital setting in which they were placed. The subsequent study (1998) was completed as a master's thesis project and revealed that student subjects, who were in their final full-time practicum placements in a variety of service facilities across North America, were an asset. They significantly increased the amount of patient care and nonpatient care in comparison to the amounts of such care provided by their supervisors alone.

It is noteworthy that the studies by Bristow and Hagler (1994, 1997), Ladyshewsky (1995), and Ladyshewsky et al. (1994) in physiotherapy and the pilot study by Hancock and Hagler (1997) in speech-language pathology were conducted in Canada and used the Workload Measurement System (1987), a statistical database system that produces workload indicators for each staff member and student and is used routinely in larger health care facilities throughout Canada. Findings as similar as these reported by different investigators, in different types of service facilities, across different disciplines, using a nationally standardized record-keeping system take on a degree of plausibility not often enjoyed by so small a cadre of research.

In summary, findings from productivity studies seem to suggest that students are an asset, but there is a need for further research in all the health sciences disciplines to discover what qualities or mix of qualities of students, supervisors, and internship environments may affect productivity. Supervisor work experience, supervisor supervision experience, and student experience are potentially high-impact variables that deserve attention as independent variables affecting patient care.

Much more extensive investigations of the impact of assistants on service delivery need to be carried out using virtually all of the same variables described for research with students. Investigators need to use actual client service records, rather than just respondents' perceptions, and they need to design studies to explore each of the many factors that might impinge on the effectiveness of assistants.

Impact of Health Care Restructuring on Supervision

The demanding nature of the supervisory process is made more challenging by health care funding cutbacks and restructured service delivery paradigms. Conservative governments have been elected on the basis of their promises to curtail escalating health care expenditures. These governments have cut funding to service providers who, in turn, have discharged large numbers of middle management, nonunion employees in their efforts to work within ever-dwindling budgets. Loss of middle management employees has made it necessary to pass their former responsibilities along to the remaining staff who are, for the most part, clinical professionals and clerical support staff. In many service environments, these new responsibilities for rehabilitation professionals have not been accompanied by a corresponding reduction in their caseloads, which has translated into a workload increase. The restructured service delivery paradigms are in such protracted states of disorganization that they are unable to respond to their employees' plight, so the dedicated but beleaguered professionals are saying, "I've had it! I'm not going to take it anymore." If they view supervision of assistants or students or even one another as "more," they are unlikely to cooperate in any but the most superficial way. Professionals themselves receive less supervision, because there are fewer program managers, of whom many are members of professions other than those they supervise. For example, it is common these days for a nurse administrator to "supervise" a cadre of audiologists, occupational therapists, physical therapists, and speech-language pathologists. Furthermore, if administrators view assistants or support workers as a partial answer to their need to continue providing the same services at a lower cost, they will hire two assistants for the price of one professional. Then, in their efforts to provide the maximum amount of clinical service, they fail to give the professionals adequate time from their busy clinical schedules to carry out their supervisory responsibilities with the assistants. To the extent to which this chain of events reflects reality, it has important implications for the quality of peer supervision, student supervision, and assistant supervision where such programs exist. It also affects decisions to implement peer supervision programs, to employ support workers, and to accept students for practicum placements.

Restructuring and Peer Supervision

In the wake of having terminated the employment of most of their middle management staff, it seems a number of service facilities have tried to respond to clinical professionals' need for supervision by implementing peer supervision programs, in which professionals monitor one another's work. Is this appealingly practical? Of course it is. Is it also problematic in some ways? Yes.

Peer supervision programs seem to meet with only limited success, probably for three reasons. One is that clinical professionals seldom have time to do their own work, much less time to monitor a colleague down the hall. This leads to minimalist supervision. Minimalist supervision is cursory feedback that is borne of a need for expediency—feedback that fulfills the letter of the law but that rarely leads to improved clinical skills for the supervisee.

Another reason peer supervision programs are problematic is that the success of a peer supervision relationship depends, in large part, on the nature of the working relationship. A close working relationship that is grounded in mutual respect can thrive in a peer supervision paradigm. Peer professionals who understand that providing the best care for their clients requires that they continue growing professionally not only tolerate peer feedback, they actively seek it. Peer supervision breaks down when the working relationship is strained. Coworkers who have other issues between them are not likely to deliver or receive feedback with the most constructive intentions.

The third reason that peer supervision programs are problematic is that peer supervisors carry little clout with their colleagues when major changes are needed. For example, if an audiologist's ability to interpret otoacoustic emissions tracings is deficient, about all the peer supervisor can do is explain the diagnostic signs present in that particular tracing and offer continued assistance with the next few patients. Peer supervisors rarely have the authority to require continuing education, caseload alterations, or anything else that might bring deficient colleagues up to speed or separate them from the clients whose needs they cannot serve. However appealing peer supervision may seem on a conceptual level, it is not a satisfactory replacement for traditional professional supervision and administration.

Restructuring and Student Supervision

It is increasingly important that professionals be accountable with regard to their ability to provide efficient, high-quality patient care. If there is a perception in public sector health care facilities that students detract from patient care by being less competent, less efficient, or requiring too much of their supervisors' time, then those facilities have every right to reassess their commitment to student education. In privatized health care facilities, where costs are often monitored even more closely, a willingness on the part of administrators to accept students may be further eroded. Each time this happens, fewer practicum options exist for students in the rehabilitation disciplines. With fewer options available, educational programs are constrained in their ability to produce graduating therapists who possess the knowledge and confidence to go directly from their educational programs to the workplace. The student's education is compromised. The employment facility—perhaps even the same one that refused to contribute to the student's education by accepting that student for a practicum placement—must now bring the student up to speed on the job, at full salary, while ensuring high standards of service. Thus, the argument can be made that service facilities will contribute to every new professional's education—it's just a matter of when. They can do it at the student's expense, or they can do it at their own expense. The responsibility lies with researchers to give health care administrators and professionals useful information that elucidates the impact of students on service delivery. With more empirical evidence, fewer decisions are made on the basis of knee-jerk reactions to anecdotal information, and more decisions are based on statistics derived from carefully collected and analyzed data.

Restructuring and Support Worker Supervision

Any responsible health care facility administrator tries to provide quality services at the lowest possible cost. Many administrators, often with the complete support of their clinical professional staff members, turn to the employment of support workers or assistants in occupational therapy, physical therapy, speech-language pathology, and nursing to accomplish this objective. Where this is done, it is sometimes overdone. Occasionally, so many assistants are hired and assigned to clinical professionals that the assistants cannot be adequately supervised. Needless to say, those administrators do not have the support of their clinical staff.

Many professionals are faced with increasing numbers of assistants whose services they are expected to skillfully manage. If they are to effectively handle this growing responsibility, they must know how to supervise assistants, and they must have the necessary time. Researchers have a responsibility to provide accurate information to help us understand how to optimize the contributions of support workers to service delivery and how to most effectively supervise their work in the rehabilitation disciplines.

In summary, information gained from research on the supervisory process with peers, students, and assistants may benefit clinical service facilities by helping administrators plan the most cost-efficient use of their human and financial resources. Findings also may influence educational programs for both assistants and professionals as their staff members plan for the clinical education process. Eventually, when all the variables are understood, academic program representatives may be able to match student educational level to practicum disorder area and supervisor level, ensuring that service delivery is complemented, not compromised. Professional associations also may use such findings when developing position and policy guidelines regarding the education, use, and supervision of students and assistants.

Supervisory Roles

The goals of the supervisory process, as they derive from the sort of person being supervised (assistant, assistant student, student professional, or professional) were discussed in a previous section. This section is aimed at identifying and achieving the more immediate goals or purposes along the way to that final objective. An important distinction exists between the (ultimate) goal of the supervisory process and the more immediate goal or purpose of a particular interaction between supervisee and supervisor. By knowing the ways in which these two types of objectives differ, a supervisor is more likely to be better positioned to specify what is desired at any given moment during a supervisory relationship. By identifying an immediate goal, a supervisor can take a specific and planned course of action to achieve that short-term objective. Clinical supervisors are called on to fill a variety of roles, each of which is responsive to a different category of needs on the part of their supervisees. Almost any need that is salient to the supervisee's progress as a learner can be conveniently pigeonholed under one of five categories. Each category of supervisee need dictates a particular supervisory role. These five supervisory roles are easy to learn and almost as easy to implement. The only real challenge is for supervisors to equip themselves to recognize the need to assume a role that is different from the one they typically find the most comfortable.

Supervisors, left to their own devices, typically take on the role of an educator, and that frequently results in feedback that is not well matched with supervisees' learning needs. The problem is that supervisees often need more than just education. A supervisor's failure to match the supervisory role with the supervisee's needs results in failure to achieve the immediate goal. Failure to accomplish an immediate or short-term objective delays the supervisee's movement along the developmental continuum toward the ultimate or overarching career goal. In short, this section is about being a good supervisor.

Anderson's Continuum

To better understand the concept of a continuum leading to an ultimate goal at the end of the supervisory process, one can examine the work of Anderson (1988). Anderson described a supervisory continuum (Figure 13.1) for use with practicum students in speech-language pathology. Although it was created to guide the work of speech-language pathology clinical educators, the continuum is applicable in virtually any rehabilitation discipline. It represents three stages of supervisee development along a horizontal bar or continuum. It begins with the evaluation-feedback stage of the supervisee's development on the left end of the bar, and it ends with the self-supervision stage of the supervisee's development on the right end

Stages

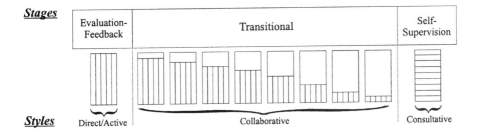

Styles

FIGURE 13.1. The supervisory continuum. (Reprinted with permission from Anderson, J. [1988]. <u>The supervisory process in speech language pathology and audiology</u> [p. 62]. Austin, TX: Pro-Ed.)

of the bar. Connecting these two stages and taking up most of the length of the continuum is the transitional stage.

Anderson viewed the evaluation-feedback stage as characteristic of the beginning supervisee, one who is ". . . unprepared for the clinical interaction, unable to problem-solve, overwhelmed by the dynamics of the situation, or accustomed to being told what to do." This supervisee tends to assume a passive role when interacting with the supervisor. Although beginning supervisees may be the most obvious examples of learners who are at the evaluation-feedback stage of development, they are not the only clinicians who may be at this stage. More advanced students and even clinical professionals with years of experience may find themselves unprepared and overwhelmed. This can happen even to experienced clinicians when they encounter new clients or change settings, programs, and jobs. In other words, the evaluation-feedback stage is not reserved for first-placement practicum students. So, when working with a supervisee who is in this stage, what should a supervisor aim for? The aim is to get the supervisee out of the evaluation-feedback stage and to move the supervisee to the right along the continuum as soon as possible.

The transitional stage is next, and it is the stage in which students spend most of their time. Supervisees in the transitional stage begin to participate more extensively in clinical decision making. They are not yet operating independently, but they are growing ever closer to that goal. They are learning to analyze clinical events to redesign their next session. Students often do this kind of analysis and planning overnight, but with experience, they become increasingly facile with their clinical problem-solving. As supervisees move along the continuum in the transitional stage, they begin to solve problems more easily, more accurately, and faster. In fact, one of the hallmarks of an outstanding clinician is an ability to quickly recognize the existence of a problem, accurately analyze the situation, and implement a new clinical strategy—all on the spot. In the natural course of events, supervisees who have progressed to the right along the continuum may move back to the left along the continuum within the transitional stage. For example, this may happen when the supervisee begins work in a new program or a different setting. Students may even move temporarily into the evaluation-feedback stage, but usually they will quickly move along the continuum again to the right. This process applies to fully qualified professionals, too. The principal difference is that when professionals find themselves in the transitional stage because of a new work environment, their return to the self-supervision stage is usually much faster.

The self-supervision stage represents the ultimate goal of the supervisory process with clinical professionals and with students in the rehabilitation professions. (The ultimate goal with assistants and student assistants is different and is discussed separately.) The self-supervision stage is the stage at which supervisees can independently analyze clinical events, plan one or more alternative strategies, and implement them. The key feature here is that this analysis is done independently, at least for the most part. Few professionals, even very experienced professionals, are completely independent in all aspects of clinical practice. All of us need the counsel of our colleagues from time to time, and when we do, we move back to the left a little way along the continuum, usually only for a short time. This, too, is a sign of a competent, self-supervising professional. A competent self-supervising professional knows when to seek help, where to find it, and how to implement it quickly and efficiently.

Participants' Interactions

Each stage of the continuum places its own demands on the participants. Although primary responsibility resides with supervisors to make the process work, supervisees must meet their share of expectations. Supervisors must be able to identify where each of their supervisees belongs on the continuum and then adopt a supervisory style that is appropriate for a learner at that particular level. Anderson points out that this is analogous to the diagnostic process used to determine the needs of clients. Supervisees must behave in ways that are consistent with their own level of development and with their particular supervisor's style. Any incongruence between the supervisee's needs and the supervisor's style or between the supervisor's style and the supervisee's response to that interactive style subverts the learning process and may even derail the relationship entirely.

The evaluation-feedback stage requires that the supervisor adopt a direct-active style of interaction with the supervisee. A direct-active style is characterized by pedantic, prescriptive, evaluative, and generally controlling behaviors on the part of the supervisor. Supervisors using a direct-active style of interaction do most of the talking while discussing clinical issues with supervisees. In turn, supervisees must behave in complementary ways. Supervisees in the evaluation-feedback stage are good listeners, feel

comfortable with their subordinate role, accept criticism, and remain generally passive during interactions with their supervisors. Note that being passive during interaction with a supervisor does not imply unresponsiveness.
Supervisees at this stage are highly responsive to their supervisors' instructions. The style "flag" hanging beneath the evaluation-feedback stage in
Figure 13.1 depicts the nature and amount of input by both parties. In this
instance, input is almost entirely from the supervisor. A direct-active teaching style is appropriate with novice clinicians, because it is effective for this
particular type of learner and very efficient. It enables a more-knowing
supervisor to pass on large amounts of information quickly to a less-know-
ing supervisee, enabling the learner to move out of the evaluation-feedback
stage as soon as possible.

As soon as the supervisee moves into the transitional stage, a new
repertoire of supervisory behaviors is required. The supervisor must adopt
a collaborative style of interaction with the supervisee. A collaborative
style is characterized by a dynamic, problem-solving series of exchanges
between supervisee and supervisor. The two parties work as partners to
plan and implement the best possible assessment and intervention with
their patients or clients and, at the same time, plan their own professional
growth and development. They do virtually everything jointly, not necessarily in the same room at the same time, but in a cooperative way, as with
a shared objective. The supervisor encourages and accepts supervisee
input, analyzes clinical events, solves problems *with* rather than *for* the
supervisee, and generally shows respect for the supervisee as a potential
contributor to clinical decision making. This style works only if the supervisee, in turn, participates actively in clinical decision making by providing input, asking thoughtful questions, self-analyzing, and working toward
clinical independence. As the supervisee gains independence and becomes
increasingly analytical and active in the decision-making process (i.e.,
moves to the right along the continuum), the supervisor provides progressively less guidance and serves more as a sounding board for the supervisee's ideas. The style flags hanging beneath the transitional stage in
Figure 13.1 depict the progressive change, over time, in the nature and
amount of input from both parties to the teaching/learning relationship.

By the time supervisees reach the self-supervision stage, they rely
only rarely on their supervisors for answers to questions and solutions to
problems. Supervisors find themselves engaging in a consultative style of
interaction; they are good listeners. Consultative supervisors give advice
when it is solicited, but they provide that advice in much the same manner as they would for a coworker down the hall. They are supportive, and
they assist with problem-solving only to the extent that the supervisee
invites them to. They allow their supervisees to accept all or part or even
none of the advice they offer. Essentially the two are interacting with one
another very much like peers. Supervisees must behave in complementary
ways; they must engage in active self-evaluation, seeking supervisory

input only when their own efforts to analyze and solve problems fail them. Supervisees must take an active role in the planning of clinical events, guiding supervisory conferences, and participating in non–patient-related activities, such as in-service sessions, institutional record keeping, and staff meetings. The style flag hanging beneath the self-supervision stage in Figure 13.1 again depicts the nature and amount of input by both parties, but in this instance shows that the supervisee is now functioning largely independently, seeking consultative input from peers only when necessary. The need for prescriptive and evaluative input from the supervisor is nonexistent, and the need for collaborative input is minimal.

Caveat

When supervising assistants and student assistants, it is *not* the ultimate goal of the process to help them reach the self-supervision stage. In fact, one of the most important understandings assistants in the rehabilitation disciplines must have when they begin working is that they must not independently alter the clinical intervention goals and strategies set out by their supervisors. Clearly, skilled assistants may be able to analyze their clinical activities and provide supervisors with valuable information that helps the supervisor modify the previously planned clinical intervention strategies, but assistants must not initiate these changes on their own. Anderson addressed this matter by saying that most assistants and their supervising professionals work in the evaluation-feedback stage of the continuum most of the time. Depending on the particular assistant's educational background, experience level, and unique personal skills, the two might move along the continuum well into the transitional stage; however, at no time would an assistant work independently. Anderson went on to point out that assistants' clear understanding of the continuum and their place on it should help them operate at their maximum potential while remaining within the acceptable boundaries of behavior for support personnel in their particular area of practice. The principles of the continuum still apply when supervising support workers, but both parties need to remember that they are working toward a modified ultimate outcome goal. They are working to form a collaborative service delivery partnership that prepares the assistant to function as efficiently and independently as possible within a carefully circumscribed scope of practice.

Adaptation of the Continuum

Anderson's continuum provided speech-language pathology practicum supervisors with a valuable guide or template for their interactions with students. It gave practicum supervisors a long-range goal. It reminded them that theirs was an important part in a much larger educational process. It helped supervisors find each student's place on a learning continuum and then provided suggestions for appropriate interactions with each student at various points along that continuum. Finally, it reminded supervisors that learners move back and forth along that continuum according to some easily discernible variables, and that understanding all these phenomena enables supervisors to provide better supervision. In short, it structured a previously unstructured process in the field of speech-language pathology and audiology.

Anderson's continuum had much to offer, but it was not a panacea for the ills of the clinical supervision process. The continuum was designed to guide the supervisory process with students only. It did not purport to work as a guide for the supervision of professionals, assistants, or assistant students, nor to be applicable in other disciplines. In spite of its narrow focus, it had a much broader practical appeal. Comments from registrants in supervision courses and at clinical education workshops that I presented with a colleague (Lu-Anne McFarlane) between 1987 and 1990 confirmed a long-held belief: that the continuum was equally applicable to the clinical education paradigms in audiology, occupational therapy, and physical therapy. In fact, a few workshop registrants from somewhat more arm's-length health sciences disciplines—such as nursing, recreational therapy, respiratory therapy, and pharmacy—reported that Anderson's continuum was applicable to the clinical education processes in their professions as well.

Unfortunately, the continuum was not responsive to certain aspects of the supervisory process in any discipline, including the one for which it was designed. Although it effectively structured the process when everything was going well, it had no inherent mechanisms to guide the behavior of supervisors whose students had gotten off track. Workshop registrants kept asking, "What about the problem student?" When McFarlane and I began searching for some supplementary strategies to guide clinical educators in their dealings with problem students, McFarlane spotted a potential resource on her husband's nightstand. It was a book (Peters & Austin, 1985) that described the principles of coaching as they applied to business management. On closer inspection, a strong parallel seemed to exist between three of the five coaching roles described by Peters and Austin and the three stages of Anderson's continuum. The two remaining roles in the coaching paradigm were directly responsive to the shortcomings of the continuum. They were the missing pieces. The remaining two roles were the roles a supervisor might assume to put a supervisee with a problem back on track. After field testing the concept of *supervisor as coach* with more interdisciplinary audiences, we wrote about their adaptation of the principles of coaching to the clinical education process in the rehabilitation disciplines (Hagler & McFarlane, 1991). Figure 13.2 depicts an overlay of the five coaching roles originally described by Peters and Austin onto Anderson's continuum to reveal the parallel structure of the two supervision models.

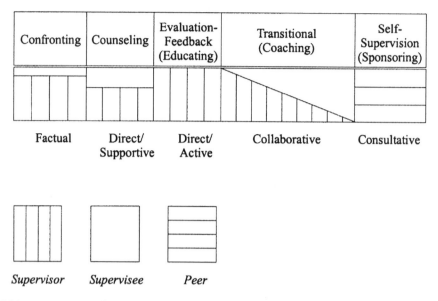

FIGURE 13.2. Coaching roles overlaid on the supervisory continuum.

Clinical Coaching

Hagler and McFarlane (1991) applied leadership theory from business management (Peters & Austin, 1985) to supervisory theory in speech-language pathology and audiology (Anderson, 1988). The goals of business and rehabilitation are obvious. The goal of business is to make money, and the goal of rehabilitation is to provide quality health care. Not so obvious is that the leadership and educational skills that help business leaders guide their employees to be successful moneymakers look amazingly like desirable clinical educator skills as they are described in the rehabilitation literature. In the beginning, this was a marriage of convenience; it gave speech-language pathologists a framework for handling problem students. A much deeper compatibility quickly became evident. The coaching paradigm became one with the supervisory continuum, and together they took on an interdisciplinary relevance that far surpassed that of either model by itself. The new model enabled clinical professionals in the rehabilitation disciplines to respond to individual supervisee needs by providing a practical framework for their interaction with supervisees at all levels of development (including problem students) and proved itself useful with all types of supervisees: student clinicians, student assistants, assistants, and professionals.

To be a good supervisor—in a clinic or in a business environment—is to be many things to those one supervises. Supervisors are teachers, skill builders, advocates, confidants, and critics. In fact, *coach* may be a better term than *supervisor*. The term *supervisor* connotes a person who ensures minimally acceptable performance from supervisees. The term *coach* connotes a person who facilitates optimal performance by an individual with promising potential. "Coaching does not mean to make less demanding, less interesting or less intense. It means to make less discouraging, less bound up with unnecessary controls and complications" (Peters & Austin, 1985). Coaching recognizes the many different roles we fill as supervisors and clinical educators. Peters and Austin (1985) outline five coaching roles: educator, coach, sponsor, counselor, and confronter. A coach's ability to recognize which role is appropriate at any given moment guides the coach during interaction with learners at all levels of development. Coaching is a process of developing excellence while recognizing that not all supervisees are excellent and that even excellent supervisees can have specific performance deficits. Although the five roles are distinct, the goal of each role and the coaching process as an overarching endeavor is to facilitate the development of an independent, creative, self-supervising clinician. Following are brief discussions of the distinguishing characteristics, applications, and outcomes of each of the coaching roles.

Educating

Educating is more than just giving information. It is a demonstration of the belief that with a little bit of information and guidance, even the new learner can contribute creatively to clinical services. It provides clear, manageable expectations, and it demands more attention to progress and reinforcement of the supervisee than other coaching roles. Educating "means giving people a chance to experiment a little bit from the start and to learn the difference between mistakes and disasters, between satisfactory and exceptional" (Peters & Austin, 1985). Educating is best suited to new learners who may be first practicum students or experienced clinicians with new clinical responsibilities. The supervisor creates an atmosphere that is positive and supportive, emphasizing the learning process and the application of academic knowledge to the clinical setting. The "educated" supervisee feels "talked with" rather than "talked at." Educating lays the foundation for later development of professional self-confidence.

Coaching

Coaching is the bread and butter of supervision in general and clinical education in particular. Supervisees need information. Coaching provides that information with questions, not exclamations. Exclamations provide information, but they do so through direct, specific suggestions or demonstrations. Questions, on the other hand, provide a pathway to information. Questions lead supervisees through a problem-solving process by helping them merge their existing knowledge with their current experiences. This skill is critical to later clinical autonomy. Students receive an abundance of exclamation points in their academic training programs. Their clinical supervisors are in the unique and enviable position of teaching in a setting that allows them to provide question marks. Coaches provide challenges and encourage risk-taking, which means they must expect and allow mistakes. Good tries that fail can be applauded, because the supervisee has learned something.

Coaching is a supervisory role best suited for supervisees who already have basic clinical skills and academic preparation. Such supervisees do not require extensive education. General guidance or minor corrections are all that is required. Coaches are encouraging, enthusiastic, and open-minded with regard to the supervisee's ability to contribute. Good coaches have the ability to listen, even to ideas that do not match their own. They are able to foster a sense of independence and accomplishment in the learner. Coaching refines skills, and skill improvements enhance confidence.

Sponsoring

Sponsoring is the ultimate expression of maximizing supervisee potential. It goes beyond coaching by arranging for supervisees to take charge of their own learning and to perform autonomously at new things. It trusts them to solicit help as necessary, reinforcing the notion that recognition of the need for help is at the heart of independence. Sponsors take a personal interest in their supervisees' development, providing feedback on yesterday's effort and opportunity for tomorrow's achievement.

A special responsibility of sponsors is to help promising learners come to grips with the subtleties of clinical practice. For example, sponsors guide learners on the best way to approach certain clients and coworkers or on how to wind their way through institutional politics. Sponsoring is not mentoring. Mentoring emphasizes "be like me;" sponsoring emphasizes "be yourself." If supervisors teach their supervisees to be like them, the result is learners limited by their own shortcomings as well as those of their supervisors. If supervisors encourage their supervisees to go beyond the supervisor's abilities, their supervisees are restricted only by their own limitations. Sponsoring requires a lot of a supervisor, because it means not being threatened by an exceptional supervisee's skills and abilities. It is difficult to remember that when a supervisor lets a supervisee shine, the supervisee does so for both of them.

As previously mentioned, not all supervisees are excellent, and not all excellent supervisees are excellent in every respect. The coaching model developed by Peters and Austin (1985) has two roles that recognize this phenomenon and guide clinical supervisors in their dealings with supervisees who have gone off track.

Counseling

The counseling role is taken up when a problem persists even after the most basic efforts to educate the supervisee about that problem have failed. It is important to note that supervisors earn the right to counsel by first educating and failing; only then can they counsel. Counseling a learner who has no problem is like putting a Band-Aid on a finger that has no cut. It's completely unnecessary and may even be a bit annoying.

Ideally, counseling is planned. It is also structured, and it follows a critical sequence of events that encourage active participation by the supervisee. Counseling helps the supervisee explore options without bias and reach a mutually agreeable understanding about what will happen, who will do it, and when it will be done. Counseling provides an opportunity for the learner to self-disclose or share the problem. It focuses on how to solve a problem that both parties recognize as real. Counseling respects the collegial nature of a healthy supervisory relationship. It encourages supervisees to participate in formulation of a solution to their own problems. Successful counseling also reflects an understanding of attributional theory—the tendency for supervisors to respond to supervisees' behaviors on the basis of their attribution or belief about the causes of those behaviors (Roberts & Naremore, 1983)—and, in the end, cultivates a closer working relationship between the supervisor and supervisee.

Counseling is needed when problems interfere with students' clinical performance. When supervisors' best attempts at educating have failed, counseling is indicated. It is a proactive response to setbacks and disappointments. Counseling puts client service first but treats the supervisee with compassion and respect. When successful, it speeds the supervisee toward improved performance. It can turn a critical situation around quickly. The counselor shows a willingness to listen and is able to give clear, useful feedback. Later payoffs include an increased sense of belonging and importance on the part of the supervisee, who enjoys a renewed commitment to learning and client care.

Confronting

A confrontation is a showdown. Confronting is needed when a supervisee's performance problems persist despite the supervisor's having previously educated and failed, and then having counseled and failed. It is done in the best interests of everyone involved. The supervisor has in mind specific, measurable standards of a behavioral nature below which the supervisee may not go. Confronting removes any remaining questions about which performance-based criteria the supervisee must meet to be able to continue with the responsibilities in question. Confronting focuses clearly on the need for some decisive action on the part of the supervisee and a deadline by which such action will take place. Results of confronting may range from the supervisee's success with current responsibilities (or success with new, less demanding responsibilities) to failure of the placement (in the case of a student) or to reassignment or even dismissal (in the case of a clinical professional).

Implementing Counseling and Confronting

Unlike educating, coaching, and sponsoring, all of which can be done on the fly and in the presence of others, counseling and confronting demand somewhat different implementation. Counseling and confronting require planning if they are to succeed, and both sequences look very much alike.

Remember that counseling comes first and that supervisors earn the right to counsel by having first tried to educate the supervisee without success. According to Peters and Austin (1985), counseling assumes that supervisees have the right to know where they stand and that supervisors have an obligation to tell them in a timely manner. Counseling is *not* hurried, angry, punitive, or intended to solve all the supervisee's problems.

The best way for a supervisor to avert these pitfalls is by planning the counseling session. Before meeting, the supervisor should determine the purpose of the counseling session. The key issue(s) must be defined and preferably written down. Usually these are quite specific aspects of clinical practice (e.g., report writing; diagnostic competence; safety issues, such as failure to follow protocol for handling medications; or intervention strategies with a particular patient/client). Objective behavioral indices of the existence of each key issue should be listed. This list may be important if the supervisee denies the existence of a problem. Also, before entering a counseling interaction, the supervisor should have some measurable results clearly in mind.

When these steps are completed, the supervisor can schedule a meeting. It is important to consider when and where. Counseling and confronting require privacy and time; neither should be compromised. At the meeting, the supervisor begins with a brief, straightforward statement of the key issue(s) accompanied by a few examples of the behavioral indices of the existence of each, and assures the supervisee that putting things back on track is the sole purpose of this meeting. Even supervisees who are unwilling to agree on what the problem is or that it is one of their own creation are likely to agree that there is something worth talking about. This is all a supervisor needs to start a successful counseling session. The next step is both the most important and the hardest to do: sit back, be quiet, and listen. Here is where supervisors can learn a great deal about their supervisee and sometimes even about themselves. Supervisees usually know when things are not going well, and most of them are highly motivated to do a good job. They simply may not know how to effect improvement. Supervisors should be prepared to learn that they are part of the problem and, if they are, to fight the tendency to be defensive about it. When the problem is finally on the table for discussion, explore it until it is understood, and then jointly devise a solution. Put together an action plan, and arrange a follow-up sequence of meetings to check on progress.

Confronting was described by Peters and Austin (1985) as a constructive, caring response to a supervisee's chronic poor performance. As with counseling, supervisors earn the right to confront their supervisees by having first counseled and failed. Confronting is a last attempt to get the supervisee back on track. It is a clear message to the supervisee that improvement is imperative and that, in the absence of improvement, there will be serious consequences. For students, these consequences may range from temporary caseload reduction to failure of the placement. For employees, consequences may range from temporary suspension of certain responsibilities to termination of employment.

Unlike counseling, the key issues already have been defined. There should be no surprises when confronting a supervisee. In fact, this offers a good check for supervisors to help them decide if confronting is the appropriate role. If they believe the supervisee might be taken back by anything they are planning to say, then perhaps counseling would be more appropriate.

The same guidelines for scheduling the meeting and maintaining an even temperament described for counseling also apply to confronting. A good way to begin a confronting sequence is with a recap of the educating and counseling that preceded it, followed by a brief account of recent behavioral evidence to indicate that the problem persists. The focus should be on behavioral matters and the value of the encounter to the supervisee. It may be advisable to follow the confrontation sequence with a letter or memo restating any expectations and consequences described during the dialogue.

There is one circumstance that most supervisors would agree justifies a departure from the "educate before counseling and counsel before confronting" rule. That is when client safety is at stake. When safety is the issue, preceptors and supervisors may jump straight from educating to confronting, without following the prescribed sequence of interactions. Rittman and Osborn (1995) provide a meaningful account of a nurse preceptor's efforts to adhere to sound principles of clinical education when confronted with a student's unsafe clinical practices. They also describe the professional dilemma preceptors face when an unsafe student is nearing graduation. Certainly unsafe practices create a special and often difficult situation, whether the supervisee is a student assistant, a student, an assistant, or a professional.

Rationale

Peters and Austin (1985) described their work as a "blinding flash of the obvious." If we view it as such, perhaps we pay them the highest possible praise, because common sense applied to human relationships is not really common at all. Furthermore, "obvious" does not translate to "easy." If it did, more supervisors in the rehabilitation professions would be responsive to the various and changing needs of their supervisees. In the case of clinical supervision of speech-language pathology students, research has shown us that clinical educators do not alter their supervisory style even to accommodate different levels of expertise among supervisees, much less to be responsive to a particular student's evolving abilities during the course of a single placement (Roberts & Smith, 1982). There is no empirical evidence to indicate that supervisors in the other rehabilitation disciplines are any better at this important skill when working with their students. Virtually all clinical professionals and their assistants are familiar with one or more clinical administrators whose supervisory style falls well short of the mark when it comes to meeting the needs of those being supervised. Is a comprehensive model—one which provides supervisors with a detailed framework for goal-oriented interaction that is responsive to supervisee's short-term and long-term needs—important in the rehabilitation professions? The answer is an emphatic *yes.*

Implementing Clinical Coaching

Dressing Right for the Occasion

Selecting the right hat (role) for a particular occasion is critical to accomplishing your supervisory purpose. In the same way that a baseball cap is a poor fit at a formal dinner, supervisory attempts to educate an advanced student fail to move that student further along the continuum to professional independence. Furthermore, it makes both parties uncomfortable in the process. If the clinical coaching model is to work, supervisors must develop the habit of always analyzing their supervisees' needs. For example, if a supervisee is beginning a first placement or is in a more advanced placement but working with a type of client never before seen, then the supervisor may want to start off as an educator, directing the supervisee's activities by giving information and suggestions. Alternatively, if a supervisee is in a more advanced placement working with one or more clients that are the same as or similar to clients previously seen in other placements, then the supervisor may want to start off as a coach. A coach, in this instance, would interact with the supervisee in ways that encourage the supervisee to participate fully in discussions and intervention planning, to analyze clinical activities, and to deductively reason from general academic information to specific problematic cases.

It is important to remember that supervisory roles are selected in response to specific learner needs. For example, a physical therapy student may have no experience with burns treatment but extensive experience with electrotherapy. The electrotherapy experience may even surpass that of the supervisor. When interacting with this particular student, the supervisor needs to adopt an educator role when discussing burns treatment and a sponsor role when addressing the student's interests and activities in the area of electrotherapy. In summary, supervisors can adopt the right role only by first identifying their supervisee's place on the adapted continuum as it applies to a particular skill and aligning their supervisory behavior with the supervisee's level of development in the target skill area. This requires that supervisors switch roles frequently in response to their students' varying needs.

Components of the Supervisory Process

Anderson (1988) adapted the work of Cogan (1973) and Goldhammer (1969) and identified five components to the supervisory process: (1) understanding, (2) planning, (3) monitoring (observing), (4) analyzing, and (5) integrating. It should be noted that monitoring is, for the most part, what supervisors do while supervisees provide some sort of clinical intervention or patient/client service. All five of these activities occur in the order in which they are listed, and with the exception of the first activity, supervisors and supervisees should cycle through them repeatedly during the course of a supervisory relationship.

The exception—understanding—refers to the supervisor's responsibility to help the supervisee understand the supervisory process. Why does the supervisee need to understand the process? An important underpinning for this chapter is that if clinical supervisors are to effectively manage the clinical work of their supervisees, they must understand the process. Likewise, supervisees are better positioned to fulfill their responsibilities as learners if they understand the process and the expectations it has of them. Unfortunately, supervisees, especially the student variety, are conditioned through years of academic course work to expect to be *educated*—that is, to be passive learners—and as a result, their natural tendency is to behave in ways that are consistent with that role. They may do this out of habit, even when they are capable of deciding for themselves what they need to know and how to learn it. If students understand that this spongelike behavior is at times inappropriate, then they are much more likely to step up and take responsibility for their own education, a habit they must develop if they are to survive as clinical professionals. Similarly, if clinical professionals understand when and how they are expected to take the initiative, especially as new employees, they make a more cost-effective contribution to service delivery and do so sooner. It may be necessary for supervisors and supervisees to return to this topic from time to time during the course of a supervisory relationship, but certainly not with the same regularity as the remaining four components.

With regard to the planning, monitoring, analyzing, and integrating components, all supervisors cycle through them multiple times in the

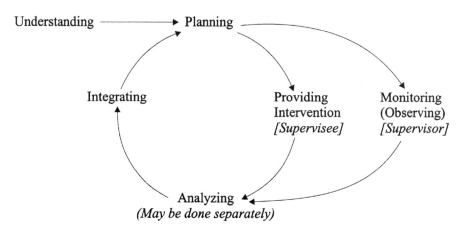

FIGURE 13.3. Components of the supervisory process.

course of a supervisory relationship, but supervisors of students cycle through them much more frequently than supervisors of rehabilitation professionals. The components are depicted in Figure 13.3 to illustrate their temporal relationship to one another.

Planning is the first activity in the four-component repeating cycle. As soon as the supervisee understands the process, it is time to begin planning. The most obvious kind of planning is for the clinical process. It includes client planning and clinician planning. Planning for clients is nothing new. Planning for the clinician may be a bit novel to some. With student clinicians, it involves structuring the clinical practicum experience to ensure that they get the most out of the placement. With assistants and clinical professionals, it involves structuring specific job responsibilities to accommodate their needs and interests. When this kind of planning is done well, assistants and professionals alike enjoy heightened job satisfaction and grow professionally and technically.

Another kind of planning is for the supervisory process. This type of joint planning is often ignored. As stated previously, the lion's share of a supervisory relationship is spent in the transitional stage with the supervisor in the coaching role. This requires that both parties share clinical decision-making responsibilities and work as partners in service delivery. If the process is truly collaborative, the supervisee solicits supervisory involvement in planned observations, session analyses, and discussions regarding assessment and intervention strategies. Similarly, supervisors may wish to plan their own professional growth as administrators, and they may ask their supervisees to help them realize those goals. For example, a supervisor might ask a supervisee to allow one or more supervisory conferences to be audio- or videotaped to afford the supervisor opportunities to self-analyze and evaluate specific supervisory skills. A supervisor might even ask a supervisee to provide evaluative feedback.

In summary, planning for clients is an essential but minimal kind of planning. Planning for specific kinds of growth for clinicians and supervisors can be a valuable complement to the supervisory process, making it far more rewarding than a partnership that is entirely client focused. This is more than many supervisors and supervisees are accustomed to. If they choose not to incorporate personal growth planning into their own partnership, that's okay, but it should be a thoughtful, jointly reached decision, not simply an oversight.

The next activity in the cycle is *observing*. Although Anderson (1988) gave this component its label, there is a somewhat better term: *monitoring*. The word *observation* seems to connote watching while the supervisee does something, but the word *monitoring* implies that more options exist, and they do. Monitoring may include editing written treatment plans, talking to other clinicians about the supervisee's performance, listening to audiotapes, reading reports, checking file notes, verifying scoring procedures on standardized tests, or seeking feedback directly from clients or their family members. Whatever form it takes, monitoring is the process by which supervisors gather information about their supervisees' work. Monitoring is the data collection part of the supervisory process. It is a dispassionate activity designed to maximize objectivity later on and to ensure that the information being collected is used in ways that encourage supervisee growth. It is *not* an activity that is intended to include evaluation. That comes later.

How does a supervisor monitor without evaluating? Evaluation-free monitoring is not particularly easy to accomplish, principally because the supervisory job, by its very nature, almost always requires evaluation. The trick is to keep evaluation in its place. Monitoring, which may include direct observation, is a time for data collection. Data may include everything from anecdotal notes to numbers. As long as the supervisor can avoid attaching a qualitative comment to the data, they are not evaluative in nature. Data, in the absence of evaluation, are potentially more useful to the supervisee.

The fourth component in the process is *analyzing*. Analysis is the part of the supervisory process in which supervisee and supervisor try to make sense of the data collected in the monitoring phase. Although analysis can be a joint effort, there are circumstances in which it is better if the two parties analyze the data separately. This is especially true in the case of practicum students who are in the early transitional stage on the continuum—that is, students who benefit mostly from being coached by their supervisors, but who are in the early stages of being coached. These students are ready to learn to be self-analytic but are not yet proficient enough to self-analyze "on line." They must be given time to contemplate their alternatives. Even as little as 20 to 30 minutes after the end of a session may be enough time for supervisees at this stage to critically evaluate their work in preparation for a supervisory conference. This is "reflection *on* action," as described by Schon (1987). Less experienced supervisees, especially students who are in the evaluation-feedback stage, may not be able to effectively analyze their own behavior in the clinic, at least not all of it. Many of these supervisees are still learning the fundamentals and are not ready to tackle the refinements. In other words, they are unable to analyze their data by themselves. Students further along the continuum, nearer the right end of the transitional stage, are able to self-analyze on the spot and then make immediate modifications to their clinical activities. This is Schon's "reflection *in* action." Of course, these supervisees are able to analyze their data separately, but they do not require that extra processing time.

Reflective practice (Schon, 1987) is a highly regarded principle in supervision, but it is probably best described not as the goal of clinical supervision but as a process within it. Fowler and Chevannes (1998) viewed the supervisory process as an environment in which reflective practice can be developed, but they emphasized that reflective practice is not the ideal for all learners, and that the supervisory process must be structured to meet the needs of each individual learner.

The fifth component in the process is *integrating*. This refers to the act of merging the information from the previous events, especially the analyses, to understand past clinical events and plan future clinical events. It is important to remember that the two parties often have different perceptions of the same data, even if their analyses of the data are on line and simultaneous. Integrating those perceptions in a collaborative manner is what clinical coaching is all about. If supervisors can train themselves to offer their supervisees only data, most supervisees are able to make partial, or even complete, sense of it through analysis. For example, after a nursing student had difficulty hearing a patient's heartbeat, her preceptor (supervisor) informed her—nonjudgmentally, of course—that her stethoscope was incorrectly placed in her ears. The student analyzed the situation and understood a number of things immediately. She recalled that the ear tips are angled slightly forward so they can be accommodated in the wearer's ear canal and that to reverse them can virtually plug the openings in the tips for some users. She reflected on why she would have forgotten this and concluded that it was probably just nervousness. Knowing that she might be nervous again, she decided that a visual reminder might avert future embarrassment. She thought she might place a red self-adhesive dot on the stainless steel tubing near the right ear tip. Red equals right. She considered all these things and verbalized them to her supervisor in a period of 20 seconds after her supervisor's comment about the stethoscope. The effect on the student was that she learned to analyze a clinical event for herself and solve a problem without relying on the preceptor to do it for her. She gained clinical self-confidence, because she found her own solution, and she was not made to feel inept or stupid by her preceptor. Contrary to what the preceptor had first thought, the student had not forgotten even the most basic facts from early in her educational program. The preceptor felt reassured that the same thing would not happen again. Both preceptor and student gained a small measure of trust and respect for one another. When events like this are played out time after time during the course of a supervisory relationship, the impact on the supervisee's clinical growth can be profound.

Documenting the Supervisory Process

There are two aspects of the supervisory process that are often documented. One is documentation of responsibilities, and the other is documentation of performance. Documentation of responsibilities for employed assistants and professionals is usually in the form of employment contracts. Even when job descriptions exist, they are often rather sketchy and lacking in detail with regard to specific responsibilities. Documentation of responsibilities for students, if they are documented at all, is usually in the form of learning contracts. Learning contracts, which seem to have originated in occupational therapy, are growing in popularity among clinical educators in the other rehabilitation disciplines. Documentation of performance, for students and practicing clinicians alike, is usually more regimented.

Employment Contracts

Documentation of the responsibilities of working assistants and professionals is usually in the form of employment contracts. Unfortunately, employment contracts do not often include much detail with regard to expectations for professional growth, program assignments, caseload mix, and other day-to-day responsibilities. Employment contracts tend to focus more on rank, salary, vacation allowance, sick leave, and a few other basic legalistic issues. Also, because of their focus, employment contracts tend not to get reviewed very often, even in the face of changing job responsibilities. Such contracts are seldom of much use when questions arise with regard to whether employees are fulfilling their job responsibilities. A supplementary, less formal, but far more detailed "contract" can be created at the departmental or program level to address this common deficiency in typical employment contracts at large institutions.

Learning Contracts

Some supervisors of practicum students require their supervisees to devise learning contracts for each placement. Learning contracts are written documents that describe the student's specific learning objectives during the placement in question. They represent a joint commitment by supervisor and supervisee to try to accomplish those objectives. The objectives listed in the contract are a marriage of three variables: (1) services and special programs in the practicum facility, (2) the supervisor's instructional objectives, and (3) the student's needs and interests. Although learning contracts can take whatever form and detail the participants want them to, it is recommended that the learning objectives be concise, measurable, time-tied, achievable, and flexible. Both participants must know exactly what is to be learned, and they must be able to identify when the learning process is complete for each objective.

Performance Evaluation

Most employment settings have performance evaluation tools that must be completed on employees, usually annually. Such evaluations take almost as many different forms as there are institutions employing rehabilitation service providers. Discussing their various merits is a task far beyond the scope of this chapter. It will suffice to say that employees usually tolerate whatever tool is currently in use in their facility and seldom campaign for modifications or replacements. They know a new one will be coming just as soon as their administrator returns from the next management seminar.

Post–secondary educational programs provide performance evaluation tools for use by the clinical educators who take their students. Although there seem to be fewer student evaluation tools than there are employee evaluation tools, there are still several. For example, in 1985, there were about 25 different tools simultaneously in use for the evaluation of clinical performance of physical therapy students and physical therapy assistant students. This created an untenable situation for clinical educators, who worked with students from many different programs and were expected to familiarize themselves with a new tool virtually every time they supervised a new practicum student. Learning and implementing so many different tools was not acceptable to busy professionals.

In response to this situation, the American Physical Therapy Association began a project to develop two clinical performance evaluation tools designed for use by all educational programs in physical therapy, one for physical therapy assistant students and one for physical therapy students. The results of the association's work are the *Physical Therapist Clinical Performance Instrument* (American Physical Therapy Association, 1998a) and the *Physical Therapist Assistant Clinical Performance Instrument* (American Physical Therapy Association, 1998b). These tools are undoubtedly the most conscientiously validated devices of their type available in any of the rehabilitation disciplines. The American Physical Therapy Association has set a standard all rehabilitation professions should try to follow.

Perhaps the most salient points that can be made about the role of evaluation in the supervisory process are that it is inevitable and important and that it has a time and a place. Evaluation in a supervisory relationship always will be required; it is one of the things supervisors do. However, evaluation by the supervisor should be kept to a minimum throughout the relationship, and it should be avoided altogether, except when it is the mutually recognized purpose during a particular encounter.

Conclusion

This chapter contains integrated information from sources so seemingly diverse as the health sciences, education, and business management, and with any luck, it provides a template with which clinical supervisors can structure the supervisory process next time they engage in it. It is intended to serve as a starting point for further study of the clinical supervisory process and to emphasize how much the rehabilitation disciplines have in common where supervision is concerned. Textbooks about rehabilitation services delivery tend to be written for discipline-specific audiences, as do textbooks about supervision. However, there may be no other topic less in need of discipline-specific discussion than clinical supervision. The reader is invited to consult some of the many references at the end of this chapter to gain additional familiarity with the principles on which this hybrid supervisory paradigm was constructed.

Clinical supervisors now have a chart (admittedly a small-scale chart) to guide them as they plan their supervisory journey. The really good ones do a little research before embarking on this demanding sojourn, and when they become lost along the way, the very astute stop to ask for directions— even the men.

Acknowledgments

I thank Dr. Jean Anderson for giving clinical educators the continuum and all its attendant theory and for granting permission to reproduce Figure 13.1 from her text *The Supervisory Process in Speech-Language Pathology and Audiology*. Thanks also to Tom Peters and Nancy Austin, whose coaching principles described in *A Passion for Excellence* are integral to the clinical supervision theory outlined in this chapter. Appreciation is extended to the *Canadian Journal of Rehabilitation* for granting permission to use text from a previously published article on the application of coaching principles in clinical supervision. Finally, I thank the *Journal of Speech-Language Pathology and Audiology* for granting permission to use text from a previously published article on the effects of students on service delivery.

References

American Physical Therapy Association. (1998a). Physical therapist clinical performance instrument. Alexandria, VA: Division of Education of the American Physical Therapy Association.

American Physical Therapy Association. (1998b). Physical therapist assistant clinical performance instrument. Alexandria, VA: Division of Education of the American Physical Therapy Association.

Anderson, J. (1988). The supervisory process in speech language pathology and audiology. Austin, TX: Pro-Ed.

Barrett, C., & Myrick, F. (1998). Job satisfaction in preceptorship and its effect on the clinical performance of the preceptee. Journal of Advanced Nursing, 27, 364–371.

Bristow, D., & Hagler, P. (1994). Impact of physical therapy students on patient service delivery and professional staff time. Physiotherapy Canada, 46(4), 275–280.

Bristow, D., & Hagler, P. (1997). Comparison of individual physical therapists' productivity to that of combined physical therapist student pairs. Physiotherapy Canada, winter, 16–23.

Cebulski, P., & Sojkowski, M. (1988). Clinical education and staff productivity. Clinical Management in Physical Therapy, 8, 26–29.

Cogan, M. (1973). Clinical supervision. Boston: Houghton Mifflin.

Fowler, J., & Chevannes, M. (1998). Evaluating the efficacy of reflective practice within the context of clinical supervision. Journal of Advanced Nursing, 27, 379–382.

Goldhammer, R. (1969). Clinical supervision. New York: Holt, Reinhart and Winston.

Hagler, P., & McFarlane, L. (1991). Achieving maximum student potential: The supervisor as coach. Canadian Journal of Rehabilitation, 5(1), 5–16.

Hagler, P., Madill, H., Warren, S., Loomis, J., Elliott, D., & Pain, K. (1993). Role and use of support personnel in the rehabilitation professions. Final report to the National Health Research and Development Program on Project #6609-1730-RP. Edmonton, AB: University of Alberta.

Hagler, P., Pain, K., & Warren, S. (1995). Impact of support workers on patient/client attendances in audiology. Paper presented at the American Speech-Language-Hearing Association Convention, Orlando, FL.

Hagler, P., Warren, S., & Pain, K. (1995). Impact of support workers on patient/client attendances in speech-language pathology. Paper presented at the American Speech-Language-Hearing Association Convention, Orlando, FL.

Halonen, R., Fitzgerald, J., & Simmon, K. (1976). Measuring the costs of clinical education in departments utilizing allied health professionals. Journal of Allied Health, 5, 5–12.

Hammersberg, S. (1982). A cost/benefit study of clinical education in selected allied health programs. Journal of Allied Health, 1, 35–41.

Hancock, J. (1997). Impact of speech pathology students on patient care. Unpublished master's thesis, University of Alberta, Edmonton, Alberta, Canada.

Hancock, J., & Hagler, P. (1998). A pilot study of the effects of S-LP practicum students on service delivery. Journal of Speech-Language Pathology and Audiology, 22(3), 141–150.

Ladyshewsky, R. (1995). Enhancing service productivity in acute care inpatient settings using a collaborative clinical education model. Physical Therapy, 75, 503–510.

Ladyshewsky, R., Bird, N., & Finney, J. (1994). The impact on departmental productivity during physical therapy student placements: An investigation of outpatient physical therapy services. Physiotherapy Canada, 46, 89–93.

Leiken, A. (1983). Method to determine the effect of clinical education on production in a health care facility. Physical Therapy, 63, 56–59.

Leiken, A., Stern, E., & Baines, R. (1983). The effect of clinical education programs on hospital production. Inquiry, 20, 88–92.

Lopopolo, R. (1984). Financial model to determine the effect of clinical education programs on physical therapy departments. Physical Therapy, 64, 1396–1402.

Peters, T., & Austin, N. (1985). A passion for excellence. New York: Random House.

Porter, R., & Kincaid, C. (1977). Financial aspects of clinical education to facilities. Physical Therapy, 57, 905–909.

Rittman, M., & Osborn, J. (1995). An interpretive analysis of precepting an unsafe student. Journal of Nursing Education, 34, 217–221.

Roberts, J., & Naremore, R. (1983). An attributional model of supervisors' decision-making behavior in speech language pathology. Journal of Speech and Hearing Research, 26, 537–549.

Roberts, J., & Smith, K. (1982). Supervisor-supervisee role differences and consistency of behavior in supervisory conferences. Journal of Speech and Hearing Research, 25, 428–434.

Schon, D. (1987). Educating the reflective practitioner. San Francisco, CA: Jossey-Bass Publishers.

Workload Measurement System. National Hospital Productivity Improvement Program, Health and Welfare Canada—Statistics Canada Health Division, 1987–88 Edition. Ottawa, Canada: Minister of Supply and Services.

CHAPTER 14

Administrative and Legal Issues

Ron Scott

Rehabilitation managers and clinical professional and support staff confront formidable legal issues in their professional practice. Most legal issues—from employment issues to health care malpractice, from patient informed consent to compliance with federal, state, and local or provincial administrative rules and regulations—simultaneously present both legal and health professional ethical concerns, because legal and health professional ethical duties have largely been melded into a unitary standard for acceptable practice. This chapter gives an overview of salient legal issues affecting rehabilitation professionals and managers in the United States.

Legal Environment

Rehabilitation professionals and managers come into contact with the legal system in four planes. First, to the extent that they are employed by governmental entities, they are directly affected by federal and state *constitutional* mandates addressing such areas as patient privacy and due process, or fundamental fairness involving patient (and provider) access to rehabilitation facilities and services. Second, all rehabilitation professionals are directly affected by governing federal and state *statutory* law, including, among many others, the Age Discrimination in Employment Act (prohibiting employment discrimination in public and private settings against workers age 40 or older), the Americans with Disabilities Act (mandating equitable treatment of physically and mentally disabled individuals in business settings), the Civil Rights Act of 1964 (prohibiting discrimination against people on the basis of race/ethnicity, gender, religion, and national origin), the Family and Medical Leave Act (mandating job-protected, unpaid leaves of absence from work for personal and family health emergencies), and the Occupational Safety and Health Act (requiring compliance by facilities with federal safety and health standards applicable to patients, staff, and others on premises). Third, *judge-made* law, in the form of civil and criminal case decisions, establishes legal precedent that must be followed by those subject to the jurisdiction, or "reach" of the court. (Health care malpractice case decisions involving rehabilitation patients and professionals fall within this category of law.) Finally, public governmental regulatory agencies at the federal, state, and local levels make and enforce *administrative rules and regulations* that directly and strongly influence rehabilitation professional practice. (A prominent example of a powerful administrative agency with broad jurisdiction is the federal Equal Employment Opportunity Commission [EEOC], which makes rules, investigates complaints, and fashions remedies concerning employment discrimination and workplace sexual harassment.)

A kind of hierarchy exists concerning legal duties incumbent on rehabilitation professionals and others (Scott, 1998). Federal constitutional law supersedes all other conflicting laws and regulations; legislative statutory law enjoys precedence over conflicting case decisions rendered by judges (except those interpreting the federal or applicable state constitution); and judge-made case law generally controls over conflicting administrative rules and regulations. As a rule of thumb, rehabilitation professionals and managers have the most contact with the base-entity on the legal totem pole—that is, regulatory agencies, whose rules most intimately and routinely affect everyday rehabilitation practice.

It has been said that we live in the most litigious of times, when people have a strong propensity to claim against and sue one another for perceived "wrongs" done by others against them. (The legal term of art for private wrongs allegedly committed by one person against another, such as in cases of alleged rehabilitation patient injury during treatment, is *tort* [French for "wrong"].) While tens of millions of civil and criminal lawsuits may come into existence each year in the United States, only tens of thousands of those formal legal cases involve allegations of wrongdoing by health care professionals against patients (Scott, 1999).

Exercise 1: Rationale and Propriety for Claims and Lawsuits

Individually or in small groups:
1. Brainstorm on possible reasons for why people have such an apparent strong propensity to claim against or sue one another.
2. Formulate possible reasons why rehabilitation health professionals may be less likely to be claimed against or sued by patients under their care.
3. Discuss the "ethics" (i.e., right and wrong) of the perceived "litigation crisis" in American society.

There are two legal systems that rehabilitation professionals need to know about: the *civil legal system*, involving largely private legal disputes, and the *criminal legal system*, involving wrongs against the public's interests. Rehabilitation professionals charged with wrongdoing may well face legal actions in both venues, as well as possible adverse administrative actions before licensure boards or certification entities, and concomitant actions before professional association ethics committees.

Exercise 2: Forums for Legal Actions Against Rehabilitation Professionals

For each representative rehabilitation profession in the class or clinical setting, or as individual professionals, as applicable, spell out in outline form all of the forums (in the United States, Canada, or elsewhere, as appropriate) in which represented rehabilitation professionals might face legal or adverse administrative action for alleged patient injury.

Besides the private/public nature differentiating civil and criminal litigation, the standards of proof for culpability and the consequences of findings of culpability differ significantly. In civil lawsuits (including health care malpractice legal actions brought by patients or their representatives against providers) and in adverse administrative actions, the standard of proof for culpability is a preponderance (or greater weight) of evidence presented in the case. This means that if a patient-plaintiff's evidence supporting a finding of liability for health care malpractice against a defendant-provider/facility in a given case is more credible than the provider's/facility's evidence, then a finding of culpability should ensue. In a criminal case, however, wherein the consequences of a finding of guilt are normally substantially more severe, the standard for proof for a public prosecutor is "beyond a reasonable doubt," meaning that the fact finder (judge or jury) can have no legitimate hesitation in finding the criminal defendant guilty.

The consequences of a finding of civil (or administrative) liability include the payment of money damages to a successful plaintiff; a declaration of rights and duties of parties to a dispute; and, in some cases, specific performance as promised by a party in breach of contract. The consequences of criminal guilt include sentencing to incarceration or the threat of incarceration through probation, as well as the imposition of a monetary fine, and, in some cases, restitution to victims of crime.

Before any rehabilitation practice issue devolves into a claim or lawsuit, providers and organizations must consult regularly and proactively with legal counsel. For providers in their individual capacity, personal legal counsel may be optimal, particularly in situations in which their legal interests might be different than those of an employing entity. For any impending claim or lawsuit, do not discuss facts of the case with those with whom you do not have a statutorily privileged relationship (i.e., discuss them only with your personal attorney). Keep in mind that an institutional attorney may not be permitted to maintain your communications in confidence.

If a rehabilitation professional requires personal legal advice and does not have a personal attorney, then the best sources for locating one are (1) through endorsement by peers who have used and recommend specific legal counsel, and (2) through the county bar association lawyer referral service, a public service in existence across the United States that provides specialized attorneys for low-cost initial consultation.

Health Care Malpractice

Health care malpractice is civil liability of a health care professional for patient injuries (physical or mental), with a legal basis for liability imposition. The term *health care malpractice* is used herein instead of medical malpractice, which affects only physicians and surgeons. Today, a larger group of primary health care providers—including physical and occupational therapists, speech and hearing professionals, nurse practitioners, physician assistants, and others—may be claimed against or sued by patients in their own capacities for malpractice.

The recognized legal bases for health care malpractice liability imposition include the following (Swisher, 1998):

- Professional negligence, or substandard care delivery (Note that non–care-related negligence [e.g., a patient "slips and falls" on a wet surface] is *not* health care malpractice, but rather *ordinary negligence*.)
- Intentional care-related misconduct, including, among other torts, *battery* (harmful or offensive patient contact) and *sexual battery* (conduct intended to arouse or gratify sexual desires of the provider or patient)
- Breach of a therapeutic contractual promise
- "Strict" (without regard to fault) liability for abnormally dangerous care-related activities or patient injury by dangerously defective care-related products or equipment (strict product liability)

The vast majority of health care malpractice claims and lawsuits involves allegations of professional negligence, or substandard care delivery (Furrow, 1997). To prevail in a professional negligence health care malpractice case, a patient must prove the existence of the following core elements by a preponderance, or greater weight, of evidence:

- A special duty owed by the defendant-provider toward the patient (This special duty becomes operational when the provider agrees to provide health professional services for the patient.)

- Violation of the special duty owed (by providing objectively sub-standard care delivery)
- "Causation" (proof that the substandard care delivery resulted in injury to the patient)
- "Damages" (proof that the patient's injuries warrant the award of money in order to restore the patient, to the extent feasible, to the *status quo ante*)

Whether a defendant–health care professional met or violated practice standards in a professional negligence legal case is established largely through expert witness testimony on the standard of care for the defendant's discipline, and expert opinion on whether the defendant met or fell below minimally acceptable practice standards. Expert witness testimony on the standard of care may be supplemented by information in authoritative and reference texts and journals, and by written practice protocols and guidelines.

Health care malpractice liability is a form of *primary liability*, that is, liability for the consequences of one's own conduct. Rehabilitation professionals and organizations may also be indirectly or *vicariously liable* for the official conduct of employees and volunteers, but not normally for the conduct of independent contractors and their staffs, so long as appropriate steps are taken to alert the public to the fact that such workers are contractors and not employees.

Corporate liability is another form of primary liability, under which a business entity, including rehabilitation clinics and other facilities, is legally responsible for certain administrative activities (Leitner, 1997). These activities include, among possible others,

- Monitoring the quality of health care service delivery in the facility or facilities, whether rendered by employees, contractors, consultants, volunteers, or others.
- Maintaining safe and secure premises for patients and others.

While a rehabilitation services administrator bears primary responsibility for implementing and executing clinical risk management program initiatives, every professional and support team member bears personal responsibility for effecting liability risk management on behalf of the organization. Clinical risk management initiatives include, among others,

- Safety programs designed to minimize injuries to patients, staff, licensees (business visitors), and others.
- Equipment calibration and ongoing safety inspections.
- Adverse incident reporting.
- Peer review and related patient care quality management processes.

- Liability awareness education processes, especially including the systematic involvement of institutional and consulting health law attorneys in in-service education programs (Metzloff, 1999).

Exercise 3: Clinical Liability Risk Management

In a small-group (3–8 people) setting (e.g., clinical department professionals from multiple disciplines), brainstorm about relevant liability concerns (based on real-life scenarios that may have occurred within the setting), and develop an action list of at least 10 liability risk management strategies and tactics to dampen liability exposure. Once validated by a larger group and approved by institutional legal counsel, implement these measures in practice.

Patient Informed Consent to Health Care Intervention

Patient informed consent is both a legal and professional ethical prerequisite to patient examination and health care intervention. The duty to make relevant disclosure of care-related information to patients and obtain their express assent to examination and intervention is grounded in respect for patient self-determination and autonomy over health care decision making (Larson, 1998). This paradigm of placing patient autonomy considerations above paternalism, or beneficence, is relatively new, and not one that health care professionals voluntarily adopted. It has been an activist judiciary in the United States during the twentieth century that has progressively and firmly mandated patient control over health care decision making.

Although the precise informed consent disclosure requirements vary from state to state, the following core information must be conveyed to patients before a health-related examination or intervention:

- Information about the nature of the physical examination
- Examination and evaluative findings
- Patient diagnosis
- Information about any recommended intervention, especially including disclosure of material risks of serious harm or complications associated with the recommended intervention
- Benefits associated with a recommended intervention ("goals")
- Information (i.e., relative benefits and risks) about reasonable alternatives to a recommended intervention

After such disclosure is made, a primary health care professional must also solicit and satisfactorily answer patient questions about the proposed examination or intervention. Finally, a provider must formally ask for and obtain patient consent to proceed. All of this communication between provider and patient (or surrogate decision maker, if the patient lacks legal capacity to consent), must take place both in a language that the patient understands and at the level of patient understanding.

Exercise 4: Informed Consent Clinic Policies and Procedures

Clinic managers, supervisors, and staff professionals are urged to review their current policies and procedures manuals to ensure that their informed consent policies are expressly and clearly stated; that such policies are universally applicable to patients seen in the clinic or by the service; and that compliance with such mandates is assured, through quality management oversight processes, such as retrospective record review or other means.

If such processes and requirements are not memorialized in existing clinic policies and procedures (or quality management) manuals, then they should expeditiously be included in these documents, subject to validation by appropriate consultants, especially including institutional or other legal advisors.

Employment Law Issues Affecting Rehabilitation Professionals, Managers, and Organizations

Workers, including rehabilitation professionals and support staff, are protected from many forms of adverse employment discrimination by federal, state, and even municipal laws, regulations, and ordinances. This section addresses several salient federal statutes protecting workers from employment discrimination. Rehabilitation managers, like all managers and administrators, should be aware of their provisions.

Title VII of the Civil Rights Act of 1964 prohibits work-related discrimination based on race/ethnicity, gender, religion, or national origin. Sexual harassment is a form of impermissible gender discrimination. Policies that help minimize its occurrence and delineate reporting and investigatory processes for sexual harassment reports are crucial to meet management responsibilities in this complex area of employment law.

Title I of the Americans with Disabilities Act of 1990 prohibits work-related discrimination of disabled employees or job applicants who can fulfill essential functions of their employment, with or without reasonable accommodation. It is similarly crucial for management to ensure that the essential functions of each job position are spelled out in writing and justifiable. (Note, too, that Title III of Americans with Disabilities Act makes nearly every health care facility, whether public or private, a public accommodation, which must be reasonably accessible to disabled and nondisabled clients alike.)

The Age Discrimination in Employment Act of 1967 and Older Worker Benefit Protection Act of 1990 prohibit work-related discrimination of employees and job applicants age 40 or older. These employment statutes are enforced by the EEOC.

Future Directions: "Managed" or "Coordinated" Care?

Managed care, the current predominant health care delivery paradigm, is characterized by both great promise and problems. Managed care may help to decrease aggregate health care expenditures (although it has not done so to date). However, legal and professional ethical duties incumbent on health care professionals and administrators and managers have not changed significantly to accommodate the business of managed care. Health professionals and managers still bear primary legal responsibility for their official actions and are held to the highest legal and ethical standards as fiduciaries—or people in special positions of trust—in relation to their patients.

Governmental initiatives—such as the Patient Bill of Rights currently tied up in political wrangling—are helping to reshape managed care into a new twenty-first century health care delivery paradigm, under which cost-containment considerations are once again subordinate to considerations of providing optimal quality patient care. Under any care delivery model, however, primary health care professionals must always simultaneously remember their coprimary duties to provide optimal quality patient care and to minimize personal and organizational liability exposure through effective clinical risk management.

Disclaimer

The material presented in this chapter is intended solely as general legal information, based exclusively on United States laws and regulations. The material herein is not intended to constitute legal advice for any particular health professional, organization, or system. Specific legal advice can only be accurately obtained from personal or institutional legal counsel, based on state or federal law, as applicable (or, for Canadians, provincial or federal law, as applicable). For those United States–based professionals in need of low-cost initial legal advice, contact the county or parish bar association Lawyer Referral Service, a public service agency in place in every locale in the nation.

Dedication

To my wife, Maria Josefa.

References

Furrow, B. R., Johnson, S. H., Jost, T. S., & Schwartz, R. L. (1997). <u>Health law: Cases, materials, and problems</u> (3rd ed.). St. Paul, MN: West Publishing Co.

Larson, E. J., & Eaton, T. A. (1998). The limits of advance directives: A history and assessment of the Patient Self-Determination Act. Wake Forest Law Review, 32(2), 249–293.

Leitner, D. L. (Ed.). (1997). Managed care liability. Chicago: American Bar Association.

Metzloff, T. B., & Sloan, F. A. (1999). Medical malpractice: External influences and controls. Law and Contemporary Problems, 60(1,2), 1–210.

Scott, R. W. (1998). Professional ethics: A guide for rehabilitation professionals. St. Louis, MO: Mosby Yearbook, Inc.

Scott, R. W. (1999). Health care malpractice: A primer on legal issues for professionals (2nd ed.). New York: McGraw-Hill, Inc.

Swisher, L. L., & Krueger-Brophy, C. (1998). Legal and ethical issues in physical therapy. Boston: Butterworth–Heinemann.

CHAPTER 15

Rehabilitation Professionals as Consultants to Business and Industry

Jean Bryan Coe

> A consultant is someone who gives professional or technical advice. A consultant is someone who borrows your watch and tells you what time it is. Really good consultants actually make you feel good about the fact that they used your watch to give you that information.

With changes in health care, the roles of rehabilitation professionals are changing and being redefined. Traditionally, we have been in the business of patient care. More and more we are working in markets outside of traditional health care. In addition, for many professionals, the focus is shifting somewhat, from taking care of patients to preventing people from becoming patients through wellness and injury-prevention programs. These programs aren't that new. What has changed is the practice setting.

As a new and rapidly growing specialization, many rehabilitation specialists—physical and occupational therapists, health educators, speech and hearing professionals—are consulting with business and industry to address the increasingly urgent need for effective programs to prevent expensive work injuries (Isernhagen, 1990a; U.S. Department of Health and Human Services, 1989). Rehabilitation professionals are now providing these programs in the world of business and industry, which is in many ways very different from a health care setting. In this role, rehabilitation professionals need to view themselves as consultants and not just as clinical subject matter experts.

Part of this new "consultant" paradigm represents nonclinical competencies that have not previously been taught in entry-level education. The purpose of this chapter is to discuss the consulting, nonclinical competencies that health professionals need and issues in working in business and industry. The chapter also provides a consulting framework as a tool for planning, implementing, and evaluating health-related programs. By understanding and developing skill in these nonclinical competencies, rehabilitation professionals can demonstrate their effectiveness as consultants. Documented effectiveness is important, because the true mark of success for consultants is repeat and referral business from satisfied customers.

> The mark of success for consultants is not getting contracts . . . the true mark of success is getting repeat business and referrals.

How Effective Are Wellness and Work Injury-Prevention Programs?

Employers are being told that wellness and work injury-prevention programs will save money and that their workers will miss fewer days because of accident or illness. However, work site–wellness (and injury-prevention) advocates often overstate the case without empirical data to back them up (Von Poppel et al., 1997). Many of the reports in business and industry journals are anecdotal, such that the implied relationship between the programs and cost savings are questionable. In addition, most organizations are more interested in decreasing injury rates as quickly as possible than in doing controlled research interventions.

Because of this situation, very few controlled studies on wellness or injury-prevention programs have been reported in the literature (Von Poppel et al., 1997). Although injury-prevention training programs emphasizing safety skill and knowledge account for more than 30% of work site–wellness programs (Green & Kreuter, 1991), most are not evaluated.

For programs that have been evaluated, the evidence is conflicting. Although a limited number of research studies have shown a reduction in disability from back injuries (Browne et al., 1984), others have shown that training programs are not an effective control for back injuries (Snook, 1988; Snook et al., 1978; U.S. Department of Health and Human Services, 1989). In a meta-analysis of the literature, von Poppel (1997) found no evidence for the effectiveness of lumbar supports, limited evidence that education does *not* help prevent back pain, and limited evidence for the effectiveness of exercise. The studies reviewed lacked control measures and appropriate measurement techniques. In spite of very limited evidence of effectiveness, organizations have increased the number of these programs, and the number of rehabilitation professionals working in this

TABLE 15.1
Direct and Indirect Costs of Work Injury

Direct costs
  Medical care
  Lost time from work
  Worker's compensation costs
Indirect costs
  Other workers working harder, with increased risk
  Recruitment, training of a replacement
  Government penalties or fines if injury rates are too high
  Increased insurance premiums
  Potential decreased employee morale, decreased productivity
  Management attitudes toward the injury that may negatively affect employee
    productivity

---

arena has increased over the past 10 years. One potential reason for this growth, especially with repeat consultant business, is satisfied customers with lower injury rates. Another reason may be that injury-prevention training programs for workers are easily implemented and organizations often view them as the least expensive approach to injury prevention (Pizatella et al., 1988).

The costs of work injury include both direct and indirect costs (Table 15.1).

Why Aren't These Programs Effective?

Intuitively, injury-prevention programs should reduce the number of injuries. After all, if workers work in a safe environment and use safe work practices, their safety record should be very good. Although training programs are popular, such programs alone are limiting. Within the work site, health behaviors are complex and deal with both the individual and the organizational environment. Therefore, attempts to change health behavior must also be multidimensional (Green & Kreuter, 1991). Experts in the field have traditionally favored a three-dimensional approach: job analysis that defines the physical requirements of the job and screens workers for specific job requirements; designing of the job to fit the worker (ergonomics); and education/training programs (Snook, 1988; Snook et al., 1978). Understanding how these dimensions fit into an organization's culture and mission is key. In addition, even multidimensional programs are not going to be effective without strong buy-in and commitment to change, from top management all the way down to individual workers. Clearly, communication is important (DeWitt, 1995).

Understanding Organizations as Systems

Rehabilitation consultants are using this three-dimensional approach to injury prevention (Isernhagen, 1990b). However, even that approach is limiting unless the consultant addresses the organization as a system. Consultants may have a limited view of the real problem(s) within an organizational, business, or industry setting. For example, an organization perceives it has a worker performance issue because they have a high incidence of a specific injury and decide they need a worker training program. Too often, consultants accept the organization's view that the problem is due to worker group behavior and provide an injury-prevention training program aimed at changing worker behaviors.

The implication is that the injury rate is caused by worker skill/knowledge deficiency. In reality, the problem may be more related to environmental factors, such as poor design of workstations or lack of reinforcement of correct skill/knowledge, than to specific worker behaviors, such as improper lifting (Komaki et al., 1990). In this case, a worker training program may temporarily decrease the incidence of injury but will not solve the real problem. However, in accepting the implied skill/knowledge deficiency as the real problem, consultants contribute to victim blaming (Green & Kreuter, 1991) and may, in fact, sabotage their own intervention programs.

> Don't contribute to the problem of victim blaming—work-related injuries are not always the worker's fault.

Victim blaming occurs when environmental (physical [such as poor job design] as well as cultural [such that safety is not emphasized]) issues are ignored and programs are targeted strictly toward the worker's responsibility for changing behavior. Both workers and unions see victim blaming as the organization's attempt to cover up other hazards. With this attitude, workers will attend mandatory training programs, but they will not be motivated to actively participate in the training or to transfer the training to their jobs. In this instance, the training program will be less effective because the organization was not analyzed as a system to identify and attempt to change the real problem(s).

Consulting Models for Rehabilitation Professionals

Rehabilitation professionals may serve as internal consultants, when they are employed by the organization, or as external consultants, when they contract with the organization for a specific project. Both forms of consulting have advantages and limitations, but working as an external consultant is the most common scenario for rehabilitation professionals (Ellexson, 1990). Those working as internal consultants often started as external consultants who built a strong relationship with that organization.

There are many variations of consulting models, but there are three basic approaches (Schein, 1969). Each has advantages and disadvantages and varying potential for success. The rehabilitation consultant needs to be aware of these models to help establish his or her style and to help organizations understand what they getting.

Purchase Model

Under the purchase model, the organization diagnoses its own problem and decides on the best solution. They then purchase the consultant's services as a prescription. For example, if the symptoms are high incidence of repetitive use syndromes, such as carpal tunnel syndrome, the organization may quickly diagnose that the problem workers are not using proper body mechanics in performing the repetitive tasks. The solution is to purchase a package deal of worker education targeted to prevent repetitive use injuries. The consultant comes in, does a canned presentation (hopefully modified so that at least the slides fit the specific organization), and exits. In the short term, the organization is happy because they got what they asked for. The purchase model works well as long as the organization does a good job of diagnosis.

One obvious limitation of this model is that the organization may have misdiagnosed its problem. In this case, the organization, as well as the consultant, may well have fallen into the victim-blaming trap. Even if injury rates do decrease initially, the lower rate will not be sustained in the long term. The organization has lost time and money and may blame the consultant for not doing an effective job. By this time, the consultant is long gone. However, the opportunity for repeat or referral business is lost.

Doctor-Patient Model

In the doctor-patient model, the organization asks the consultant to diagnose the problem and prescribe a treatment/solution. This model has advantages over the purchase model in that the consultant is often more objective in defining the problem. The consultant has the opportunity to get input from multiple levels within the organization to make a diagnosis and recommendations for a program to address the problem(s). This model can work well, assuming that the consultant makes a correct diagnosis, and, perhaps more critical, that the organization accepts the diagnosis and treatment. However, if the primary problem is the ergonomics of equipment on the line, and the organization isn't ready to retool the line, they most likely will not accept the diagnosis. They may then go consultant shopping until they get a diagnosis and treatment plan they like better.

Consensus Model

Under the consensus model, the consultant and the organization work together to correctly assess/diagnose the symptoms and the real problem(s) and develop strategies to address them. Ideally, the consultant works with a stakeholder group—with members from all levels within the organization—to help understand and validate the data from both the workers' as well as management's perspective. Because they participated in the diagnosis and treatment decision via the stakeholder group, the organization is much more likely to accept the consultant's recommendations. With this buy-in and active support for the total program, the potential for effective change is much higher (Isernhagen, 1990b).

In the consensus model, the consultant is working as a change agent. Obviously, the level of trust between the organization and the consultant has to be much higher. The time required for implementation of the model is longer, because correct diagnosis takes longer and the program usually includes long-term evaluation of changes. Implementing the consensus model may cost more up front, but it has much greater potential for success as measured in the bottom line. This model is more difficult for the consultant to sell up front. Often the consultant will start with an organization on a small project, which builds the requisite trust, and then move toward this model. Additionally, the consensus model has tremendous potential for repeat and referral business for the consultant.

Issues for Rehabilitation Consultants

Objectivity

To be effective as change agents, consultants must be objective. The consultant needs to remember that management and workers perceive issues and needs differently, and both perspectives need to be addressed (Geroy & Wright, 1988; Green & Kreuter, 1991). Concerning injury-prevention programs, management's perspective is primarily the bottom line: decrease injury rates to cut workers' compensation claims, which in turn reduces health care costs and workers' compensation insurance premiums (Asfahl, 1990; Green & Kreuter, 1991). The workers' perspective may include distrust of management, attitudes about injury as part of the risks of the job, or their supervisor's lack of concern for them as injured workers.

Organizational Knowledge

Rehabilitation professionals must realize that they do not have all the expertise within the organization. Most large organizations have occupational health and safety staff who can offer excellent insights into the organization and help the consulting process. The consultant definitely needs the support of these experts. In addition, consultants need to view an organization as a system of interrelated parts and understand how changes in one part can affect other parts. For example, a seemingly simple work station adaptation may cause problems for workers on another shift because they are using a different process. Part of understanding an organization is identifying its culture, both formal and informal (Lippitt & Lippitt, 1986).

Formal culture embodies written policies and procedures, corporate philosophy (including return-on-investment philosophy), strategic plans, and job descriptions. How formal culture is interpreted and actually practiced constitutes an organization's informal culture. Examples of informal culture include ways to get around the system, power and influence patterns, and workers' attitudes and perceptions. Consultants can identify an organization's formal and informal culture by review of written documents, interviews with employees at various levels, and direct observation.

> Whatever organization you are trying to consult with, if you speak their language, you have already begun to win them over. Always remember that very few organizations speak "medicalese."

Formal and informal cultures do not always agree. In terms of injury prevention, an organization's formal culture may identify a safe work environment as a high priority, but informally, supervisors do not emphasize or reinforce safe work practices and workers do not think safety is a high priority. Understanding an organization's culture, especially as it relates to safe work practices and injury prevention, helps rehabilitation professionals identify causes of work injuries and plan appropriate interventions to address those problems.

Consultants need to have basic information about the organization before making a proposal for a contract. At a minimum, they need to know (1) what product or service the organization is selling and where they see themselves in the market; (2) their return-on-investment philosophy; (3) strategic plans; (4) bottom-line strength; (5) production problems; (6) injury history, including costs and Occupational Safety and Health Administration (OSHA) violations; and (7) their compensation system (Ellexson, 1990). Some of this information is available as a matter of public record, but most of the information can be gathered during the initial contact with the organization. Once the proposal is accepted, the consultant needs additional, specific information about the organization. This information may be garnered from stakeholders, as well as through both formal and informal methods, such as reviewing policies and procedures and talking with/interviewing employees at all levels.

Ethics

Consulting may present some ethical challenges for rehabilitation professionals in conflicting loyalties to the workers and to the organization.

These challenges include avoiding victim blaming, labeling, or coercion of individuals, and preserving confidentiality of information. Many of these issues can be addressed or prevented through the initial contract negotiation and through worker participation in identifying problems and planning appropriate program intervention(s) (Green & Kreuter, 1991; Lippitt & Lippitt, 1986). Consultants must also decide how they will handle situations in which the organization wants a training program, but the consultant knows that a training program will not meet the organization's need to lower injury rates, except perhaps in the short term to remove an OSHA or government violation.

Communication

To effect change, consultants need collaborative communication skills. An important part of this process is the establishment of the stakeholder group (Geroy & Wright, 1988). Terminology is another key to communication—consultants need to relay information that is meaningful to the decision makers in terms that they understand (Geroy & Wright, 1988; Orlandi, 1986). Often, specific information that is important to the therapist in the medical model is not important or meaningful to decision makers in the organization, and vice versa. Learning the organization's culture, language, and objectives early in the consulting relationship will prove invaluable in future communication.

Negotiation

Consultants need negotiation skills on two levels. The first level is to negotiate entry into the organization; the second is to then help the organization negotiate the best solutions for their problems. To effectively negotiate entry into the organization, consultants have to know in advance what they need in a contract agreement. For example, consultants need to insure that they have access to specific information and access to workers as well as management. They also need to negotiate for top management support, as evidenced by management's active participation in the process and support of the stakeholder group.

Based on initial information about the organization, such as injury histories, rehabilitation consultants may choose to limit their consulting to the part of the organization with the greatest injury rate. They also need to establish joint guidelines concerning confidentiality of information and define their responsibilities and their authority to make changes within the organization. Guidelines for regular feedback of findings should be determined to keep the organization informed throughout the consulting process. These issues need to be negotiated at the beginning of the consulting relationship to, in effect, establish the rules of engagement. Effective negotiation of these points is dependent on knowing which points are essential to the consultation situation and being sensitive to the needs and constraints of the organization, such as with information that is highly proprietary.

Once entry into the organization is accomplished and the ground rules have been laid, the consultant needs to negotiate with management and workers to find the best fit of solutions and strategies. This concept of *best fit* represents another shift from the traditional medical model (with the therapist being the patient advocate) to the consultant, who represents both the workers and the organization (management). The use of the stakeholder model helps insure finding this best fit.

Consultants may find themselves in the role of mediating between differing factions or groups within an organization. This mediation role requires special skills. When groups disagree, the tendency is to become defensive and argue positions rather than the interests on which those positions are based. The skilled negotiator needs to help these groups separate the people from the problem and focus on their interests rather than their positions. The negotiator also needs to facilitate the groups' development of a variety of possible solutions and of objective standards to evaluate each possibility before making a decision (Fisher & Ury, 1992).

Basic Principles for Consensus Consulting

Because each organization has a different culture and different rules, there are very few, if any, absolute rules that consultants must follow. However, each of the preceding five issues should serve as guidelines. In addition, two basic principles should always be applied.

First, program interventions must fit the organization conceptually, philosophically, and logistically. This principle emphasizes the need to learn and understand the culture and the need for negotiation skills. Interventions must be adapted to the organizational situation. This concept of fit identifies a significant problem with using completely prepackaged programs. What worked well for a group of office workers does not work well for a group of industrial machinists.

Second, interventions must have support from all levels of the organization to ensure success (Bullock, 1988; Green & Kreuter, 1991; Orlandi, 1986). Unless management is an integral part of industrial injury-prevention programs, and unless workers understand the problem and how the program will help, even the best interventions are doomed to failure. This requisite support should be negotiated during the consultant's entry into the organization and highlights the importance of collaborative communication between the consultant and the organization.

Consulting Framework for Rehabilitation Professionals

The consulting framework for program planning and evaluation (Figures 15.1 and 15.2) is based on rehabilitation professional consultants working with a stakeholder group, but it does not assume that any particular

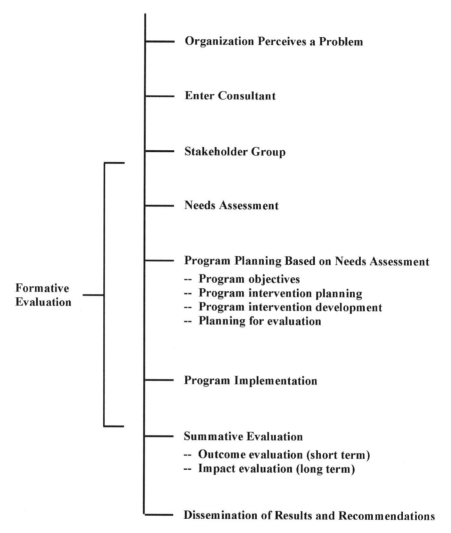

FIGURE 15.1. Program Planning and Evaluation Model (Part I).

program intervention will be implemented. The term *intervention* refers to a specific activity, such as training programs or workplace modification projects. *Program* refers to the entire package of interventions, which are designed, developed, and implemented to meet the overall objectives. The consulting process uses a specific needs assessment to identify the real (rather than expressed) problems relating to injury prevalence and builds on the multidisciplinary approach. It is important for consultants to recognize their own limits of expertise. Setting limits while offering comprehensive programs often results in multidiscipli-

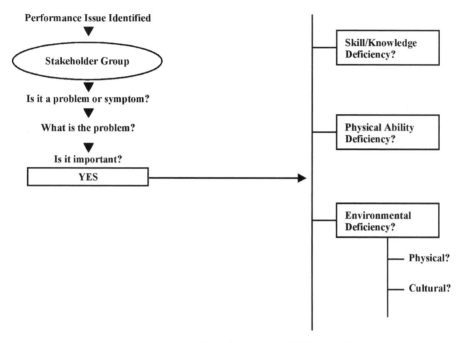

FIGURE 15.2. Program Planning and Evaluation Model (Part II).

nary consulting. In addition, the process includes ongoing (formative) and final (summative) evaluation.

Needs Assessment

The fourth component of the framework shown in Figure 15.1 is needs assessment. Needs assessment is a systematic attempt to define needed change by determining the problem(s) and the cause(s) (Geroy & Wright, 1988). Needs assessment is the most critical stage in the design of any program, because it provides a basis for developing objectives and specific program interventions (Gilley & Eggland, 1989). For example, an organization perceives a problem of high injury rates caused by workers' unsafe work practices. In reality, the cause may be lack of reinforcement of correct behaviors on the job or workstation design that prevent workers from using proper body mechanics. If the cause is poorly designed workstations, training workers in proper body mechanics will not be an effective solution. A thorough needs assessment identifies an organization's needs based on the real cause(s) of the problem(s).

Rehabilitation professionals cannot complete this assessment without help; a successful needs assessment uses the stakeholder group to get an accurate picture of what is happening. The stakeholder group should include representatives of any group either affected by a work injury problem or potentially affected by solutions. For example, members would include representatives of workers, supervisors, union officials, safety or health personnel, managers, top management, and decision makers. Stakeholders serve the important function of helping to gather and validate information about a problem and should be actively involved in identifying causes as well as solutions. They are also responsible for keeping their constituents informed about the assessment and planning process.

Although each needs assessment is organization and situation specific, a systematic approach is essential. The majority of designs pose a sequence of questions that must be answered to determine causes of a problem. Information to identify and answer specific questions can come from many sources, including consultant interviews at different levels within the organization; surveys; direct observation of workers on the job; and review of records, such as injury reports. Consultants might also use specific job task analyses and workers' fitness screening results.

A needs assessment model for rehabilitation professionals based on the three-dimensional injury-prevention approach of training, job site analysis, and preplacement screening is shown in Figure 15.3 (Ellexson, 1990; Isernhagen, 1988; Rodgers, 1988). Following this model, the consultant would attempt to identify (1) worker skill/knowledge deficiencies, (2) worker physical ability deficiencies compared with job analysis, (3) organization physical and cultural environmental deficiencies, or (4) any combination of the three as they relate to work injury.

As an example, follow Figure 15.3. Consider that an organization has a problem of a high incidence of back injury in jobs that require heavy lifting. The following are examples of questions consultants would need to answer in various areas to determine causes and thus organizational needs:

Skill or knowledge deficiencies. Do workers know proper lifting and handling techniques? If not, an education/training program is appropriate with specific program content based on identified skill/knowledge deficiencies. If the answer is yes, have workers had an opportunity to practice safety skills in job-related settings? If not, a program incorporating appropriate practice is appropriate. If workers have the knowledge and skill, and have had practice, skill/knowledge deficiency is not causing the problem.

Physical ability deficiencies. Based on job task analysis, can workers physically do the job safely? If not, can workers be physically conditioned, or can the job be adapted, such as using an assistive device for lifting? If the worker cannot be trained and the job cannot be changed, reassignment of some workers may be an alternative.

Physical and cultural environmental deficiencies. Concerning the physical environment, does job design prevent use of good body mechanics or require poor body mechanics, such as lifting heavy objects from floor level? Does a job require constant repetitive motion? Is equipment

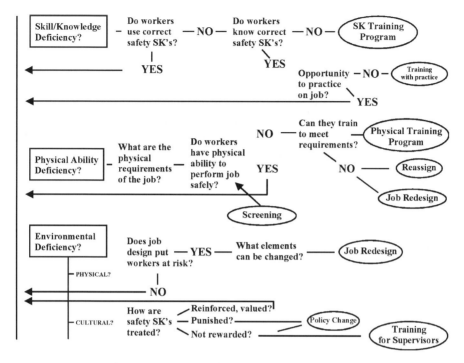

FIGURE 15.3. Needs Assessment Model. (SK = skills and knowledge.)

poorly designed, such as a work surface that is too low? If the answers to these questions are yes, equipment and job design should be carefully considered to identify appropriate changes to adapt jobs to fit the worker(s). Managers are often concerned that job redesign will be costly in terms of money for equipment and lost productivity. However, many job redesigns are very low cost and actually increase productivity over time, especially if injury rates decrease. Obviously, especially in industry with expensive equipment, some jobs are not easily redesigned, but job rotation could address some issues like repetitive motions. An organization's cultural environment takes into account worker motivation to perform a job correctly, using proper body mechanics and lifting techniques. Does proper performance matter? Is correct work behavior reinforced, or is it punished, with supervisors pushing for higher output with less time for safety? If supervisors don't emphasize/reinforce safe lifting practices and teamwork, learned behaviors, such as correct body mechanics, are quickly forgotten. In such a case, an appropriate intervention may be a policy change with increased management commitment to safety from top management down to supervisors. An additional strategy may be a supervisor training program to review safety practices and discuss ways to reinforce workers' safety behaviors.

This example does not cover every possibility, but it does present a systematic approach, address organizations as systems, and fit closely with rehabilitation professionals' clinical expertise. However, a needs assessment may identify causes of work injury for which the consultant does not have the appropriate training and expertise to develop appropriate programs. Although some rehabilitation consultants would have the expertise to address psychosocial problems as well as ergonomic interventions, some would not. Consultants have an ethical obligation to clearly identify their expertise and strengths (high potential for success) and their limitations (when to refer to another expert). They must also feel comfortable telling an organization that they cannot meet the organization's needs and to offer other referral sources.

In summary, rehabilitation professionals need to develop their needs assessment skills to systematically identify causes of work injury. Identifying causes is crucial to developing effective programs. As shown in this needs assessment model, when causes are identified, potential solutions are also identified.

Program Planning Based on Needs Assessment

By identifying causes, needs assessment provides a crucial basis for planning a program to effectively meet an organization's needs. Borrowing from the precede/proceed model for health behavior change (Green & Kreuter, 1991), the stakeholder group can also identify the relative importance as well as the potential for change of identified predisposing, enabling, and reinforcing factors. These factors are as follows:

- *Predisposing factors* include knowledges, attitudes, beliefs, or values that either facilitate or hinder a behavior change.
- *Enabling factors* are vehicles or barriers to change that are created by the organization, the culture, or the environment.
- *Reinforcing factors* include intrinsic and extrinsic rewards, such as safety contests or feedback from supervisors concerning use of the correct behaviors.

Examples of predisposing, enabling, and reinforcing factors related to injury prevention are shown in Table 15.2.

These factors can be rated according to importance (based on the findings of the needs assessment) and changeability (based on feasibility, cost, and management support of and commitment to the program). This rating helps prioritize the factors as target areas for change. Addressing all three types of factors helps insure a balanced approach between education/learning and environmental changes.

TABLE 15.2
Examples of Predisposing, Enabling, and Reinforcing Factors

Predisposing Factors
    Workers know how to correctly perform the tasks.
    Workers think the safety skills are not important.
    Supervisors do not think the safety skills are worthwhile.
    Workers view injury as part of the job.
    Workers question organization's level of commitment to change.
Enabling Factors
    Workers have not had an opportunity to practice skills on the job.
    Union supports the training program.
    Speed takes precedence over safety.
    Top management is committed to change.
Reinforcing Factors
    Safety skills are not reinforced on the job.
    No penalty is assigned for avoidable work injuries.
    Supervisors serve as role models for safety on the job.
    Supervisors push for production at the expense of safety.

Effective program planning based on the needs assessment starts with developing goals and objectives. After clearly identifying the problems and causes, as well as the predisposing, enabling, and reinforcing factors, consultants can then work with the stakeholders to prioritize causes of a problem and set program goals and objectives. Injury-prevention program objectives may target changes in worker or supervisor behaviors, policies related to cultural environment, or the physical environment. Goals relate to final, long-term program outcomes and are rather global. Organizations usually set injury-prevention program goals as decreasing incidence of work injury and decreasing health care costs related to injury. Program objectives should support the goals and address identified needs. Objectives should be reasonable and state how much of what outcome is expected by when (Anderson & Ball, 1983; Gelatt, 1989; Green & Lewis, 1986). They should also be meaningful to an organization's decision makers.

Objectives should be measurable, but some changes are easier to measure than others. For example, if an objective is "By a certain date, improve design of work stations in department X to prevent workers from having to lift from floor level," the change is easy to measure. The workstations were either appropriately modified within the time frame or they were not. Behavioral changes are more difficult to assess, but rehabilitation professionals can measure change—such as increased use of proper lifting techniques—through use of direct behavioral observation against a set standard (Reber & Wallin, 1984). Once a standard is set, consultants can observe workers either doing a procedure correctly or incorrectly and then assign a safety score as the percentage of workers performing correctly during the observation period. Using such an approach, an objective for increasing safe work practices would be "By a specific date, the 100 workers in department X will increase compliance of personal safety procedures on the job from 30% to 90% as measured by behavioral observation against a standard set for this department." Behavioral observations are nothing new for rehabilitation professionals; however, using safety scores can make those observations more meaningful to an organization and facilitate evaluation of injury-prevention programs.

Once program objectives are established and agreed on, the consultant and stakeholder group should determine specific program interventions to meet those objectives. Possible interventions—such as formal injury-prevention training with practice or less formal, on-the-job training—should be ranked based on potential effectiveness, practicality, and feasibility. Rehabilitation professionals have the clinical expertise and experience to make specific recommendations concerning effectiveness. In addition, effectiveness of any intervention is immediately improved if people who are affected have had some input into decisions (Gilley & Eggland, 1989), further emphasizing the value and importance of using a stakeholder group. Issues of practicality and feasibility include costs, as defined by an organization; logistics, such as scheduling; and organization policy restrictions and guidelines.

At this stage, rehabilitation professionals need to negotiate the best fit of possible program interventions for the entire organization, from top management to line workers. Final choice of program interventions should address all of the agreed-on program objectives. Plans for each intervention should include, at a minimum, a timeline for implementation, a budget, a responsible individual, and some mechanism for monitoring progress. Such plans are especially important for nontraining interventions, such as policy changes, for which rehabilitation professionals may not have direct responsibility.

Training

Most injury-prevention programs include training interventions. Training is perhaps the nonclinical/consulting competency with which rehabilitation professionals are most familiar. Therapists certainly have background in both individual and group patient education, but may have received little formal education on how to plan and teach training programs in organizational settings. Consultants will want to consider expanding their background in the field of adult education, which views learners as self-directed and responsible for their own actions and recognizes adults' experiences as important resources for learning (Knowles, 1984; Knowles et al., 1998). In a training situation, adults actively participate in learning (as opposed to passively attending a mandatory class) when they experience a specific need. Research also shows that adults look for practical applications, learn by doing (rather than just listening), and prefer a problem-centered rather than content-centered approach (Cross, 1983; Knowles et al., 1998).

> Don't do an education program for construction workers using slides of office workers . . . you immediately lose credibility. They may look like they are awake, but they are not listening.

Adult education has significant implications for rehabilitation professionals as trainers in injury prevention. Perhaps most important, they must motivate the employees (learners) and make their presentations meaningful. Motivation starts by helping workers realize that they need the information (Wlodkowski, 1988) and teaching them skills/knowledge they can use on the job. Effective, motivating instructors need expertise, enthusiasm, empathy, and clarity. Rehabilitation professionals have clinical expertise in injury prevention to share with workers and are typically enthusiastic about their subject. In terms of empathy, they may need to develop more understanding and consideration for workers as learners and specifically the work site conditions and requirements. Examples include personalizing training to help workers apply new skills and knowledge to particular job situations, adapting a training presentation to participants' learning and experience levels, and considering situations from a worker's perspective. The last essential is presenting information so that workers can easily understand and apply the knowledge and skills. To increase clarity, consultants need to use terminology participants understand and allow for practice and follow-up on the job instruction as needed.

Another important concern is transfer of the training back to the job (Michalak, 1981). Correct bending and lifting is not exactly difficult, but learning correct body mechanics does not immediately translate into on-the-job performance (St-Vincent et al., 1989). To help insure transfer of training, consultants must provide more than just didactic information. Workers must become active participants and be challenged to think critically and apply the information to their own work setting. Beware of turning down the lights for a passive slide show or video. Instead, try to involve participants and make learning more applicable. Consultants might use slides depicting both correct and incorrect behavior and ask "What's wrong with this picture?" Other possibilities include role playing, problem-solving scenarios, and on-the-job consultation.

Transfer of training is both acquisition of new behaviors and maintenance of those behaviors on the job. Anything the consultant, an organization, or workers do to keep that new skill up to some performance standard maintains the behavior. For example, an opportunity to use new, safe work practices, followed by positive feedback (reinforcement) from a supervisor would help maintain those practices (Bandura, 1982; Bryan et al., 1993). Transfer of training to the work site should be a consideration in any training intervention.

Program Evaluation

> Consultants must be able to demonstrate the effectiveness of their health promotion or injury-prevention programs . . . that's more than a one-day training program, that's a long-term commitment to the organization.

With increased emphasis on accountability, program evaluation is another important nonclinical competency for rehabilitation professionals. Evaluation should be accurate, practical, and feasible within organizational constraints, and should protect rights of individuals (Anderson & Ball, 1983). Rehabilitation professionals need to be familiar with and skilled in both types of evaluation—formative and summative, as shown in Figure 15.1.

Formative evaluation occurs throughout the consulting process and allows for midcourse corrections to be made as needed. Monitoring progress of an intervention, troubleshooting a new workstation design, and pilot testing a training presentation are examples of such evaluation. Rehabilitation professionals can use formative evaluation, such as participant feedback of early intervention efforts, to modify subsequent interventions. Formative evaluation often occurs spontaneously during program planning. However, consultants can use this type of evaluation more effectively in program intervention design and development by carefully planning.

Summative evaluation occurs toward the end of the process to address both outcomes (short-term objectives) and impact (long-term goals) (Anderson & Ball, 1983; Green & Kreuter, 1991). Exactly what is measured as outcomes and impact (lower injury rates, fewer sick days, higher productivity) needs to be clearly defined early in the process. Being as specific as possible about what and how to measure is very much like defining long- and short-term patient treatment goals. If you don't have clear goals, you don't know where you are going, and you won't know when you arrive.

Rehabilitation professionals should plan summative evaluation procedures as part of overall program planning, including timelines, type of information to be collected, and responsible individuals. Short-term effects address how well program objectives were met. For example, were workstations modified, or did workers increase their compliance of safety behaviors as measured by safety scores? Information used to determine long-term program impact has to be meaningful to an organization's decision makers and often reflects the bottom line. Rehabilitation professionals need to determine what information decision makers want and understand that each organization views injuries and costs of injuries differently (Swanson & Gradous, 1989). For example, information collected over a set period of time may include injury rates; direct medical costs related to injuries; indirect costs related to injuries such as overtime, lost production, or training a new worker; and number/size of insurance claims.

Health and safety or finance personnel are normally responsible for tracking information for summative evaluation. However, consultants need to help plan the evaluation and need to understand what information is being monitored and how it is being analyzed. Although injury-prevention programs may have been completed by this time, consultants should maintain contact with an organization in a consultant role during summative evaluation to answer any questions or make recommendations for ongoing interventions. Results of summative program evaluation are important for an organization's decision makers in terms of continuing or modifying programs and strategic planning. Ideally, summative evaluation indicates that program objectives were met and that an organization's goals of decreased injuries and decreased costs were also met. Final evaluation results of programs can also be very effective future marketing tools for successful consultants. Based on successful outcomes of a well-planned program evaluation, rehabilitation professionals can present a strong case for a direct cause-and-effect relationship between an injury-prevention program and a decrease in injury and costs.

> A consultant has to understand that there is no such thing as one corporate culture. It is heterogeneous out there. Create a discipline whereby you can frame the right kinds of questions, be a good listener, and be able to tailor your approach to fit the needs and circumstances of the organization.

Summary

As consultants to business and industry, rehabilitation professionals need to understand the consulting process and develop specific nonclinical competencies. As discussed, competencies in needs assessment, program planning, training, and program evaluation are important tools for rehabilitation professionals as consultants. This review has been a general overview of consulting—highlighting the consensus model—and is by no means exhaustive. Rehabilitation professionals who want to do consulting will want to expand their knowledge of organizations and develop their nonclinical skills. Rehabilitation professionals may benefit from further literature review based on cited references; from pursuing continuing education opportunities or degrees within the fields of business, safety, adult education, and human resources development; and from spending time with other consultants and in different organizations. The result of such efforts will be improved consultation with business and industry to help organizations effectively reduce work injury rates and lower costs.

References

Anderson, S. B., & Ball, S. (1983). The profession and practice of program evaluation. San Francisco: Jossey-Bass Publishers.

Asfahl, C. R. (1990). Industrial safety and management (2nd ed.) (pp. 22–50). Englewood Cliffs, NJ: Prentice Hall.

Bandura, A. (1982). Self-efficacy mechanism in human agency. American Psychologist, 37(2), 122–147.

Browne, D. W., Russell, M. L., Morgan, J. L., et al. (1984). Reduced disability and health care costs in an industrial fitness program. Journal of Occupational Medicine, 26(11), 809–816.

Bryan, J. M., Beaudin, B. P., & Greene, D. S. (1993). Increasing self-efficacy and outcome expectations: A model to facilitate transfer of learning. Journal of Vocational and Technical Education, 9, 24–30.

Bullock, M. I. Health education in the workplace. (1988). In S. J. Isernhagen (Ed.), Work injury: Management and prevention (pp. 1–6). Rockville, MD: Aspen Publishers.

Cross, K. P. (1983). Adults as learners. San Francisco: Jossey-Bass Publishers.

DeWitt, J. (1995). Ergonomics: Bigger is better. Apparel Industry Magazine, 56(5), 62–66.

Ellexson, M. (1990). Consulting with industry: Providing services to employers (pp. 1–15). Irvine, CA: Roy Matheson & Associates, Inc.

Fisher, R., & Ury, W. (1992). Getting to yes: Negotiating agreement without giving in (2nd ed.). New York: Houghton-Mifflin.

Gelatt, J. P. (1989). Planning for excellence: How to position and fund rehabilitation and education programs. Rockville, MD: Aspen Publishers.

Geroy, G. D., & Wright, P. C. (1988). Evaluation research: A pragmatic strategy for decision makers. Performance Improvement Quarterly, 1(3), 32–38.

Gilley, J. W., & Eggland, S. A. (1989). Principles of human resource development. Reading, MA: Addison-Wesley and University Associates.

Green, L. W., & Kreuter, M. W. (1991). Health promotion planning: An educational and environmental approach (2nd ed.). Mountain View, CA: Mayfield Publishing.

Green, L. W., & Lewis, F. M. (1986). Measurement and evaluation in health education and health promotion. Palo Alto, CA: Mayfield Publishing.

Isernhagen, S. J. (1988). The therapist. In S. J. Isernhagen (Ed.), Work injury: Management and prevention (pp. 331–337). Rockville, MD: Aspen Publishers.

Isernhagen, S. J. (1990a). Special interest group in industrial physical therapy, February 1990, New Orleans. Orthopedic Physical Therapy Practice, 2(4), 17.

Isernhagen, S. J. (1990b). There is no magic answer . . . but there are effective methods. Orthopedic Physical Therapy Practice, 2(4), 13–14, 21.

Knowles, M. S. (1984). Andragogy in action. San Francisco: Jossey-Bass Publishers.

Knowles, M. S., Holton, E. F., & Swanson, R. A. (1998). The adult learner (2nd ed.). Houston, TX: Gulf Publishing.

Komaki, J., Heinzmann, A. T., & Lawson, L. (1980). Effect of training and feedback: Component analysis of a behavioral safety program. Journal of Applied Psychology, 65(3), 261–270.

Lippitt, G., & Lippitt, R. (1986). The consulting process in action. San Diego, CA: University Associates.

Michalak, D. F. (1981). The neglected half of training. Training and Development Journal, 35(5), 22–28.

Orlandi, M. A. (1986). The diffusion and adoption of worksite health promotion innovation: An analysis of barriers. Preventive Medicine, 15(3), 522–536.

Pizatella, T. J., Nelson, R. M., Nestor, D. E., et al. (1988). The NIOSH strategy for reducing musculoskeletal injuries. In S. J. Isernhagen (Ed.), Work injury: Management and prevention (pp. 39–53). Rockville, MD: Aspen Publishers.

Reber, R. A., & Wallin, J. A. (1984). The effects of training, goals setting, and knowledge of results on safe behavior: A component analysis. Academy of Management Review, 27(3), 544–560.

Rodgers, S. H. (1988). Matching worker and worksite: Ergonomic principles. In S. J. Isernhagen (Ed.), Work injury: Management and prevention (pp. 39–53). Rockville, MD: Aspen Publishers.

Schein, E. H. (1969). Process consultation: Its role in organization development (pp. 4–10). Reading, MA: Addison-Wesley.

Snook, S. H. (1988). Approaches to the control of back pain in industry: Job design, job placement and education/training. Occupational Medicine: State of the Art Reviews, 3(1), 45–59.

Snook, S. H., Campanelli, M. S., & Hart, J. W. (1978). A study of three preventive approaches to low back injury. Journal of Occupational Medicine, 20(5), 478–481.

St-Vincent, M., Tellier, C., & Lortie, M. (1989). Training in handling: An evaluative study. Ergonomics, 32(2), 191–210.

Swanson, R. A., & Gradous, D. B. (1989). Forecasting financial benefits of human resource development. San Francisco: Jossey-Bass Publishers.

U.S. Department of Health and Human Services, Public Health Service. (1989). Promoting health/preventing disease: Year 2000 objectives for the nation. Washington, DC: U.S. Government Printing Office.

Von Poppel, M. N. M., Mireille, N. M., Koes, B. W., et al. (1997). A systematic review of controlled clinical trials on the prevention of back pain in industry. Occupational and Environmental Medicine, 54(12), 841–847.

Wlodkowski, R. J. (1988). Enhancing adult motivation to learn. San Francisco: Jossey-Bass Publishers.

Suggested Readings

Bryan, J. M., Geroy, G. D., & Isernhagen, S. J. (1993). Nonclinical competencies for physical therapists consulting with business and industry. Journal of Orthopaedic and Sports Physical Therapy, 18(6), 673–681.

Isernhagen, S. J. (1988). Work injury: Management and prevention. Rockville, MD: Aspen Publishers.

Journal of Orthopaedic and Sports Physical Therapy (special issue on trends in occupational health). (1994). 19(5).

CHAPTER 16

Health Promotion

Vivien Hollis

In basic terms, health promotion involves enabling individuals and communities to increase control over the determinants of health, and thereby improve their health (Stachtchenko & Jenicek, 1990). However, health promotion is a developing field, and definitions of health promotion are inconsistent. Because there are different views about what constitutes health, this affects how health promotion is understood, the approach and process to be taken, and the outcomes to be achieved. In this chapter, historical perspectives are profiled, the meaning that people attribute to the term *health* is discussed, and health care issues that shaped the development of health promotion are identified. Cultural and ethical issues are reviewed, and a framework for multidisciplinary health promotion is presented. Finally, the challenges to health promotion are outlined.

Why Health Promotion? A Story

Approximately 15 years ago, an occupational therapist interested in the development of health education was spending a day with a health educator. During the day, they called on an elderly scholarly man who had a long-standing diagnosis of emphysema. As they approached the front door, they heard his hacking cough. Waiting for him to open the door, the health educator quickly told her colleague how she had spent a lot of time explaining the condition and the consequences of continued smoking, and how she had left him a lot of reading material including summary leaflets, apparently to no avail. The occupational therapist asked to have a try, approaching it this time from an occupational perspective.

She asked the elderly man about his daily routine. He talked about a lack of activity, attributing this to shortness of breath. As she worked systematically through his daily living activities, he told how he had little appetite and therefore did not cook much, although once was a good eater; how he was constantly tired; and how coughing pained and exhausted him. When prompted regarding visitors, he said that his daughter seldom visited and when she did, she complained of the smell of smoke and dirty ashtrays in the house, saying that her hair and clothes reeked of tobacco and had to be washed after each visit. His main visitors were the health care professionals, like the doctor and nurse who called regularly. The picture emerged of an elderly man, with few pastimes except for the television, who could not get out because of poor health. Slowness, inactivity, and lack of company contributed to feelings of helplessness and dependency. Lack of stimulation led to lack of interest and in turn to reduced motivation to do much. Inactivity bred inactivity and a downward spiral.

Back in the car on the way to the next visit, the health educator and occupational therapist discussed the situation: the incongruity between a government that collects huge tax revenues from cigarette sales to support a health care system that deals with the potential results of cigarette smoking; the incompatibility of providing costly therapeutic interventions that may be no more effective than providing transport for an outing with friends; the dependency on professional services that were devised to encourage independence and promote a better quality of life; the medical nature of the intervention that placed this man in a sick role as someone who required expert help, when some problems could have been improved by himself and an interested community; the waste of his potential reinvestment in that community. This man's health problems were more than medical, and the solutions were diverse and specific to his personal needs and circumstances. Thus began an interest for the two in the scope of health promotion.

Historical Perspectives

Ancient Greek physicians believed that health was a perfect balance of body, mind, and spirit, a concept very much in line with the original World Health Organization's (WHO, 1946) definition:

> Health is a state of complete physical, mental, and social well-being and not merely the absence of disease or infirmity.

This definition was, and still is, appealing. In contrast to the view that health means not being sick, lack of ailments, or freedom of disease, WHO signified the importance of well-being as having a number of components. The foundations were laid for thinking about the health needs of people as being multifaceted. Some rehabilitation professions incorporated this concept into practice.

The WHO (1946) definition has been criticized on a number of fronts. The term *state* was felt, by some, to be inappropriate and that *process* would have been better. The argument raises issues about whether health promotion is viewed as the journey or the destination. Others have challenged the ideal state, as described, as being neither absolute for all nor indeed achievable. Many criticisms, however, centered on what others celebrated, the issue of health being more than "the absence of disease." The essence of the argument is that such a broad definition has no parameters to what are the legitimate concerns of health providers and thus no limit on potential expenditure. The WHO definition set the scene for continuing debate regarding health boundaries, and importantly, it changed perceptions for service users and professionals concerning expectations. The issue is much more than an academic debate, because the way in which health is defined affects how resources are allocated and to some extent determines the people employed to deliver those services.

During the 1950s and 1960s, public health approaches to promoting health focused on preventing disease and were based on immunization and screening programs. Concern was raised regarding the failure of people to participate in these programs, the escalating costs of health care, and the realization that increased investment in health care produced limited outcomes as measured by health status. This provided an impetus for public policy to change in the 1970s. It occurred at the same time as challenges to the biomedical approach, or "medical model," to education and health care.

For many years, the delivery of health care and the education of health care professionals continued to concentrate, to varying degrees, on sickness, illness, disease, and disability when the focus was changing to wellness and ability. Educational curricula were often taught in a reductionist way—as elements of normal and abnormal functioning—even when the world included people with severe disabilities living what they knew to be normal lives. Treatment was based on diagnosis and therapy for specific "conditions," when it was known that social conditions contributed to, if not caused, many health problems (Black et al., 1982). Imrie (1997) denounced rehabilitation programs as being driven by professional elites, who shape and construct the meanings of disability around technical, psychosocial, and medical concerns.

By fostering a doctrine that people with disabilities have conditions that can be treated and cured, the medical model was seen as a way for health care professionals to retain power, status, and control, while at the same time deflecting attention from questions regarding these issues. Consequently, traditional didactic education programs were viewed as limited in their ability to produce educated professionals with skills to empower, facilitate, and support communities and individuals in health promotion strategies. This gap in provision led in the 1990s to a plethora of courses aimed at multidisciplinary education and collaboration in health promotion, consequently bringing together a number of fields of study under one umbrella. Although medicine and cure are undoubtedly important approaches, they are recognized as being limited for people whose determinants of health are complex and, according to various directives such as the *Black Report* (Black et al., 1982), include sociopolitical factors.

Two opposing themes developed in the 1960s and 1970s. The first was the reforms of the 1960s, which included such things as civil rights, human potential, women's movements, and disability rights movements. Many groups demanded increased knowledge and authority so as to decrease dependency on others (Morgan & Marsh, 1998). Despite the former, the second theme was the expansion of the medical framework to include not only the customary physical and mental impairments but also problem drinking, child abuse, learning disabilities, delinquency, and crime (Dubos, 1969). It is these groups of people, often with long-term or continuing problems, with whom rehabilitation professionals have greatest input.

A Paradigm Shift

Imrie (1997) argued that the conception of disability as a biomedical problem and the difficulties that face disabled people as being the result of their physical or mental impairments does not take into account disabling environments and the wider attitudinal strictures of prejudice and discrimination. The Lalonde report (1974) countered the biomedical model of health by presenting the argument that health is affected by many factors, including genetics, lifestyle, social and physical environments, and access to health care. Marc Lalonde, then Canadian Minister of Health and Welfare, issued "A New Perspective on the Health of Canadians" and identified health promotion as a term and a key strategy of national government policy. As a result, Canadian public health policy shifted from treatment to prevention. International interest was stimulated, and a range of health promotion policy documents was produced by many countries, including Australia, Sweden, the United Kingdom, and the United States. In 1986, as a response to the new health movement, WHO, Health and Welfare Canada, and the Canadian Public Health Association convened the First International Conference on Health Promotion. The conference was held in Ottawa, Canada, and 212 participants from 38 countries met to exchange and share experiences. This conference resulted in the Ottawa Charter (WHO, 1986) and redefined health promotion as:

> [T]he process of enabling people to increase control over, and to improve, their health. To reach a state of complete physical, mental, and social well-being, an individual must or group must be able to identify and realize aspirations, to satisfy needs, and to change or cope with the environment. Health is therefore seen as a resource for everyday life, not the objective of living. Health is a positive concept emphasizing social and personal resources, as well as physical

capacities. Therefore, health promotion is not just the responsibility of the health sector, but goes beyond healthy lifestyles to well-being.

Following hard on the heels of, and based on, the concepts set down in the Ottawa Charter, the Epp report (1986) "Achieving Health for All," kept the health promotion pot boiling. This health promotion framework outlined the formidable challenges of reducing inequalities in health, increasing prevention, and enhancing coping with chronic disease and disability. These were powerful themes. While including the aspect of "prevention" of the earlier programs, this framework encouraged the creation of more inclusive strategies of fostering public participation, strengthening community health services, and coordinating healthy public policy.

The *Jakarta Declaration on Leading Health Promotion into the Twenty-First Century* (WHO, 1997) identified five priorities:

1. Promote social responsibility for health
2. Increase investments for health development
3. Expand partnerships for health promotion
4. Increase community capacity and empower the individual
5. Secure an infrastructure for health promotion

Health: A Summary

As already stated, conceptions of health vary. At one end of the spectrum who described health as being "a resource for everyday life, not the object of living," and as such, social and personal resources are stressed, as well as physical capabilities (Nutbeam, 1998). The occupational therapy profession was founded on this holistic principle, and the nursing profession has embraced this approach, often defining many components of health in nursing texts. The other end the medical model emphasizes normality, the state of being whole, lack of physical and mental disease, and freedom from pain.

Studies in the late 1980s and early 1990s indicated that adult populations defined health as the absence of illness, a functional capacity, and a positive condition (Edelman & Mandle, 1994). Blaxter (1990), in a survey of 9,000 adults in the United Kingdom, had similar results. She too found that absence of disease and illness was important. This is not surprising. It is easier for people to agree on the concept of health when it is defined narrowly and negatively, such as the absence of disease and illness. People value health in this sense because pain, damage to the body, dependency, and death are feared. Blaxter also identified the conceptionalization of health as being a multidimensional concept, which also included physical fitness, energy and vitality, social relationships, functional ability, healthy lifestyle behavior, and having a reserve to combat problems and psychosocial well-being. By 1990, the focus of health was on well-being and wellness and included the absence of illness.

Health Promotion Explained

In some countries, notably Canada, two separate concepts labeled *health promotion* and *population health* dwell together. *Population health* originated from medical epidemiology, which seeks to understand the distribution and determinants of disease and dysfunction so as to target and control health risks in specified populations. Policy makers have favored this quantitative, technical, and preventive approach that makes use of epistemologic methodologies. Health promotion, having originated in community and public health, is thought to be qualitative, to emphasize a social policy approach, and to incorporate the health education of individuals and communities. In other countries, health promotion incorporates elements of what is understood in Canada to be *population health*.

Health promotion is acknowledged to generate differences in opinion because of different societal needs, the wide range of health promotion activities, and the different backgrounds of health promotion professionals. For the sake of clarity, and because, quite simply, the promotion of health should be all encompassing, the term *health promotion* is used in this chapter to encapsulate both concepts and so represents a broad base. However, it is acknowledged that researchers and practitioners are inclined to one of the two concepts, in varying degrees, and that health improvement concentrates on either preventive medicine or the promotion of positive health.

In this chapter, the medical model and social models of health are intertwined and incorporate political and economic dimensions. This is illustrated as follows. People's understanding of health emphasizes the absence of illness and pain. Therefore, therapeutic intervention that helps reduce disease and control symptoms—as well as preventive medicine measures, such as screening, early diagnosis, and treatment for particular high-risk groups—is an essential element. Living and working conditions and the inequalities of disadvantaged groups are known to affect health, so public policy, environmental change, and community action are other elements. Personal lifestyle choices affect health, so health promotion also embraces the concept of self-responsibility. Consequently, health promotion is not simply about relying on medical care, or changing attitudes and behavior of individuals or groups, but making the environment conducive to supporting healthy behavior. Health promotion is, in itself, a holistic concept.

Health promotion can be explained as *a process* of

- Protecting and promoting health, through reducing risk behaviors and promoting health behaviors.
- Providing a strategy for better health as opposed to a strategy for better health services.

- Realigning the focus to the production of health rather than on the consumption of health services and health care.
- Adding life to years rather than only adding years to life.
- Enhancing health, not only maintaining the status quo by preventing problems.

Health promotion can be explained in terms of *outcome* as changes to

- Knowledge (measured by questionnaires and individual interviews, which can determine what had been understood).
- Attitude (measured by questionnaires using *strongly agree* to *strongly disagree* or in focus groups; more difficult than measuring knowledge).
- Behavior (measured by self-reporting, which is subject to inaccuracy by people stating what they know they *should be* doing, rather than what they *are* doing; use of diaries or log books, which have been effective in measuring people's diet, alcohol intake, smoking habits, compliance with medication; observation when appropriate; commodity sales such as cigarettes, condoms).
- Health status (measured through the use of self-administered health status measures indicating physical ability, social interaction, anxiety, depression, family and work roles; through the use of mortality and morbidity indicators; by decreased number of people with late-stage disease).
- Social support (measured by self-completed questionnaires and interview schedules that are available, some of which designed specifically for particular groups, such as adolescents and the elderly).
- Quality of life (measured by a range of self-administered quality-of-life measures).

Outcome evaluation can be qualitative or quantitative. Qualitative methods are useful for ascertaining the meaning and experience of the program for participants, staff, and sometimes those not directly involved. Detailed information usually can be obtained, but from a smaller group. Quantitative measures are useful for rating, in numeric terms, the extent of changes occurring as a result of the program and determining changes in outcomes such as health status and health behavior.

For more information on evaluation measures and further details of the range of health measures, see Hawe et al. (1990).

Values, Beliefs, and Culture

Canada, the United States, and the United Kingdom consist of a heterogenous group of people with roots from across the world. This makes the articulation of common values difficult, if not impossible. There are many communities and many subcultures based on occupational class, geo-graphic origin, ethnicity, religion, and age group. Values emanate from sacred texts, such as the Koran and the Bible, as well as from history recorded as stories, song, and dance. These cornerstones provide the pride and solidarity (as well as humiliation) that individuals—and, by deed of membership, groups of people—share. Values also emanate from collective standards and understanding.

Recognizing and respecting the cultural understandings, values, knowledge, and meaning of participants is essential when planning health promotion programs. Firstly, the association between illnesses or medical problems and particular groups needs to be understood but not taken as absolutely binding. Bhat et al. (1998) indicate that there may be diseases, such as sickle-cell anemia, tuberculosis, and heart disease that are more common among certain racial or cultural groups. However, the often cited, higher incidence of tuberculosis in the United Kingdom among those from Asian origins may have little to do with race and biological predisposition and more to do with social—particularly living—conditions. Similarly the link between those from particular ethnic backgrounds who move to a new country and then experience mental health problems may be due to disen-franchisement, isolation, and lack of opportunities rather than to genetics or cultural predisposition.

Second, family structures, religion, and beliefs often dictate medical convictions and practices that are incongruent with western culture. Thirdly, compliance with medical advice will be limited if there is dispar-ity between medical practice and cultural understanding, or the experience of reality.

Hilary Graham (1987) in her study of smoking mothers of young chil-dren found that programs did not take account of the realities of their lives. The mothers agreed that it would be desirable to give up smoking, but because a physical break was impossible in the care of young children, having a cigarette with a cup of coffee was the only respite available to break the routine that did not cost a lot and was not fattening (Bunton and Macdonald, 1992). Likewise, in an attempt to preserve their sense of self worth young people from working class and ethnic minority groups, who were rated as low achievers, have tended to respond by constructing an identity that is at odds with those who rated them as such. These young people are at risk for smoking and abusing drugs as a way of retaliating at an education system that failed them (Fuchs, 1968; Coard, 1971). Advising people not to engage in a certain behavior will have little effect unless it is rooted in an understanding of real situations and circumstances.

It is therefore vitally important to be creative and find an approach that is culturally appropriate. In other words, ask the question "What envi-ronmental factors support the particular behavior?" and start from there. Environment refers to the physical, social, economic, political, and cul-tural elements that closely interact and that make up the whole.

The Themes of Health Promotion

A consumer-orientated approach represents an attempt to make services more responsive to service users. Advocacy, empowerment through partnership, enabling, choice, and mediation between the different interests in pursuit of health are all strategies that attempt to achieve this end. This is in line with the Jakarta Declaration (WHO, 1997) to expand partnerships for health promotion, increase community capacity, and empower the individual, thus promoting social responsibility for health and increasing investments for health development.

Advocacy means speaking for the service users—who because of a range of communication problems cannot understand the issue in question or cannot express their opinions—to represent their views and make the best decision about his or her life. Often a relative, friend, or volunteer is appointed to act in this capacity.

Empowerment is the process of enabling individuals or communities to take control of health promotion activities. The responsibility is for health professionals to share knowledge and give appropriate and timely information in a variety of ways that are understandable and acceptable. It is also required that they help and support communities to develop their own strategies that are directed to their needs. It has often been said that empowerment, as fundamental to health promotion, is about making healthy choices easy choices.

Choice, however, is often determined by financial and social circumstances, and therefore is not equally available to all. Also, many choices are not within users' scope of control but rather are dependent on a wider political and sociologic realm. Nevertheless, individuals and communities can be supported in lobbying for change. Thus health professionals can find that health promotion efforts are directed to curative, preventive, and salutary approaches. The salutogenic model (Antonovsky, 1996) stresses an orientation that actively promotes health rather than just being low on risk factors.

Ethical Dilemmas

The difficulty for health professionals is to balance the need to prevent disease, protect and maintain health, and promote healthy behavior with a respect for freedom of choice, including the freedom to adopt an unhealthy lifestyle (Tones, 1997). Although health education informs choices by critically raising awareness, it cannot coerce, persuade, or otherwise try to manipulate users. Choice allows for people to continue taking risks, such as smoking, driving without seat belts, and eating unhealthy foods.

Empowerment is a heady concept. Thibeault and Hébert (1997) raise the question of what happens when groups have conflicting agendas. How would a professional react if community empowerment turned into radical political action? Would indeed the professional be compromised if he or she had supported such action or, more contentiously, if he or she had been actively involved? There is also the concern that through empowerment, old conflicts between groups could be stirred and confrontations ignited (Robertson & Minkler, 1994).

By the very nature of professional education and training, professionals do have power. However, this may encourage the abrogation of responsibility for health from users to health professionals who "know best." In delegating this power, users allow health professionals to maintain control of programs. Those who do become involved in partnerships may be the most active and vociferous but may not represent wider views. Limited time and finances may exclude some demographic groups altogether.

The term *healthy lifestyle* has become almost synonymous with the term *risk evasion*. Accordingly, if individuals do not comply with such evasion, might they be blamed for any ill health resulting and perhaps vulnerable to a withholding or forfeiting of treatment? Further, to promote a healthy lifestyle, risks have to be minimized by creating an environment that allows, facilitates, and encourages people to stay well. However, this is incompatible with some professional principles, which value self-efficacy, the acquisition of coping strategies, and adaptation to a changing environment. How can this be achieved without the necessary prerequisites of tolerance to and acceptance of risk and uncertainty?

A Health Promotion Framework for the Multidisciplinary Team

Some authors have argued that professions should adopt the health promotion concept only if it has congruence with professional practices and beliefs. Others have studied the concepts and found that the basic health promotion philosophy and principles generally do relate well to the values and beliefs of certain professions (Thibeault & Hébert, 1997). However, as has been described, there are various definitions of health, and thus a range of understandings of health promotion. Some professionals, working in both community and curative care settings, have used the concept to develop and evaluate particular programs based on their expertise, perhaps focusing on a certain aspect, such as education, lifestyle behavior, or physical activity (DeMars, 1992; Owen, 1996; Pert, 1997; Richardson & Eastlake, 1994; Rothman & Levine, 1992).

Approaches may be directed toward any, or a combination of, methods, including health education, social change, empowerment, and community. The focus may be on individuals, groups, or the environment (including the social and political environment). Goals may be to facilitate adjustments to lifestyle, enable people to develop knowledge and skills, explore attitudes, support social and political changes, make healthy choices easy choices, increase power and ability of communities, and help people to work together. The tenor is that prevention is supported by coping strategies, that environments evolve to meet changing needs, that communities benefit from combined experiences and skills, and that people have both the ability to make decisions and the freedom to make choices.

The two most recent and persuasive models are the salutogenic model (Antonovsky, 1996) and the population health promotion (PHP) model (Hamilton & Bhatti, 1996). The salutogenic model provides a theory to guide health promotion based on a unique combination of cognitive, behavioral, and motivational rationale, and thus provides a basis for research and indicates how action could proceed. In contrast, the PHP model is an all-inclusive conceptualization based on forward-thinking ideas and experiential knowledge. As such, it provides a framework for action.

The following is intended as a guide for multidisciplinary teams wishing to investigate how to proceed. Examples for both the salutogenic model and the PHP model are based on the Ottawa Charter. The Ottawa Charter (WHO, 1986) called for action in five areas:

1. Build healthy public policy (e.g., legislation to support community action, equitable distribution of income).
2. Create supportive environments (physical, social, economic, cultural, spiritual) that recognize the changing nature of society (e.g., clean air and water, accessible buildings, comfortable housing, healthy workplaces).
3. Strengthen community action so that communities have the capacity to determine priorities, make decisions, and take action on issues that affect their health.
4. Develop personal skills (e.g., increased knowledge).
5. Reorient health services to create a real partnership between service providers and users.

Population Health Promotion Model

The PHP is usually depicted as the model in Figure 16.1. The figure is explained as a rubric cube, which means that each of the elements may correspond with all of the others. However, to clarify the themes, they are presented as linear; but this might also be thought of as a multifaceted, three-dimensional model.

Each of the elements on one column can relate to any number of the elements on other columns (Table 16.1). Stakeholders, such as health service commissioners, providers, and service users, need to address the full spectrum, but particular organizations may wish to target a particular health determinant. Thus, healthy child development can be promoted by working at the community level and using the strategy of reorienting health services to ensure, for example, that community clinics focus on

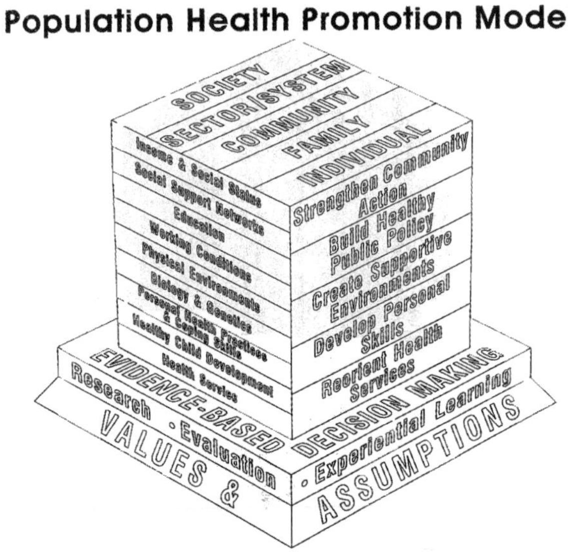

Population Health Promotion Model

FIGURE 16.1. Population health promotion model. (Source: Hamilton, N., & Bhatti, T. [1996]. Population health promotion: An integrated model of population health and health promotion [Report]. Ottawa, ON: Health Promotion Development Division.)

primary care services for young children. Another example, as quoted by Hamilton & Bhatti (1996), indicates that social support networks can be targeted to the family level using the strategy of creating supportive environments. Thus, the goal might be the creation of family situations that help children learn to develop positive social relations.

This example can be taken further for a multidisciplinary team approach. If at all possible, the team should include representatives from the target group, or in PHP terms, "level." The first step is to consider the issues, difficulties, or problems with family situations, being careful that these considerations are well grounded and not based on assumptions and prejudices. If appropriate, priorities should be agreed on, and these should be based on good evidence and supported by the target group representatives. All members of the team could decide how, individually and collectively, they could best support the creation of learning opportunities for positive social relations. Initially, discussions might address professional perspectives and what each member, from his or her particular background and expertise, could contribute. Decisions regarding purpose, action, and outcomes have greater potential for success if grounded on research and agreed to by the team. The focus need not be direct, as there are many ways in which messages can be conveyed, such as discussion groups in nursery and preschools. To involve the older children in secondary schools,

TABLE 16.1
Population Health Promotion Model

Determinants of health
   Income and social status
   Social support networks
   Education
   Working conditions
   Physical environments
   Biology and genetics
   Personal health practices and coping skills
   Healthy child development
   Health services
Levels of action
   Society
   Sector/system
   Community
   Family
   Individual
Strategies (based on the Ottawa Charter)
   Strengthen community action
   Build health public policy
   Create supportive environments
   Develop personal skills
   Reorient health services

---

messages can be conveyed through media such as free videos, leaflets, articles in newspapers, and learning packages. The community should be fully involved and committed to the project and empowered to carry out many of the tasks themselves in a sensitive manner.

However, a word of caution. The PHP model is not unidimensional. It is recommended that all of the strategies be reviewed against all the levels as they all have an impact on each other, rather than dealing with any in isolation. This does not mean that the team has the resources to deal with all strategies, but that important factors should not be neglected or overlooked.

Salutogenic Model

Antonovsky (1996) suggested a continuum that visualizes people to be somewhere along a "healthy/dis-ease" spectrum at given points in time. Personal, collective, or situational resources facilitate successful coping with the inherent stressors of human existence and explain a movement along the continuum. These resources he calls *generalized resistance resources*, and he concludes that these are fostered through a sense of coherence (SOC) emanating from repeated life experiences. An SOC enables people to make sense of and cope with life. People are able to cope because it is believed that the challenge is understood (comprehensible), that resources are available to cope (manageable), and that it has particular meaning for them (meaningful). So, confronted with a stressor, the person or collective with a strong SOC is able to reach out in any given situation and apply the resources appropriately to that stressor. The strength of one's SOC, Antonovsky concludes, has a strong impact in facilitating movement toward health. To that end, he developed a 29-item scale to measure SOC (Antonovsky, 1987).

Antonovsky (1996) did not propose particular programs but suggested that the question be asked: "What can be done in this community—factory, geographical community, age or ethnic or gender group, chronic or even acute hospital population, those who suffer from a particular disability, etc.— to strengthen the sense of comprehensibility, manageability, and meaningfulness of the persons who constitute it?"

In this model, the emphasis is on active health promoters (salutary factors) rather than on risk factors. Hence the name *salutogenesis*, meaning the origins of health.

Taking this further for a multidisciplinary team approach, and importantly to determine what can be done in this community, try the following exercise. Select a group—for example, those people with a history of back pain—and ask the following questions:

Comprehensibility. What is the range of predispositions, circumstances, and environmental factors that cause the problem, maintain it, or exacerbate it? Consider the response in terms of the five action areas of the Ottawa Charter: community action, public health policy, environments, personal skills, and health services.

Manageability. What are the short- and long-term changes that need to be made, and what existing resources are available? Consider the response in terms of the five action areas of the Ottawa Charter.

Meaningfulness. What helps to influence motivation or sustain it? Consider the response in terms of the five action areas of the Ottawa Charter.

Asking these questions would be compatible with the principles that Antonovsky advocated. It would prevent health promotion strategies from becoming submerged in preventive or curative medicine, dwelling on risk factors and particular diseases. It would provide a collective response, but one that would be tailored to individual needs.

Challenges to Health Promotion

An important theme of health promotion is the need to develop interventions that do not resort to institutionalized and medical forms of care. There is also a commitment to multisectoral collaboration and action. However, the justification for funding inevitably falls on trying to do the greatest good for the greatest number of people with limited public money.

Arguments are therefore inclined to concentrate on biomedically oriented prevention related to cancer, stroke, and heart disease. Thus, the tendency is to be focused on prevention rather than wellness. This is supported by arguments about reality and achievable goals based on evidence and well-rehearsed theory, versus ideology and rhetoric. The challenge, then, is to provide the evidence through a sound theoretic underpinning that promotes program development and research.

Suspicion is aroused when health promotion appears to be an off-loading of responsibility for escalating health care costs to individuals and their unhealthy lifestyles—what has become known as "victim blaming." There are those who have rejected health promotion, fearing that it is a conspiracy to contain health expenditure by shifting the culpability and costs to consumers who are deemed not to have led a healthy life. A belief that savings can be made to the health care budget has encouraged many providers to try and use it for this purpose. Conversely, there are those who used to see health promotion as a panacea for a sick health service and are now disenchanted with the relative ineffectiveness of progress to date. Still others, seeing marketing opportunities, have redefined services in health promotion terms to access funds and attract users. The responsibility is to demonstrate cost utilization as long-term efficiency and effectiveness, and to challenge the quick-fix answers provided by inconclusive short-term outcomes promising financial savings—in other words, to make the argument in *value* rather than in the market-oriented term of *cost*.

Conclusion

In the past, the emphasis was adding years to life. Now the emphasis is adding life to years. Definitions of *healthy* and *normal* are recognized as not being fixed, although the concept of health continues to be debated. Health promotion is characterized by a number of guiding values, including an emphasis on social justice, empowerment, and equity. However, the ideologic principles—such as a broad view of the determinants of health; the holistic notion of physical, mental, social, and spiritual well-being; and the effect of social and environmental influences—appear to offer continual themes for debate and "navel gazing." Those who debate semantics and principles have described the failings of health promotion, and the notion of a healthy lifestyle has become almost synonymous with a lifestyle that is characterized by risk evasion.

We have now passed the stage of describing health promotion as the metaphor of preventing people from falling into the river, as opposed to pulling them out downstream—the old "prevention is better than cure" argument. As Antonovsky (1996) stated, by virtue of being a living system, we are all in the river, and none of us are on the shore. Therefore, we are all vulnerable. The question for him was how dangerous is the river and how well can we swim? The identification of criteria of elements of effective health promoters, as well as the strategies, is the current and future objective.

References

Antonovsky, A. (1987). Unraveling the mystery of health. San Francisco: Jossey-Bass.

Antonovsky, A. (1996). The salutogenic model as a theory to guide health promotion. Health Promotion International, 11(1), 11–18.

Bhat, A., Carr-Hill, Ohn, S. (1988). Britain's black population. Aldershot: Gown.

Black, D. , Morris J. N., Smith, C. (1982). In P. Townsend & N. Davidson (Eds.), Inequalities in health: The Black report. Harmondsworth, England: Penguin.

Blaxter, M. (1990). Health and lifestyles. London: Tavistock/Routledge.

Bunton, R., Macdonald, G. (Eds.) (1992). Health Promotion: Disciplines and Diversity (p. 57). London, England: Routledge.

Coard, B. (1971). How the West Indian child is made educationally subnormal in the British school system. London: New Beacon Books.

DeMars, P. A. (1992). An occupational therapy life skills curriculum model for a native American tribe: A health promotion program based on ethnographic field research. American Journal of Occupational Therapy, 46(8), 727–736.

Dubos, R. (1969). Human ecology. WHO Chronicles, 23, 299.

Edelman, C. L., Mandle, C. L. (1994). Health promotion throughout the lifespan (p. 13). St. Louis, MO: Mosby–xYear Book, Inc.

Epp, J. (1986). Achieving health for all: a framework for health promotion. Ottawa, ON: Health and Welfare Canada.

Fuchs, E. (1968). How teachers learn to help pupils fail. In N. Keddie (Ed.), Tinker, tailor: The myth of cultural deprivation. Harmondsworth, England: Penguin.

Graham, H. (1987). Women's smoking and family health. Social Science and Medicine and Family Health, 1, 47–56.

Hamilton, N., Bhatti, T. (1996). Population health promotion: An integrated model of population health and health promotion (Report). Ottawa, ON: Health Promotion Development Division.

Hawe, P., Degeling, D., Hall, J. (1990). Evaluating health promotion. Artarmon, Australia: MacLennan & Petty Pty. Ltd.

Imrie, R. (1997). Rethinking the relationships between disability, rehabilitation, and society. Disability and Rehabilitation, 19(7), 263–271.

Lalonde, M. (1974). A new perspective on the health of Canadians. Ottawa, ON: Health & Welfare Canada.

Morgan, I. S., & Marsh, G. (1998). Historic and future health promotion contexts for nursing. Image: Journal of Nursing Scholarship, 30(4), 379–383.

Nutbeam, D. (1998). Health promotion glossary. Health Promotion International, 13(4), 349–364.

Owen, N. (1996). Strategic initiatives to promote participation in physical activity. Health Promotion International, 11(3), 213–218.

Pert, V. (1997). Exercise for health. Physiotherapy, 83(9), 453–460.

Richardson, B., Eastlake, A. (Eds.). (1994). Physiotherapy in occupational health: Management, prevention and health promotion in the work place. Oxford: Butterworth–Heinemann.

Robertson, A., Minkler, M. (1994). New health promotion movement: A critical examination. Health Education Quarterly, 21(3), 295–312.

Rothman, J., Levine, R. (Eds.). (1992). Prevention practice: Strategies for physical therapy and occupational therapy. Philadelphia: Saunders.

Stachtchenko, S., Jenicek, M. (1990). Conceptual differences between prevention and health promotion: Canadian and international perspectives. Toronto, ON: Centre for Health Promotion, University of Toronto.

Thibeault, R., Hébert, M. (1997). A congruent model for health promotion in occupational therapy. Occupational Therapy International, 4(4), 271–293.

Tones, K. (1997). Health education as empowerment. In M. Sidell, L. Jones, & A. Peberdy (Eds.), Debates and dilemmas in promoting health: A reader (pp. 33–42). Buckingham, UK: Macmillan (The Open University).

World Health Organization. (1948). Constitution. Geneva: Author.

World Health Organization. (1986). Ottawa charter for health promotion. Health Promotion, 1(4), iii–v.

World Health Organization. (1997). Jakarta declaration on health promotion in the 21st century. Geneva: Author.

Additional Reading

Bercovitz, K. L. (1998). Canada's active living policy: A critical analysis. Health Promotion International, 13(4), 319–328.

Evans, R. G., & Stoddart, G. L. (1990). Producing health, consuming health care. Social Science and Medicine, 31, 1347–1363.

Førde, O. H. (1998). Is imposing risk awareness cultural imperialism? Social Science and Medicine, 47(9), 1155–1159.

Fraser, E., Bryce, C., Crosswaite, C., McCann, K., & Platt, S. (1995). Evaluating health promotion: Doing it by numbers. Health Education Journal, 54, 214–225.

Health Promotion Development Division, Health Canada. (1996). Report of the roundtable on population health and health promotion. Ottawa, ON: Author.

Mastravic, R. S. (1999, January–February). Demonstrating value: Healthcare organizations can document positive outcomes from their community-benefit services. Health Progress, 54–57.

Mount, J. (1991). Evaluation of a health promotion program provided at senior centers by physical therapy students. Physical & Occupational Therapy in Geriatrics, 100(1), 15–24.

Norton, L. Health promotion and health education: What role should the nurse adopt in practice? Journal of Advanced Nursing, 28(6), 1269–1275.

Pederson, A., O'Neill, M., & Rootman, I. (Eds.). (1994). Health promotion in Canada: Provincial, national & international perspectives. Toronto, ON: W. B. Saunders, Canada.

Pike, S., & Forster, D. (Eds.). (1995). Health promotion for all. New York: Churchill Livingstone.

Renwick, R., Brown, I., & Nagler, M. (1996). Quality of life in health promotion and rehabilitation. Thousand Oaks, CA: Sage.

Rootman, I., & Goodstadt, M. (1996). Health promotion and health reform in Canada (Position Paper). Toronto, ON: University of Toronto, Centre for Health Promotion.

Waxler-Morrison, N., Anderson, J., & Richardson, E. (Eds.). (1990). Cross-cultural caring: A handbook for health professionals. Vancouver: University of British Columbia Press.

Webb, P. (Ed.). (1994). Health promotion and patient education: A professional's guide. London: Chapman & Hall.

Woolf, S. H., Jonas, S., & Lawrence, R. S. (Eds.). (1996). Health promotion and disease prevention in clinical practice. Baltimore, MD: Williams & Wilkins.

Index

Page numbers followed by *f* refer to figures; those followed by *t* refer to tables.

Ability, cultural effects of, 133
Abstinent, defined, 183
Accreditation, defined, 6
Activity, defined, 21
Activity(ies) of daily living (ADLs)
  defined, 7
  goals for, 236, 238–239
Acute care of the elderly units, 169
Administrative rules and regulations, 320
Age, cultural effects of, 132
Age Discrimination in Employment Act
  of 1967, 319, 325
Aging
  effects on sexuality, 192–193
  of U.S. population, 123
Alexander, P.A., in clinical reasoning
  and decision making, 71
Americans with Disabilities Act of
  1990, 319
  Title I, 325
Amok, 141
Anderson, J., in supervision of rehabilitation delivery, 287,
  296–298, 297f, 309, 310f, 311
Anderson's continuum, in supervision
  of rehabilitation delivery,
  296–298, 297f
  adaptation of, 300–301
Annon, J.S., in sexual health discussion,
  193, 194t
Antonovsky, A., in health promotion,
  363–364, 365–366
Anxiety
  "aesthetic," in formulation of attitudes
  toward disability, 115–116

"existential," in formulation of attitudes toward disability,
  115–116
Anxiety reduction, sources of, cultural
  variations of, 146–147
Aphasia, defined, 7
Arthroplasty, defined, 11
Assessment, needs, by rehabilitation
  professionals, 338f, 339–342,
  339f, 341f
Assisted living, defined, 16
Assisted Living Federation of America, 16
Assisted suicide, ethical issues related
  to, 57
Assisted-living facilities
  benefits of, 16
  persons served by, 16
  rehabilitation services in, 16–17
    case study, 17
  residents of, typical, 16
  services provided by, 16
  in U.S., number of, 16
Assistive technology, defined, 19
Attitude(s)
  defined, 110
  of health professionals, treatment
    models influencing, 112–113
  health promotion, related changes
    in, 357
  toward disability, 109–121. *See also*
    Disability(ies), attitudes
    toward
"Attraction template," 179
Augmentative communication,
  defined, 19

Austin, N., in supervision of rehabilitation delivery, 303, 306, 307–308

Babineau, J., in vocational rehabilitation, 263
Baillie, H.W., in ethical issues in rehabilitation, 46
Balla, J., in vocational rehabilitation, 263, 264, 265f
Barrett, T.M., in ethical issues in rehabilitation, 46
Basmajian, J.V., in rehabilitation ergonomics, 255
Beauty, culturally defined, 137
Behavior(s)
    health, cultural diversity and, 123–154
    health promotion, related changes in, 357
    sexual, diversity among, 177
Belief(s), health promotion effects of, 357–358
Bellini, J., in vocational rehabilitation, 263–264
Benner, P., in clinical reasoning and decision making, 70
Berkowitz, M., in vocational rehabilitation, 261
Bhat, A., in health promotion, 358
Bias, reproductive, 178
Biomedical model, health professionals' attitudes toward disability influenced by, 113
Body, social dimensions of, cultural interpretation of, 137–138
Body functioning, cultural interpretation of, 136–137
Body image, cultural interpretation of, 135–136
Body space, cultural interpretation of, 138–139
Boshuizen, H.P.A., in clinical reasoning and decision making, 68, 70
Breadth, in case management, 90
Bristow, D., in supervision of rehabilitation delivery, 291, 292
Burton, K., in rehabilitation ergonomics, 257
Business, goal of, 302–303

California Critical Thinking Skills Test, 77

Campanella, T., in vocational rehabilitation, 267, 275
Carnevali, D., in clinical reasoning and decision making, 76–77
Case management, 87–107. *See also* Case manager(s)
    breadth in, 90
    case manager's role in, 87–88
    case studies, 94–95, 99–101
    client-centered, 93
    core activities of, 93
    defined, 87, 89, 90
    delivery models of, 90–91
    duration in, 90
    gatekeeping in, 93
    goals achieved through, 87
    goals of, 91–93
    historical background of, 87, 88–89
    intensity in, 90
    internal, 91
    literature related to, 91, 92
    organizational arrangements in, 90–91
    origins of, 87, 88–89
    preparation in, 102–103
    process of, 93–102
    professional opportunities in, 102–103
    research in, 102–103
    system-centered, 93
    terminology related to, 89–90
Case manager(s). *See also* Case management
    clients requiring services by, 97
    coordinating assessment and access to services by, 93–98
        case study, 94–95
        goals of, 96
        integration of services, 98
        "single point of entry" to services, 97–98
    coordinating planning, delivery, and monitoring of services by, 98–102
        case study, 99–102
    external, 91
    preparation by, 102–103
    professional opportunities for, 102–103
    research by, 102–103
    role of, 87–88, 93–102
Cebulski, P., in supervision of rehabilitation delivery, 291, 292
Celibate, defined, 183

Certification, defined, 5
Chevannes, M., in supervision of rehabilitation delivery, 312
Chi, M.T.H., in clinical reasoning and
decision making, 75
Churches, cultural diversity effects
on, 124
Civil legal system, 321
Civil Rights Act of 1964, Title VII, 325
Class structure, cultural effects of,
133–134
Client-centered therapy, 112
Clinical decision making, multidisciplinary, 79–82
Clinical reasoning
context of, 65–67, 66t, 67f
in context-oriented research, 68
and decision making, 63–86
defined, 63, 64
effectiveness of, 74
errors in, 77–79
ethical/pragmatic, defined, 71
expertise in, 75–77
insensitivity in, 78
interpretive and critical research in, 68
irrationality in, 78
models of, 69–75, 72f, 73f
hypothetico-deductive
reasoning, 69
inductive reasoning, 69
integrated, client-centered, 71–75
interpretive, 70–71
knowledge-reasoning integration,
69–70
pattern recognition, 69
models used in different health professions, 68–69
mystery in, 78
narrowness in, 78
nature of, 64–67, 66t, 67f
in nursing, 65
in occupational therapy, 64
in physiotherapy, 64
process of, 74
in process-oriented research, 67
rigidity in, 78
social ecology model of health and
interactional professional,
80–81
in speech and hearing sciences, 65
vagueness in, 78
wastefulness in, 78
Clinical reasoning loop, 72, 72f

Coaching
clinical
confronting in, 305–306
counseling in, 305–306
dressing for the occasion, 308–309
educating in, 303
implementation of, 308–313, 310f
rationale for, 307–308
sponsoring in, 304–305
in supervision of rehabilitation
delivery, 302–308, 302f
defined, 303–304
Cogan, M., in supervision of rehabilitation delivery, 309
Cognitive styles, cultural, 142–144
abstractive processing, 143–144
associative processing, 143–144
closed-minded, 142–143
open-minded, 142–143
in processing information, 143–144
Collaborative reasoning, defined, 71
Commission on Accreditation of
Rehabilitation Facilities
(CARF), 6
Commitment, in development of long-
term relationship, 182
Communication
augmentative, defined, 19
styles of, cultural, 144–145
Communication skills, of rehabilitation
professionals, 336
Communication/cognition, goals
for, 237
Community, in cultural identity,
129, 130f
Comorbidities, defined, 7
Comprehensive care, defined, 28
Comprehensive outpatient rehabilita-
tion facilities (CORFs), 16
defined, 18
vs. other ambulatory rehabilitation
settings, 18–19
Comprehensive services, in rehabilita-
tion, 209
"Compression of morbidity," 157–158
Conditional reasoning, defined, 71
Confronting, in supervision of rehabili-
tation delivery, 305–306
Congenital impairments, defined, 1
Consensus consulting, principles
for, 337
Consensus model, for rehabilitation
professionals, 334

Consent, informed, patient, to health
    care intervention,
    324–325
Consultant(s), defined, 329
Consulting
    consensus, principles for, 337
    framework for, for rehabilitation
        professionals, 337–339,
        338f, 339f
Consulting models, for rehabilitation
    professionals, 332–333
Context, in explanatory model of sick-
    ness, 140
Context (knowledge)-oriented research,
    clinical reasoning and deci-
    sion making in, 68
Continuing Care Accreditation Com-
    mission, 17
Contract(s)
    employment, in supervision of reha-
        bilitation delivery, 313
    learning, in supervision of rehabilita-
        tion delivery, 313–314
Convalescent services, rehabilitation and,
    9–10. *See also* Rehabilitation-
    based subacute programs
Cooper, J.E., in vocational rehabilita-
    tion, 271–272
CORFs. *See* Comprehensive outpatient
    rehabilitation facilities
    (CORFs)
Corporate liability, 323
Cost containment, in rehabilitation, 209
Counseling
    sexual, P-LI-SS-IT model for, 194t
    in supervision of rehabilitation deliv-
        ery, 305–306
Crepeau, E.B., in clinical reasoning and
    decision making, 70
Criminal legal system, 321
Cultural diversity
    church transitions due to, 124
    family organizational and structure
        affected by, 123–124
    global economic effects of, 123
    and health behavior, 123–154
    schools affected by, 124
    in U.S. by 2056, 123
Cultural environmental deficiencies,
    rehabilitation professional's
    role in assessment of,
    340–3441, 341f
Cultural identity, sources of, 129–130, 130f
Cultural miscommunication, 145

Cultural misunderstandings, causes of,
    128–129
Cultural sensitivity, in rehabilitation
    process, 148–151, 149t, 151t
Culture. *See also* Culture learning,
    health associated; Culture-
    learning process
    ability and, 133
    age and, 132
    anxiety reduction and, 146–147
    assumptions associated with, 126–128
    boundaries of, vagueness of, 128–129
    class structure and, 133–134
    cognitive styles of, 142–144. *See also*
        Cognitive styles, cultural
    communication styles affected by,
        144–145
    conscious, 127–128
    decision making and, 146
    defined, 126–128
    disability and, 133
    dynamic nature of, 128
    effect on health status, 125
    equality/inequality issues and, 147
    ethnicity and, 131
    gender and, 131–132
    health and, 133
    health promotion effects of, 357–358
    language and, 132–133
    learning of, 128–134. *See also* Cul-
        ture-learning process
    objective elements of, 127
    race and, 130–131
    reflection questions for rehabilitation
        practitioners associated
        with, 149t
    religion and, 132
    as shared identification, 127
    as social construct, 126, 127
    social levels within, 129–130, 130f
    socioeconomic factors and, 134
    spirituality and, 132
    subconscious, 127–128
    subjective elements of, 127
    time use and, 147–148
    values systems and, 145–148
Culture learning, health-associated
    beliefs about body in, 135–139
    beliefs about health and healing in,
        139–142
    body functioning in, 136–137
    body image in, 135–136
    body space in, 138–139
    communication styles in, 144–145

context in, 140
edible vs. nonedible food in, 139–140
social dimensions of body in, 137–138
thinking styles in, 142–144. *See also*
    Cognitive styles, cultural
truth in, 145–146
value systems in, 145–148
Culture-learning process, 128–134, 130f
  ability in, 133
  age as factor in, 132
  boundaries of culture in, 128–129
  class structure in, 133–134
  contexts within which people social-
    ly construct culture in,
    129–130, 130f
  disability in, 133
  ethnicity in, 131
  gender in, 131–132
  health in, 133
  language in, 132–133
  race in, 130–131
  religion in, 132
  social levels within, 129–130, 130f
  socioeconomic factors in, 134
  spirituality in, 132
Cunnilingus, defined, 202

Dailey, D., in sexuality, 179–180
Decision making
  clinical, multidisciplinary, 79–82
  clinical reasoning and, 63–86
  in context-oriented research, 68
  defined, 63
  interpretive and critical research in, 68
  locus of, cultural variations of, 146
  meeting of professional cultures and
    models of, 81–82
  nature of, 64–67, 66t, 67f
  in process-oriented research, 67
Diagnostic reasoning, defined, 70–71
Direct costs, defined, 157
Disability(ies)
  attitudes toward, 109–121
    aesthetic and existential anxiety
      in, 115–116
    ethnic influences on, 111–112
    factors contributing to, 109
    "person first" language in,
      117–118, 118t
    research on, 110–111
    study questions, 119–120
    treatment models influencing,
      112–113
  care for persons with, types of, 211

cultural effects of, 133
defined, 117
in the elderly, causes of, treatment
  of, 164t
ethical issues related to, 58
prevalence of, 258
sexuality effects of, 186,
  192–193, 192t
stigma associated with, 113–115
Disclaimer(s), legal, 326
Doctor-patient model, for rehabilitation
  professionals, 333
Duration, in case management, 90
Dynamic frailty, defined, 161
Dysarthria, defined, 7

Economy, global, cultural diversity
  and, 123
Elderly
  acute care of the elderly units for, 169
  determinants of health for, 156t
  disabilities in, causes of, treatment
    of, 164t
  disease presentation in, 162–163, 162f
  frail, needs of, 158
  health care costs of, 156–157
  health maintenance in, barriers to,
    159, 160f
  home care for, 171–172
  long-term institutional care for, need
    for, 155–156
  nursing home care for, 172–173
  outpatient care for, 173
  pain in, elements of, 159, 160f
  population of, in U.S., 123, 155
  quality of life of, preserving of, 158
  rehabilitation for, 155–175. *See also*
    Geriatric rehabilitation
  sexuality in, 192–193
Empathy, in formulation of attitudes
  toward disability, 116
Employment contracts, in supervision of rehabilitation
  delivery, 313
Enculturation, 126
Epp, J., in health promotion, 355
Equality/inequality issues, cultural variations of, 147
Ergonomics
  complementary role of, 252–253, 252f
  defined, 243
  goals of, 249, 250, 250t
  origin of, 246
  philosophy of, 247–248, 248f

Ergonomics (continued)
  rehabilitation, 243–260
    application of, 253–258, 254f–256f
    components of, 256f
    divergence between, 251–252
    need for, 258–259
    patient-environment interface
      in, 258
    therapist-patient interface in,
      255–258
  rehabilitation and
    parallelism between, 249–251,
      250t, 251f
    reasons for, 244–245
    theoretical model of, 255f
Ethic(s)
  defined, 46
  research, 53–55
  of self-care, 48–51, 49t–50t
Ethical issues
  health promotion–related, 359–360
  in rehabilitation, 43–61
    assisted suicide, 57
    case studies, 44, 45, 51, 52
    consultant-related, 335–336
    cultural sensitivity related to, 56–57
    disability, 58
    ethical principles, 46–47, 48–53,
      49t–50t
    euthanasia, 57
    mercy killing, 57
    responsibilities associated with,
      45–47, 47f
    responsibility to clients, 51
    responsibility to rehabilitation dis-
      ciplines, 52–53
    responsibility to society as a
      whole, 53
    research-related, 53–55
Ethical/pragmatic reasoning, defined, 71
Ethnicity
  cultural effects of, 131
  defined, 131
  effect on attitudes toward disability,
    111–112
  vs. nationality, 131
Euthanasia, ethical issues related to, 57
Evaluation-feedback stage, in supervi-
    sion of rehabilitation deliv-
    ery, 297, 297f, 298–299
Excitement, in sexual response, 184
Explanatory model of illness, 140–141
  client's, eliciting of, 151t
External case managers, 91

Fadiman, A., in ethical issues in rehabil-
    itation, 56
Family(ies)
  in cultural identity, 129, 130f
  organizational and structural changes
    in, 123–124
Family and Medical Leave Act, 320
Family care, future implications for, 211
Fellatio, defined, 202
Female-superior (woman-on-top)
    position, in sexual inter-
    course, 201
Feuerstein, M., in vocational rehabilita-
    tion, 264, 264f
Fisher, S., in clinical reasoning and deci-
    sion making, 70
Fleming, M.H., in clinical reasoning and
    decision making, 64
Fonteyn, M., in clinical reasoning and
    decision making, 70, 76
Food, cultural interpretation of, 139–140
Fowler, J., in supervision of rehabilita-
    tion delivery, 312
Frailty
  defined, 158
  dynamic, defined, 161
  stable, defined, 161
Function
  assessment of, 211–212
  defined, 211–212
Functional assessment, 209–241
  activity analysis in, 219–221, 220t,
    222f–226f
  assessment of function in, 221, 226,
    227t
  case studies, 219, 234, 235
  changes in, 209–211, 210f
  client-centered interview in,
    215–218, 217f–218f
  clinical perspective of, 212–215,
    214f–215f
  common language in, 227–229, 228t,
    230t–231t, 232f
  components of, 215–229, 217f–218f,
    220t, 222f–226f, 227t, 228t,
    230t–231t, 232f
  contextual observation in, 226–227
  discipline contributions in, 218–219
  documentation of, 233–234
  functional goal writing in, 234–237
  future trends in, 237–238
  implementation of, 229, 233
  occupational therapists' role in, 213,
    214f, 219

physical therapists' role in, 213–215, 214f, 218–219
speech therapists' role in, 215, 215f, 219
standardized, 229, 230t–231t
in vocational rehabilitation, 263–264
vs. standardized assessment, 213
Functional Independence Measure (FIM), 228
Functional status, in the elderly, evaluation of, 161–162

Gardner, J., in vocational rehabilitation, 267, 275
Garrett, R.M., in ethical issues in rehabilitation, 46
Gastrostomy, defined, 19
Gatekeeping, in case management, 93
Gender
    cultural effects of, 132–133
    defined, 131
Generalized resistance resources, 363–364
Geographic region, in cultural identity, 129, 130f
Geriatric home care, 171–172
Geriatric medicine
    challenges in, 155–158, 156t, 157t
    opportunities in, 155–158, 156t, 157t
Geriatric rehabilitation. *See also* Elderly
    factors influencing, 163t
    home care, 171–172
    in outpatient setting, 173
    programs for, 169–171
    settings for, 169–173
    team approaches to, 155–175
        assessment, 159, 161–162
            dynamic vs. stable frailty in, 161
            functional status in, 161–162
            multidisciplinary, 162
        critique of, 166, 168, 168f
        examples of, 164–166, 167t
        functional teams in, 164–165, 167t
        goals in, 158–159
        interdisciplinary teams in, 165–166, 167t
        leadership styles in, 168, 168f
        multidisciplinary teams in, 165, 167t
        transdisciplinary teams in, 166, 167t
Glaser, R., in clinical reasoning and decision making, 75

Global economy, cultural diversity and, 123
Goal(s)
    defined, 21
    functional, writing of, 234–237
    long-term, defined, 21
    short-term, defined, 21
Goldhammer, R., in supervision of rehabilitation delivery, 309
Gould, S.J., in ethical issues in rehabilitation, 54
Graham, H., in health promotion, 358
Groen, G.J., in clinical reasoning and decision making, 69

Haddad, in rehabilitation teamwork, 28–29
Hagler, P., in supervision of rehabilitation delivery, 291, 292, 302
Hall, E.T., in cultural effects on communication styles, 144
    in space surrounding bodies, 138
Hallam, R., in vocational rehabilitation, 268
Hancock, J., in supervision of rehabilitation delivery, 292
Handicap(s), defined, 117
Harkappa, K., in rehabilitation ergonomics, 255
Healing, cultural interpretation of, 139–142
Health
    conceptions of, 355–356
    cultural effects of, 133
    cultural interpretation of, 140
    culture-learning associated with, 134–148. *See also* Culture learning, health-associated
    defined, 352–353
    maintaining of, cultural interpretation of, 139–142
    population, health promotion and, 356
    population determinants of, 156t
Health behavior, cultural diversity and, 123–154
Health care
    changes in, 209–211, 210f
    managed care, 209
    medical model of, 209–210, 210f
    overlapping sectors of, 141–142
    physician-centered, 134

Health care (continued)
  prospective payment systems, 209
  quantitative, 134
  restructuring of, effect on supervision
      in rehabilitation delivery,
      293–295
  sexual, 180–181
  single-case–centered, 134
  specialist-oriented, 134
Health care malpractice, 322–324
Health care teams
  benefits to health care, 30t
  history of, 27–28
  purpose of, 28–29
Health consciousness, rehabilitation
      resulting from, 1–2
Health maintenance, barriers to, in the
      elderly, 159, 160f
Health professionals, attitudes of, treat-
      ment models influencing,
      112–113
"Health Professionals as Contributors to
      Attitudes Towards Persons
      with Disabilities," 111
Health promotion, 351–368
  beliefs and, 357–358
  challenges to, 364–365
  changes related to, 357
  culture and, 357–358
  defined, 351, 354–355, 356
  ethical issues related to, 359–360
  explanation of, 356–357
  framework for, for multidisciplinary
      team, 360–364, 362f, 363t
  historical perspectives on, 352–354
  paradigm shift in, 354–355
  population health and, 356
  population health promotion model,
      361–363, 362f, 363t
  priorities of, 355
  process of, 356–357
  reasons for, 351–352
  salutogenic model, 363–364
  themes of, 359
  values and, 357–358
Health status
  factors affecting, 125
  health promotion–related changes in,
      357
Hébert, R., in health promotion,
      359–360
Hemiparesis, defined, 7
Heruti, R., in rehabilitation teamwork,
      37–38

Heterosexual intercourse, positioning
      for, 200–202
HICAP program logic model, 275, 276f
Higgs, J., in clinical reasoning and deci-
      sion making, 68
Home care, for the elderly
  goals of, 171–172
  types of, 171
Home health rehabilitation services, 12–16
  case study, 13–15
  criteria for, 13
  defined, 12
  indications for, 12–13
  interdisciplinary communication in, 15
  referral for, 13–14
  time frame for, 15–16
Hot-cold theory, in cultural beliefs
      about structure and function
      of body, 136, 139–140
Human factors, vs. ergonomics, 244
Humanism
  defined, 12
  health professionals' attitudes toward
      disability influenced by,
      112–113
Hypothetico-deductive reasoning, 67f, 69

Identity, defined, 179
Impairment(s)
  congenital, defined, 1
  defined, 1, 21, 117
  prevalence of, 27
Imrie, R., in health promotion, 354
Individual, in cultural identity, 129, 130f
Inductive reasoning, 69
Informed consent, patient, to health
      care intervention, 324–325
Inpatient rehabilitation, 6–9, 8f
  accredited hospital–based rehabilita-
      tion units, 6–7
  acute rehabilitation units, 6
  defined, 21
  length of stay in, 7
  process of, 7–9, 8f
  types of, 6
Insensitivity, in clinical reasoning and
      decision making, 78
Intensity, in case management, 90
Interactive reasoning, defined, 71
Intercourse, heterosexual, positioning
      for, 200–202
Interdisciplinary, defined, 21
Interdisciplinary teams, defined, 4
Internal case management, 91

Interpretive and critical research, clinical reasoning and decision making in, 68
Intervention, defined, 338
Intimacy, defined, 179
Irrationality, in clinical reasoning and decision making, 78
Isernhagen, S.J., in vocational rehabilitation, 261, 272

Jakarta Declaration on Leading Health Promotion into the Twenty-First Century, in health promotion, 355
Jensen, G.M., in clinical reasoning and decision making, 70
Joint Commission on Accreditation of Healthcare Organizations (JCAHO), defined, 6
Jones, in attitudes toward disability, 114
Judge-made law, 320
Judy, J.E., in clinical reasoning and decision making, 71

Kaplan, H.S., in sexual response, 184
Kaufman, D.R., in clinical reasoning and decision making, 70
Keith, R.A., in functional assessment, 213
Kemp, B., in rehabilitation teamwork, 28
Kleinman, A., in explanatory model of sickness, 140
Knowledge
    health promotion–related changes in, 357
    organizational knowledge of, 334–335
Knowledge deficiencies, rehabilitation professional's role in assessment of, 340, 341f
Knowledge-reasoning integration, 69–70
Koch, L.C., in vocational rehabilitation, 263
Koro, 141
Krefting, D., in social construct of culture, 129
Krefting, L., in social construct of culture, 129
Kumar, S., in rehabilitation ergonomics, 255, 257

Ladyshewsky, R., in supervision of rehabilitation delivery, 291, 292

Lalonde, M., in health promotion, 354
Language
    cultural effects of, 132–133
    "person first," 117–118, 118t
Lateral-entry (side-entry) position, in sexual intercourse, 201–202
Law, M., in vocational rehabilitation, 265, 266f
Leach, J., in vocational rehabilitation, 268
Learning contracts, in supervision of rehabilitation delivery, 313–314
LeBlanc, M., in rehabilitation ergonomics, 259
Lefier, L., in rehabilitation ergonomics, 259
Legal issues
    affecting rehabilitation professionals, managers, and organizations, 325
    rehabilitation-related, 319–327
        disclaimer in, 326
        future directions in, 326
        health care malpractice, 322–324
        patient informed consent, 324–325
Legal system, components of, 319–322
Level of service, defined, 5
Liability
    corporate, 323
    primary, 323
Licensure, defined, 5–6
Lifestyle(s), sexual, diversity among, 177
Ling, C., in rehabilitation teamwork, 29
Livneh, in defining "aesthetic" and "existential" anxiety, 115
Long-term goal, defined, 21
Love, and relationships, 181–183

Mainstreamed, defined, 19
Mal de ojo, 141
Male-superior (man-on-top) position, in sexual intercourse, 201
Malpractice health care, 322–324
Managed care, 209
    functional outcomes in, 212
    reimbursement in areas of, focus for, 212
Masturbation
    attitudes toward, 183–184
    defined, 183
Matrix structures, defined, 165
McClelland, R.W., in case management, 93
McFarlane, L., in supervision of rehabilitation delivery, 301, 302

McKay, M., in vocational rehabilitation, 262, 268–269

McMahon, B.T., in vocational rehabilitation, 266

Medicine, new goals of, 157, 157t

Men, sexual dysfunction in, 187t, 190t–191t

Mercy killing, ethical issues related to, 57

Miscommunication, cultural, 145

Missionary position, in sexual intercourse, 201

Misunderstanding(s), cultural, causes of, 128–129

Mobility, goals for, 236, 238–239

Moglowsky, N., in vocational rehabilitation, 263, 266

Multidisciplinary, defined, 21

Multidisciplinary teams, defined, 2–4

Murrell, K.H.F., in ergonomics, 243

Mystery, in clinical reasoning and decision making, 78

Narrative reasoning, defined, 71

Narrowness, in clinical reasoning and decision making, 78

Nationality, vs. ethnicity, 131

Needs assessment
  enabling factors in, examples of, 342, 343t
  predisposing factors in, examples of, 342, 343t
  program planning based on, 342–344, 343t
  by rehabilitation professionals, 338f, 339–342, 339f, 341f
  reinforcing factors in, examples of, 342, 343t

Needs assessment model, 341f

Negotiation, by rehabilitation professionals, 336–337

Noe, S.R., in ethical issues in rehabilitation, 53

Nonambulatory, defined, 11

Nonverbal, defined, 19

Nursing
  clinical reasoning in, 65
  skilled, defined, 21

Nursing home
  geriatric care in, 172–173
  in nursing home, 172–173

Objectivity, rehabilitation consultants' role in, 334

Occupational Safety and Health Act, 320

Occupational therapist, role in functional assessment, 213–215, 219

Occupational therapy, clinical reasoning in, 64

Ohry, A., in rehabilitation teamwork, 37–38

Older Worker Benefit Protection Act of 1990, 325

Opportunity costs, defined, 157

Organizational knowledge, rehabilitation consultants' role in, 334–335

Orgasm, in sexual response, 184

Osborn, J., in supervision of rehabilitation delivery, 307

Ottawa Charter, action called for by, 361

Outpatient rehabilitation, defined, 21

Outpatient rehabilitation services, 17–20
  case study, 19–20
  defined, 17
  freestanding facilities, 18
  hospital-based, 18
  physician-based rehabilitation facilities, 18
  private practice clinics, 18
  single-therapy clinics, 18
  vs. CORFs, 18–19

Outpatient setting, geriatric care in, 173

Pain, elements of, in the elderly, 159, 160f

Paraphilia(s), defined, 185

Participipation, defined, 21

Patel, V.L., in clinical reasoning and decision making, 69, 70

Patient informed consent, in health care intervention, 324–325

Patient interview
  in functional assessment, 215–218, 217f–218f
  in sexual health, 193–198, 194t, 196t–197t

Pattern recognition, 69

Peat, M., in rehabilitation ergonomics, 255

Peer supervision programs, in supervision of rehabilitation delivery, 293–294

Performance evaluation, in supervision of rehabilitation delivery, 314–315

Perron, J., in vocational rehabilitation, 262, 268–269

Perrow, C., in case management, 89–90
"Person first" language, 117–118, 118t
Personal boundaries, cultural interpretation of, 138–139
Personal knowledge, clinical reasoning and decision making in, 68
Person-centered therapy, 112
Personhood, in attitudes toward disability, 118
Peters, T., in supervision of rehabilitation delivery, 303, 306, 307–308
Physiatrist(s), defined, 2
Physical ability deficiencies, rehabilitation professional's role in assessment of, 340, 341f
Physical environmental deficiencies, rehabilitation professional's role in assessment of, 340–341, 341f
Physical therapist, role in functional assessment, 213–215, 214f, 218–219
Physical Therapist Assistant Clinical Performance Instrument, 314
Physical Therapist Clinical Performance Instrument, 314
Physician-centered health care, 134
Physiotherapy, clinical reasoning in, 64
Pity, in formulation of attitudes toward disability, 116
Plateau stage, in sexual response, 184
Pomeroy, W.B., in sexuality history taking, 193, 195
Population health, health promotion and, 356
Population health promotion model, 361–363, 362f, 363t
Power struggles, in development of long-term relationship, 182
Predictive reasoning, defined, 71
Primary liability, 323
Process-oriented research, clinical reasoning and decision making in, 67
Professional craft knowledge, clinical reasoning and decision making in, 68
Professional socialization, defined, 81
Professionalization, defined, 81
Program, defined, 338
Propositional knowledge, in clinical reasoning and decision making, 68

Prospective payment systems, in health care, 209
Purchase model, for rehabilitation professionals, 333
Purtillo, R., in rehabilitation teamwork, 28–29

Quadriplegia, defined, 19
Quality of life
of elderly, preserving of, 158
health promotion–related changes in, 357
Quantitative health care, 134

Race
cultural definition of, 130–131
in culture-learning process, 130–131
Reasoning
clinical, and decision making, 63–86. *See also* Clinical reasoning
collaborative, defined, 71
conditional, defined, 71
diagnostic, defined, 70–71
hypothetico-deductive, 67f, 69
inductive, 69
interactive, defined, 71
narrative, defined, 71
predictive, defined, 71
teaching as, defined, 71
Rehabilitation
administrative issues in, 319–327
costs of, 2
defined, 1–2, 55–56
ethics in, 43–61. *See also* Ethical issues, in rehabilitation
final outcome of, 253
functional assessment in, 209–241. *See also* Functional assessment
goals of, 248–249, 250, 250t, 302–303
health consciousness and, 1–2
health promotion in, 351–368. *See also* Health promotion
historical background of, 1
inpatient, 6–9, 8f. *See also* Inpatient rehabilitation
legal issues in, 319–327. *See also* Legal issues, rehabilitation-related
origin of, 245–246
philosophy of, 246–247, 247f
sexual health services in, 177–208
goals of, 177–178

Rehabilitation (continued)
  sexuality in, 177–208. *See also* Sexuality, in rehabilitation
  subacute, defined, 22
  supervision of service delivery in, 285–317. *See also* Supervision of rehabilitation delivery
  teamwork in, 27–42. *See also* Rehabilitation team
  for traumatic injuries, 2
  vocational, 261–283. *See also* Vocational rehabilitation
Rehabilitation ergonomics, 243–260. *See also* Ergonomics
Rehabilitation process, cultural sensitivity in, 148–151, 149t, 151t
Rehabilitation professionals
  changing roles of, 329
  communication by, 336
  consensus consulting by, principles for, 337
  as consultants to business and industry, 329–349
    in physical ability deficiencies, 340, 341f
    in physical and cultural environmental deficiencies, 340–341, 341f
    program evaluation, 346–347
    in skill or knowledge deficiencies, 340, 341f
    training for, 344–346
  consulting framework for, 337–339, 338f, 339f
  consulting models for, 332–334
    consensus model, 334
    doctor-patient model, 333
    purchase model, 333
  ethical issues facing, 335–336
  issues facing, 334–337
  needs assessment by, 338f, 339–342, 339f, 341f
  negotiation skills of, 336–337
  objectivity of, 334
  organizational knowledge of, 334–335
  in understanding organizations as systems, 332
Rehabilitation settings, 1–26
  application activities in, 20–21
  assisted-living facilities, 16–17
  home health rehabilitation services, 12–16
  inpatient services, 6–9, 8f. *See also* Inpatient rehabilitation
  outpatient services, 17–20. *See also* Outpatient rehabilitation services
  study questions, 22
  terminology related to, 21–22
  transitional care, 9–12, 12f
Rehabilitation team, 2–5, 3f, 27–42
  approaches of, 34–35
    interdisciplinary, 34–35
    multidisciplinary, 34
    transdisciplinary, 35
  benefits of working on, 29–31, 29t, 30t
  benefits to health care provider, 30t
  benefits to patients, 29, 29t
  case studies, 39–41
  creation of, guidelines for, 35–37, 36f
  ethics for, 43–61. *See also* Ethical issues, in rehabilitation
  evolution of, stages of, 37
  future considerations for, 38
  history of, 27–28
  meetings of, 37–38
  purpose of, 28–29
  questions related to, 27
  study questions, 38
  team members, 2, 32–33, 32f, 33t
    clients, 37
    consultants, 36, 36f
    core members, 35–36, 36f
    extended members, 36, 36f
    levels of, 35–36, 36f
    process of becoming, 31
    resource persons, 36, 36f
  team settings, 33, 34t
Rehabilitation-based subacute programs, 9–10
  indications for, 10
  types of, 10
Relationship(s)
  long-term, development of, stages in, 182–183
  love and, 181–183
Religion, cultural effects of, 132
Reproductive bias, 178
Research ethics, 53–55
Resolution, in sexual response, 184
Rigidity, in clinical reasoning and decision making, 78
Rittman, M., in supervision of rehabilitation delivery, 307
Rogers, C., in attitudes toward disability, 112
Romance, in development of long-term relationship, 182

Rousch, S.E., in attitudes toward disability, 111
Rumrill, P.D., in vocational rehabilitation, 263, 266, 268, 270

Schmidt, H.G., in clinical reasoning and decision making, 68, 70
Schon, D., in supervision of rehabilitation delivery, 312
School(s), cultural diversity effects on, 124
Scorzelli, J.F., in ethical issues in rehabilitation, 53
Scott, I., in clinical reasoning and decision making, 77, 78
Self-care, ethics of, 48–51, 49t–50t
Self-supervision stage, in supervision of rehabilitation delivery, 297f, 298, 299–300
Sensitivity, cultural, in rehabilitation process, 148–151, 149t, 151t
Sensual awareness, sexual, 199–200
    activities for, 199–200
Sensual pleasure, 183
Sensuality, defined, 179
Sexual behaviors, diversity among, 177
"Sexual beingness," 180
Sexual counseling, P-LI-SS-IT model for, 194t
Sexual desire, 184
Sexual dysfunction, 185–186, 187t–191t
    causes of, 185
    defined, 185
    types of, 185
    in women, 187t–189t
Sexual excitement, 184
Sexual fantasy, 183
Sexual function, 183–185
    enhancement of, options and alternatives in, 194t, 198–203
Sexual health
    defined, 177
    discussion of, guidelines for, 193–198, 194t, 196t–197t
Sexual health care, in rehabilitation, need for, 180–181
Sexual health services
    goals of, 177–178
    in rehabilitation, 177–208
Sexual lifestyles, diversity among, 177
Sexual orientation, in development of long-term relationship, 183
Sexual pleasure, 183–185
Sexual response, stages in, 184

Sexuality
    defined, 178–180
    in rehabilitation, 177–208
        case studies, 203–205
        disabilities effects on, 186, 192–193, 192t
        discussion guidelines, 193–198, 194t, 196t–197t
        in the elderly, 192–193
        emotional aspects of, 178
        health professionals' attitudes toward, 181
        illness effects on, 186, 192–193, 192t
        knowledge and beliefs concerning, 178
        in men, 187t, 190t–191t
        options and alternatives in, 194t, 198–203
        patient history in, 193, 195
        patient interview in, 193, 195
        positioning for heterosexual intercourse in, 200–202
        positive vs. negative aspects of, 180
        sensual awareness in, 199–200
        sexual health record keeping in, 195–198, 196t–197t
    reproductive aspects of, 179–180
Sexualization, defined, 180
Sherman, R., in defining culture, 126
Shervington, J., in vocational rehabilitation, 263, 264, 265, 265f
Short-term goal, defined, 21
Simmonds, M., in rehabilitation ergonomics, 255, 257
Single-case–centered health care, 134
Sitting coital position, in sexual intercourse, 202
Skill deficiencies, rehabilitation professional's role in assessment of, 340, 341f
Skilled nursing, defined, 21
"Skin hunger," 179
Smith, P., in vocational rehabilitation, 271
Social class, cultural effects of, 133–134
Social support, health promotion–related changes in, 357
Socialization, professional, defined, 81
Socioeconomic factors, cultural effects of, 134
Sojkowski, M., in supervision of rehabilitation delivery, 291, 292
Specialist-oriented health care, 134

Speech and hearing sciences, clinical
    reasoning in, 65
Speech therapist, role in functional
    assessment, 215, 215f, 219
Spirituality, cultural effects of, 132
Sponsoring, in supervision of rehabilita-
    tion delivery, 304–305
Stability, in development of long-term
    relationship, 182
Stable frailty, defined, 161
Standardized assessment, vs. functional
    assessment, 213
Statutory law, 319
Stigma
    defined, 113
    disability as, 113–115
Strong, S., in vocational rehabilita-
    tion, 263
Student supervision, in supervision of
    rehabilitation delivery,
    294–295
Subacute care, defined, 9–10
Subacute rehabilitation, defined, 22
Subacute rehabilitation units, 10
    case study, 10–12, 12f
    examples of, 10
Suicide, assisted, ethical issues related
    to, 57
Supervisee(s)
    defined, 286
    types of, 288
Supervision of rehabilitation delivery,
    285–317
    analyzing in, 310f, 311–312
    Anderson's continuum in,
        296–298, 297f
        adaptation of, 300–301
    clinical coaching in, 302–308, 302f
    components of, 309–313, 310f
    documentation of, 313–315
    employment contracts in, 313
    evaluation-feedback stage in, 297,
        297f, 298–299
    goals of, 287–289
    impact of assistants and students on,
        289–293
        cost-benefit studies of, 290–291
        productivity studies in, 291–293
    impact of health care restructuring
        on, 293–295
    integrating in, 312–313
    learning contracts in, 313–314
    monitoring in, 310f, 311
    need for, 287

observing in, 310f, 311
participants' interactions in, 297f,
    298–300
peer, restructuring and, 293–294
performance evaluation in, 314–315
planning in, 310–311, 310f
process of, goals in, 296
self-supervision stage in, 297f, 298,
    299–300
student, restructuring and, 294–295
supervisory roles in, 296–301,
    297f, 302f
support worker, restructuring
    and, 295
transitional stage in, 297–298,
    297f, 299
Supervisor(s), defined, 286
Supervisory continuum, 296–298, 297f
Support worker supervision, in supervi-
    sion of rehabilitation deliv-
    ery, 295
Susto, 141

Tabanka, 141
Talo, S., in vocational rehabilitation,
    264, 273, 274f
Taylor, E.B., in defining culture, 126
Teaching as reasoning, defined, 71
Team(s), defined, 27
Teamwork, in rehabilitation, 27–42. *See
    also* Rehabilitation team
    geriatric, 155–175. *See also* Geriatric
        rehabilitation
*The Spirit Catches You and You Fall
    Down*, 56
Thibeault, R., in health promotion,
    359–360
"Thinking in Practice" study, 76
Thought patterns, cultural, 142–144.
    See also Cognitive styles,
        cultural
Time usage, cultural variations of,
    147–148
Titchen, A., in clinical reasoning and
    decision making, 68
Toffler, A., in cultural diversity and
    health care, 124–125
Trach, J.E., in vocational rehabilita-
    tion, 269
Transdisciplinary, defined, 22
Transdisciplinary teams, defined, 4
Transitional care, rehabilitation services
    in, 9–12, 12f
Transitional movements, defined, 11

Transitional stage, in supervision of rehabilitation delivery, 297–298, 297f, 299
Traumatic injuries, rehabilitation for, 2
Truth, cultural variations of, 145–146

Vagueness, in clinical reasoning and decision making, 78
Value(s), health promotion effects of, 357–358
Value systems, cultural, 145–148
Vocational rehabilitation, 261–283
    assessment in, 262–264, 273–275, 274f
        components in, 263
        functional, 263–264
    case studies, 279–280
    emerging themes in, 275–277
    literature review of, 262
    plan for
        development of, 264–267, 264f–266f
        implementation of, 267–271
            components in, 267–268
            context/site in, 268–270
            staff roles and functions in, 270–271
            train-then-place method in, 268
    work hardening in, 271–272

Wachter, M.D., in ethical issues in rehabilitation, 51

Wastefulness, in clinical reasoning and decision making, 78
Watts, N., in clinical reasoning and decision making, 78
Wealth and Health, Health and Wealth, in identifying factors that determine health, 277
Webb, R., in defining culture, 126
Wellness programs, work site–related, effectiveness of, 330–331, 331t
Westmorland, in vocational rehabilitation, 263
Women, sexual dysfunction in, 187t–189t
Work hardening, in vocational rehabilitation, 271–272
Work injury, direct and indirect costs of, 331t
Work injury-prevention programs effectiveness of, 330–331, 331t inefficiency of, causes of, 331
Work injury–prevention programs, inefficiency of, 331
Work site–wellness programs effectiveness of, 330–331, 331t inefficiency of, causes of, 331

Zborowshki, in attitudes toward disability, 111